Shape Memory Polymers for Biomedical Applications

Related titles

Shape memory alloys for biomedical applications
(ISBN 978-1-84569-344-2)

Natural-based polymers for biomedical applications
(ISBN 978-1-84569-264-3)

Biomedical polymers
(ISBN 978-1-84569-070-0)

Woodhead Publishing Series in Biomaterials: Number 97

Shape Memory Polymers for Biomedical Applications

Edited by

L'Hocine Yahia

ELSEVIER

AMSTERDAM • BOSTON • CAMBRIDGE • HEIDELBERG
LONDON • NEW YORK • OXFORD • PARIS • SAN DIEGO
SAN FRANCISCO • SINGAPORE • SYDNEY • TOKYO
Woodhead Publishing is an imprint of Elsevier

WP WOODHEAD PUBLISHING

Woodhead Publishing is an imprint of Elsevier
80 High Street, Sawston, Cambridge CB22 3HJ, UK
225 Wyman Street, Waltham, MA 02451, USA
Langford Lane, Kidlington OX5 1GB, UK

British Library Cataloguing-in-Publication Data
A catalogue record for this book is available from the British Library

Library of Congress Control Number: 2014957594

ISBN 978-0-85709-698-2 (print)
ISBN 978-0-85709-705-7 (online)

For information on all Woodhead Publishing publications
visit our website at http://store.elsevier.com/

Typeset by SPi Global
www.spi-global.com
Printed and bound in the United Kingdom

Contents

List of contributors

S. Bertoldi Materials and Chemical Engineering 'G. Natta', Milano, Italy

N. Chirani École Polytechnique, Montréal, QC, Canada

S.W. Crowder Vanderbilt University, Nashville, TN, USA

L. De Nardo Materials and Chemical Engineering 'G. Natta', Milano, Italy

R.O. do Nascimento Laboratory for Innovation and Analysis of Bio-Performance, École Polytechnique, Montréal, QC, Canada

K. Dyamenahalli University of Colorado, Aurora, CO, USA

A. Famili University of Colorado, Aurora, CO, USA

S. Farè Materials and Chemical Engineering 'G. Natta', Milano, Italy

Y.Q. Fu Northumbria University, Newcastle upon Tyne, United Kingdom

J.C. Griffis MedShape, Inc., Atlanta, GA, USA

M.K. Gupta Vanderbilt University, Nashville, TN, USA

S. Hayashi SMP Technologies Inc., Tokyo, Japan

W.M. Huang Nanyang Technological University, Singapore

T. Javanbakht Biomedical Engineering Institute, Ecole Polytechnique, Montreal, QC, Canada

G. Li Louisiana State University, Baton Rouge, LA, USA

H. Lu Harbin Institute of Technology, Harbin, China

J.K. Luo University of Bolton, Bolton, United Kingdom

R. Matsui Aichi Institute of Technology, Toyota, Japan

D.A. Mbeh Laboratory for Innovation and Analysis of Bio-Performance, École Polytechnique, Montréal, QC, Canada

H. Meng Southern University, Baton Rouge, LA, USA

R. Rath Vanderbilt University, Nashville, TN, USA

D.L. Safranski MedShape, Inc., Atlanta, GA, USA

R. Shandas University of Colorado, Aurora, CO, USA

W. Sokolowski California Institute of Technology, Pasadena, CA, USA

J. Song University of Massachusetts Medical School, Worcester, MA, USA

S. Strandman University of Montreal, Montreal, QC, Canada

H.-J. Sung Vanderbilt University, Nashville, TN, USA

K. Takeda Aichi Institute of Technology, Toyota, Japan

M.C. Tanzi INSTM, Politecnico di Milano, Italy

H. Tobushi Aichi Institute of Technology, Toyota, Japan

J. Xu University of Massachusetts Medical School, Worcester, MA, USA

L. Yahia École Polytechnique de Montréal, Montréal, QC, Canada

X.X. Zhu University of Montreal, Montreal, QC, Canada

Woodhead Publishing Series in Biomaterials

1 **Sterilisation of tissues using ionising radiations**
Edited by J. F. Kennedy, G. O. Phillips and P. A. Williams
2 **Surfaces and interfaces for biomaterials**
Edited by P. Vadgama
3 **Molecular interfacial phenomena of polymers and biopolymers**
Edited by C. Chen
4 **Biomaterials, artificial organs and tissue engineering**
Edited by L. Hench and J. Jones
5 **Medical modelling**
R. Bibb
6 **Artificial cells, cell engineering and therapy**
Edited by S. Prakash
7 **Biomedical polymers**
Edited by M. Jenkins
8 **Tissue engineering using ceramics and polymers**
Edited by A. R. Boccaccini and J. Gough
9 **Bioceramics and their clinical applications**
Edited by T. Kokubo
10 **Dental biomaterials**
Edited by R. V. Curtis and T. F. Watson
11 **Joint replacement technology**
Edited by P. A. Revell
12 **Natural-based polymers for biomedical applications**
Edited by R. L. Reiss et al
13 **Degradation rate of bioresorbable materials**
Edited by F. J. Buchanan
14 **Orthopaedic bone cements**
Edited by S. Deb
15 **Shape memory alloys for biomedical applications**
Edited by T. Yoneyama and S.Miyazaki
16 **Cellular response to biomaterials**
Edited by L. Di Silvio
17 **Biomaterials for treating skin loss**
Edited by D. P. Orgill and C. Blanco
18 **Biomaterials and tissue engineering in urology**
Edited by J. Denstedt and A. Atala
19 **Materials science for dentistry**
B. W. Darvell
20 **Bone repair biomaterials**
Edited by J. A. Planell, S. M. Best, D. Lacroix and A. Merolli
21 **Biomedical composites**
Edited by L. Ambrosio

22 **Drug–device combination products**
Edited by A. Lewis
23 **Biomaterials and regenerative medicine in ophthalmology**
Edited by T. V. Chirila
24 **Regenerative medicine and biomaterials for the repair of connective tissues**
Edited by C. Archer and J. Ralphs
25 **Metals for biomedical devices**
Edited by M. Ninomi
26 **Biointegration of medical implant materials: Science and design**
Edited by C. P. Sharma
27 **Biomaterials and devices for the circulatory system**
Edited by T. Gourlay and R. Black
28 **Surface modification of biomaterials: Methods analysis and applications**
Edited by R. Williams
29 **Biomaterials for artificial organs**
Edited by M. Lysaght and T. Webster
30 **Injectable biomaterials: Science and applications**
Edited by B. Vernon
31 **Biomedical hydrogels: Biochemistry, manufacture and medical applications**
Edited by S. Rimmer
32 **Preprosthetic and maxillofacial surgery: Biomaterials, bone grafting and tissue engineering**
Edited by J. Ferri and E. Hunziker
33 **Bioactive materials in medicine: Design and applications**
Edited by X. Zhao, J. M. Courtney and H. Qian
34 **Advanced wound repair therapies**
Edited by D. Farrar
35 **Electrospinning for tissue regeneration**
Edited by L. Bosworth and S. Downes
36 **Bioactive glasses: Materials, properties and applications**
Edited by H. O. Ylänen
37 **Coatings for biomedical applications**
Edited by M. Driver
38 **Progenitor and stem cell technologies and therapies**
Edited by A. Atala
39 **Biomaterials for spinal surgery**
Edited by L. Ambrosio and E. Tanner
40 **Minimized cardiopulmonary bypass techniques and technologies**
Edited by T. Gourlay and S. Gunaydin
41 **Wear of orthopaedic implants and artificial joints**
Edited by S. Affatato
42 **Biomaterials in plastic surgery: Breast implants**
Edited by W. Peters, H. Brandon, K. L. Jerina, C. Wolf and V. L. Young
43 **MEMS for biomedical applications**
Edited by S. Bhansali and A. Vasudev
44 **Durability and reliability of medical polymers**
Edited by M. Jenkins and A. Stamboulis
45 **Biosensors for medical applications**
Edited by S. Higson
46 **Sterilisation of biomaterials and medical devices**
Edited by S. Lerouge and A. Simmons
47 **The hip resurfacing handbook: A practical guide to the use and management of modern hip resurfacings**
Edited by K. De Smet, P. Campbell and C. Van Der Straeten
48 **Developments in tissue engineered and regenerative medicine products**
J. Basu and J. W. Ludlow

49 **Nanomedicine: Technologies and applications**
Edited by T. J. Webster
50 **Biocompatibility and performance of medical devices**
Edited by J-P. Boutrand
51 **Medical robotics: Minimally invasive surgery**
Edited by P. Gomes
52 **Implantable sensor systems for medical applications**
Edited by A. Inmann and D. Hodgins
53 **Non-metallic biomaterials for tooth repair and replacement**
Edited by P. Vallittu
54 **Joining and assembly of medical materials and devices**
Edited by Y. (Norman) Zhou and M. D. Breyen
55 **Diamond-based materials for biomedical applications**
Edited by R. Narayan
56 **Nanomaterials in tissue engineering: Fabrication and applications**
Edited by A. K. Gaharwar, S. Sant, M. J. Hancock and S. A. Hacking
57 **Biomimetic biomaterials: Structure and applications**
Edited by A. J. Ruys
58 **Standardisation in cell and tissue engineering: Methods and protocols**
Edited by V. Salih
59 **Inhaler devices: Fundamentals, design and drug delivery**
Edited by P. Prokopovich
60 **Bio-tribocorrosion in biomaterials and medical implants**
Edited by Y. Yan
61 **Microfluidic devices for biomedical applications**
Edited by X-J. James Li and Y. Zhou
62 **Decontamination in hospitals and healthcare**
Edited by J. T. Walker
63 **Biomedical imaging: Applications and advances**
Edited by P. Morris
64 **Characterization of biomaterials**
Edited by M. Jaffe, W. Hammond, P. Tolias and T. Arinzeh
65 **Biomaterials and medical tribology**
Edited by J. Paolo Davim
66 **Biomaterials for cancer therapeutics: Diagnosis, prevention and therapy**
Edited by K. Park
67 **New functional biomaterials for medicine and healthcare**
E.P. Ivanova, K. Bazaka and R. J. Crawford
68 **Porous silicon for biomedical applications**
Edited by H. A. Santos
69 **A practical approach to spinal trauma**
Edited by H. N. Bajaj and S. Katoch
70 **Rapid prototyping of biomaterials: Principles and applications**
Edited by R. Narayan
71 **Cardiac regeneration and repair Volume 1: Pathology and therapies**
Edited by R-K. Li and R. D. Weisel
72 **Cardiac regeneration and repair Volume 2: Biomaterials and tissue engineering**
Edited by R-K. Li and R. D. Weisel
73 **Semiconducting silicon nanowires for biomedical applications**
Edited by J.L. Coffer
74 **Silk biomaterials for tissue engineering and regenerative medicine**
Edited by S. Kundu
75 **Biomaterials for bone regeneration: Novel techniques and applications**
Edited by P. Dubruel and S. Van Vlierberghe

76 **Biomedical foams for tissue engineering applications**
Edited by P. Netti
77 **Precious metals for biomedical applications**
Edited by N. Baltzer and T. Copponnex
78 **Bone substitute biomaterials**
Edited by K. Mallick
79 **Regulatory affairs for biomaterials and medical devices**
Edited by S. F. Amato and R. Ezzell
80 **Joint replacement technology Second edition**
Edited by P. A. Revell
81 **Computational modelling of biomechanics and biotribology in the musculoskeletal system: Biomaterials and tissues**
Edited by Z. Jin
82 **Biophotonics for medical applications**
Edited by I. Meglinski
83 **Modelling degradation of bioresorbable polymeric medical devices**
Edited by J. Pan
84 **Perspectives in total hip arthroplasty: Advances in biomaterials and their tribological interactions**
S. Affatato
85 **Tissue engineering using ceramics and polymers Second edition**
Edited by A. R. Boccaccini and P. X. Ma
86 **Biomaterials and medical-device associated infections**
Edited by L. Barnes and I. R. Cooper
87 **Surgical techniques in total knee arthroplasty (TKA) and alternative procedures**
Edited by S. Affatato
88 **Lanthanide oxide nanoparticles for molecular imaging and therapeutics**
G. H. Lee
89 **Surface modification of magnesium and its alloys for biomedical applications Volume 1: Biological interactions, mechanical properties and testing**
Edited by T. S. N. Sankara Narayanan, I. S. Park and M. H. Lee
90 **Surface modification of magnesium and its alloys for biomedical applications Volume 2: Modification and coating techniques**
Edited by T. S. N. Sankara Narayanan, I. S. Park and M. H. Lee
91 **Medical modelling: The application of advanced design and rapid prototyping techniques in medicine Second Edition**
Edited by R. Bibb, D. Eggbeer and A. Paterson
92 **Switchable and responsive surfaces for biomedical applications**
Edited by Z. Zhang
93 **Biomedical textiles for orthopaedic and surgical applications: Fundamentals, applications and tissue engineering**
Edited by T. Blair
94 **Surface coating and modification of metallic biomaterials**
Edited by C. Wen
95 **Hydroxyapatite (HAP) for biomedical applications**
Edited by M. Mucalo
96 **Implantable neuroprostheses for restoring function**
Edited by K. Kilgore
97 **Shape memory polymers for biomedical applications**
Edited by L. Yahia

Part One

Fundamentals of shape-memory polymers for biomedical applications

Introduction to shape-memory polymers for biomedical applications

1

L. Yahia
École Polytechnique de Montréal, Montréal, QC, Canada

1.1 Introduction

The ability of polymers to respond to external stimuli is of high scientific and technological significance. Such stimuli include heat (thermo-responsive materials), stress/pressure (mechano-responsive materials), electrical current/voltage (electro-responsive materials), magnetic field (magneto-responsive materials), pH-change/solvent/water/moisture (chemo-responsive materials), light (photo-responsive materials), and ultrasound-responsive materials (Sun et al., 2012).

Shape-memory polymers (SMPs) are a class of mechanically functional "smart" materials that have generated substantial interest for biomedical applications. SMPs have most notably been promoted for their potential in minimally invasive surgery, where a compacted device could be passed through a smaller incision and deployed to its full shape once inside the body. In addition, SMPs offer the ability to provide structural support, exert stabilizing forces, elute therapeutic agents, and biodegrade.

As new SMPs are developed for medical applications, it is important to consider the potentially harmful effects the SMPs could have when implanted in the body, and the resulting immune response that is elicited. *In vivo* testing of materials must be conducted to evaluate the local and systemic interactions of the SMPs with the native tissue. Implanted materials elicit a complex wound-healing process, including hemostasis, inflammation, and repair and remodeling. Typically, materials are implanted subcutaneously in soft tissue to determine the inflammatory response, as has been done for some SMPs (Filion et al., 2011), followed by implantation in an animal model to the target site for functional *in vivo* testing. A safety consideration unique to SMPs for medical applications is the effect the triggering mechanism may have on the body. Heat-triggered SMPs must be triggered at a cytocompatible temperature at or above 37 °C. SMPs with a triggering temperature lower than body temperature may recover prematurely before implantation, whereas SMPs with triggering temperature above 37 °C may cause cell and tissue damage upon triggering. This provides one motivation for the study of non-thermal triggering mechanisms, such as light, solvent, and magnetic/electric fields.

Shape Memory Polymers for Biomedical Applications. http://dx.doi.org/10.1016/B978-0-85709-698-2.00001-5

1.1.1 Shape-memory effect

Since its discovery in alloys in 1932 by Chang and Read (1951), the shape-memory effect (SME) has been extensively investigated in metal alloys for its potential use in medicine (Lipscomb and Nokes, 1996). The fundamental phenomenon of the memory effect governed by thermoelastic behavior of the martensite phase was widely reported by Kurdjumov and Khandros (1949). This phenomenon was later observed in polymers (Kim et al., 1996; Lendlein et al., 2001), thus introducing a variety of materials with stimuli responsiveness, which represented a less expensive and more efficient alternative to established shape-memory alloys (Yahia and Ryhänen, 2000; Yahia et al., 2009). More recently, the synthesis of SMPs has found inspiration in biological substances, as naturally occurring bile acids have been used to fabricate amorphous, thermoplastic polyesters with shape-memory properties (Gautrot and Zhu, 2006, 2009). Interestingly, these bioinspired polymers displayed rubber-like elasticity, glass transitions close to body temperature, high strains at low temperatures, and low systemic toxicity. In addition, these natural biodegradable polymers have several advantages inside the body, such as the capacity for the complete dissolution of the implant. The advantage of biodegradable SMPs is the same as traditional biodegradable materials, except that the shape-memory effect imparts additional functionality to the material by easing minimal invasion and self-actuation inside the body (Lu et al., 2007).

1.1.2 Biocompatibility of SMPs

As mentioned above, the development of metallic or polymeric shape-memory materials for biomedical applications is progressing rapidly because of the unique properties of these materials. However, they must fulfill the basic criterion of biocompatibility before they can be fabricated into medical implants or scaffolds for tissue engineering. The period during which a biomaterial remains inside the human body is important to consider in terms of its use. Though the shape-memory alloy nitinol (NiTi) has typically been successfully used in biomedical devices, its biocompatibility remains controversial due to its high content of potentially carcinogenic nickel. Among the numerous studies that have assessed the biocompatibility of NiTi, several have demonstrated the potential cytotoxicity of NiTi-based devices (Berger-Gorbet et al., 1996). Observed cellular death and severe tissue damage were associated with the release of nickel ions from NiTi alloys. However, other studies agree on the safety of NiTi alloy (Yahia and Ryhänen, 2000). Therefore, caution is required when NiTi-based devices are used long term because of the possibility that dissolved nickel ions will be released into the human body and cause both toxic and allergic reactions (Yahia et al., 2009). In contrast to shape-memory alloys, SMPs have been generally accepted as biocompatible. Many research groups have assessed the biocompatibility of various SMPs. Numerous early studies focused on the biocompatibility of commercially polyurethane SMPs, which in general display low cytotoxicity and *in vivo* inflammatory response. In 2003, Metcalfe et al. tested cold hibernated elastic memory foams for the treatment of lateral wall aneurysms in carotid arteries by using an *in vivo* model in dogs (Metcalfe et al., 2003). These materials were fabricated from polyurethane-based SMP in the form of open cellular structures (foams) by Mitsubishi Heavy Industry and Jet Propulsion Laboratory (California Institute of Technology, Pasadena, CA, US) and behaved as self-deployable structures by means of the shape-memory properties and the elastic recovery of the foam. After confirming the absence of both cytotoxic effects on L929 fibroblast cultures and mutagenicity with strains of Salmonella typhimurium, *in vivo* aneurysm embolization showed satisfactory occlusion with improved angiographic results at 3 weeks. Furthermore, the inherent porosity of these foams allowed for cellular invasion and induced neointima formation. Unfortunately, residual aneurysm necks and recurrences were observed when incomplete lumen filling occurred. In addition to the long-established polyurethane SMP materials, the evaluation today of many other SMPs for biocompatibility in biomedical applications is opening the door for further application of SMPs in medicine. Despite some positive data indicating good biocompatibility in SMPs, the biocompatibility of biomaterials depends on many factors (e.g., the implantation site, level of wear, and duration of the implantation). More systematic studies both *in vitro* and *in vivo* are required to better address the concern of biocompatibility before fabricating biomaterials into implants.

1.1.3 Sterilization of SMPs

All medical devices must undergo sterilization before they can be used clinically. Conventional methods of sterilization listed in the U.S. FDA guide include exposure to steam, ethylene oxide, and irradiation (gamma or e-beam), and plasma treatment (Moisan et al., 2001; França et al., 2013). All proposed SMP medical devices must eventually be validated with a designated *sterilization method* before they can be used clinically; it can influence the biocompatibility and performance of a device and can also alter the thermomechanical properties that directly affect the shape-memory properties. For example, Nardo et al. (2010) have reported the effects of sterilizations by plasma and ozone on the chemico-physical, thermomechanical, and shape-memory performance of polyurethane foams. Therefore, identifying an appropriate process that can achieve the required sterility without compromising the properties of SMP is challenging.

In summary, the main requirements for SMP as envisioned for biomedical use are: (i) actuation, preferentially remote, within biologically safe ranges to avoid damage of surrounding tissues; (ii) biocompatibility; (iii) safe sterilization method; (iv) compressed temporary shape to facilitate minimally invasive deployment; (v) and biodegradability by gradual erosion to avoid explantation.

Multidisciplinary research, including efforts from chemists, physicians, biologists, engineers, and clinicians, will contribute to significant advances in the biomedical use of SMP from bench to bedside.

The book consists of 14 chapters. This chapter briefly introduces the most important problems related to the biocompatibility, sterilization, and safety of SMPs. The next three chapters (Chapters 2–4) present the mechanical properties and experimental techniques for the mechanical characterization of SMPs. Chapter 5 provides more details related to different aspects of biocompatibility assessment through *in vitro* and *in vivo* experimental procedures. One of the significant driving forces for research into SMPs is their biomedical applications. Biological evaluation is mandatory prior to their applications as biomaterials. Some types of SMP fillers meant to achieve novel functions are toxic.

Chapter 6 is devoted to the underlying mechanism and physico-chemical requirements of chemo-responsive shape change/memory polymers. A phenomenological thermodynamic model studies the constitutive relations and working mechanism of the chemo-responsive SME in SMPs. In real implementation, according to the magnitude of volume expansion in polymers, there are three categories of chemo-responsive SME: softening, swelling, and dissolving.

In Chapter 7, the authors discuss three different processing methods to obtain SMP-based cellular solids. The three-dimensional structures obtained via different processing methods resulted in a broad spectrum of size, dimension, shape, distribution, and interconnection of pores, preserving the shape-memory properties of the investigated materials. These different properties may meet the needs of various medical applications and be effectively used in the design of novel devices for mini-invasive surgical procedures.

Chapter 8 introduces the use of thiol-ene photopolymers as SMP systems. The thiol-ene polymer networks have been compared to a commonly utilized acrylic SMP and shown to have significantly improved properties for two different thiol-ene-based polymer formulations. Thiol-ene-based SMP systems have comparable thermomechanical properties while also exhibiting a number of advantageous properties due to the thiol-ene polymerization mechanism, which results in the formation of a homogenous polymer network with low shrinkage stress and negligible oxygen inhibition.

Chapter 9 deals with shape-memory polyurethane (SMPU), which is one emerging class of the SMPs. This chapter deals with the SMPs, including their chemical properties, thermodynamic immiscibility, and biomedical applications. The authors have explained some of the properties of SMPs, such as their microstructure and thermo-mechanical behavior as well as some techniques for activating them, including thermal, electric, magnetic, water and solution, and light triggering. They have also explained the facility of the production of composite SMPUs. The biocompatibility of SMPUs has also been mentioned in this chapter.

Chapter 10 introduces poly(lactic acid): a biodegradable aliphatic polyester that has the advantage of being not only biodegradable but also renewable because the raw material (lactic acid) can be produced by microbial fermentation of biomass.

In Chapter 11, the authors introduce naturally occurring bile acids that are ideal building blocks for a new generation of biomaterials displaying low systemic toxicity and engineered properties. They report the synthesis of bile acid-based polyesters using entropy-driven ring-opening metathesis polymerization and characterization of the structure of the resulting polymers.

In the final three chapters (Chapters 12–14), the authors present a few examples of medical applications, including vascular and coronary devices, dental, and sutures.

The scope of the book is to discuss recent progress and challenges in the SMPs for biomedical applications and to provide a comprehensive review of their properties and applications.

With great pleasure, we take this opportunity to thank the authors for their time and hard work, which has enabled us to complete the current volume *Shape-Memory Polymers for Biomedical Applications*. We believe that with the authors' excellent contributions, this book will provide a common platform for both biomaterials specialists and clinicians—not only those involved in research on smart biomaterials, but anyone else planning to do research in this area (especially graduate students).

References

Berger-Gorbet, M., Broxup, B., Rivard, C., Yahia, L.H., 1996. Biocompatibility testing of NiTi Screws using Immunohistochemistry on sections containing metallic implants. J. Biomed. Mater. Res. 32 (2), 243–248.

Chang, L.C., Read, T.A., 1951. Plastic deformation and diffusionless phase changes in metals—the gold-cadmium beta phase. Trans. AIME 189, 47–52.

Filion, T.M., Xu, J., Prasad, M.L., Song, J., 2011. In vivo tissue responses to thermal-responsive shape memory polymer nanocomposites. Biomaterials 32, 985–991.

França, R., Mbeh, D.A., Samani, T.D., Tien, C., Mateescu, M.A., Yahia, L.H., Sacher, E., 2013. The effect of ethylene oxide sterilization on the surface chemistry and in vitro cytotoxicity of several kinds of chitosan. J. Biomed. Mater. Res. B Appl. Biomater. 101 (8), 1444–1455.

Gautrot, J.E., Zhu, X.X., 2006. Main-chain bile acid-based degradable elastomers synthesised via entropy-driven ring-opening metathesis polymerization. Angew. Chem. Int. Ed. 45 (41), 6872–6874.

Gautrot, J.E., Zhu, X.X., 2009. Shape memory materials based on naturally occurring bile-acids. Macromolecules 42, 7324–7733.

Kim, B.-K., Lee, S.-Y., Xu, M., 1996. Polyurethanes having shape memory effects. Polymer 37 (26), 5781–5793.

Kurdjumov, G.V., Khandros, L.G., 1949. First reports of the thermoelastic behaviour of the martensitic phase of Au-Cd alloys. Dokl. Akad. Nauk SSSR 66, 211–213.

Lendlein, A., Schmidt, A.M., Langer, R., 2001. AB-polymer networks based on oligo (ε-caprolactone)-segments showing shape-memory properties. Proc. Natl. Acad. Sci. U. S. A. 98, 842.

Lipscomb, P., Nokes, L.D.M., 1996. The Application of Shape Memory Alloys in Medicine. Mechanical Engineering Publications, Limited, Suffolk, UK.

Lu, X.L., Cai, W., Gao, Z.Y., Tang, W.J., 2007. Shape memory effects of poly(L-lactide) and its copolymer with poly(ε-caprolactone). Polym. Bull. 58, 381–391.

Metcalfe, A., Desfaits, A.C., Salazkin, I., Yahia, L., Sokolowski, W.M., Raymond, J., 2003. Cold hibernated elastic memory foams for endovascular interventions. Biomaterials 24 (3), 491–497.

Moisan, M., Barbeau, J., Moreau, S., Pelletier, J., Tabrizian, M., Yahia, L.H., 2001. Low-temperature sterilization using gas plasmas: a review of the experiments and an analysis of the inactivation mechanisms. Int. J. Pharm. 226 (1), 1–21.

Nardo, L.D., Moscatelli, M., Silvi, F., Tanzi, M.C., Yahia, H., Fare, S., 2010. Chemico-physical modifications induced by plasma and ozone sterilizations on shape memory polyurethane foams. J. Mater. Sci. Mater. Med. 21, 2067–2078.

Sun, L., Huang, W.M., Ding, Z., Zhao, Y., Wang, C.C., Purnawali, H., Tang, C., 2012. Stimulus-responsive shape memory materials: a review. Mater. Des. 33 (1), 577–640.

Yahia, L.H., Ryhänen, J., 2000. Bioperformance of shape memory alloys. In: Yahia, L.H. (Ed.), Shape Memory Implants. Springer, Berlin, Heidelberg, pp. 3–23.

Yahia, L.H., Rayes, F., Warrak, A.O., 2009. Regulation, orthopedic, dental, endovascular and other applications of TiNi shape memory alloys. In: Yoneyama, T., Miyazaki, S. (Eds.), Shape Memory Alloys for Biomedical Applications. CRC/Woodhead Publishing Limited, England, pp. 306–320.

Mechanical properties of shape-memory polymers for biomedical applications

2

D.L. Safranski, J.C. Griffis
MedShape, Inc., Atlanta, GA, USA

2.1 Introduction

Shape-memory polymers (SMPs) are mechanically active polymers, representing one class of stimuli-responsive polymers along with electro-active polymers, hydrogels, and pH-sensitive polymers (Lendlein and Kelch, 2005; Bar-Cohen, 2004; He et al., 2008; Qiu and Park, 2001). Typically, SMPs have a one-way shape change between a temporary programmed shape and a final permanent shape (Figure 2.1). Starting with the original shape, the SMP is heated to or above the activation temperature (T_a), which may be a glass transition temperature (T_g) or a melting temperature (T_m). After heating, the SMP is deformed into a temporary shape and cooled below the T_a, while maintaining the temporary shape. This first part of the shape-memory cycle is often referred to as programming. The SMP is now stored in its temporary shape until it is heated back to the vicinity of T_a, where the SMP will change back to its original shape. The second part of the shape-memory cycle is referred to as recovery. Classically, SMPs recover by thermal activation via direct or indirect heating. Direct heating tends to be the dominant activation method for recovery (Lendlein and Kelch, 2002; Yakacki et al., 2008a). Indirect heating has been accomplished by using various fillers and particles, which allow for resistive, induction, light, and laser heating (Yakacki et al., 2009a; Lendlein et al., 2005a; Maitland et al., 2007; Yang et al., 2005; Mohr et al., 2006). Activation by solvents or immersion in water has also been shown (Pierce et al., 2011). Besides one-way activation between a temporary shape and a final shape, triple-shape and multi-shape SMPs have been studied as well as two-way SMPs that change shape directly between two shapes (Xie, 2010; Behl et al., 2010; Ware et al., 2012a; Chung et al., 2007; Luo and Mather, 2010; Qin and Mather, 2008). A variety of activation methods exist, allowing for the use of SMPs in numerous potential applications.

The effects of water on the SMP's mechanical properties have been thoroughly studied (Pierce et al., 2011; Yu et al., 2011; Yang et al., 2004, 2006; Smith et al., 2009, 2011). Briefly, the uptake of water into the polymer relaxes the polymer chains, resulting in a decrease in T_g. The water molecules are either "bound" type, which directly interact with polymer chains, or "free" type, which swell the polymer, causing interruption of intermolecular bonding. "Plasticization," a mechanical softening, is often thought to be the only result when a polymer interacts with water; however,

Shape Memory Polymers for Biomedical Applications. http://dx.doi.org/10.1016/B978-0-85709-698-2.00002-7

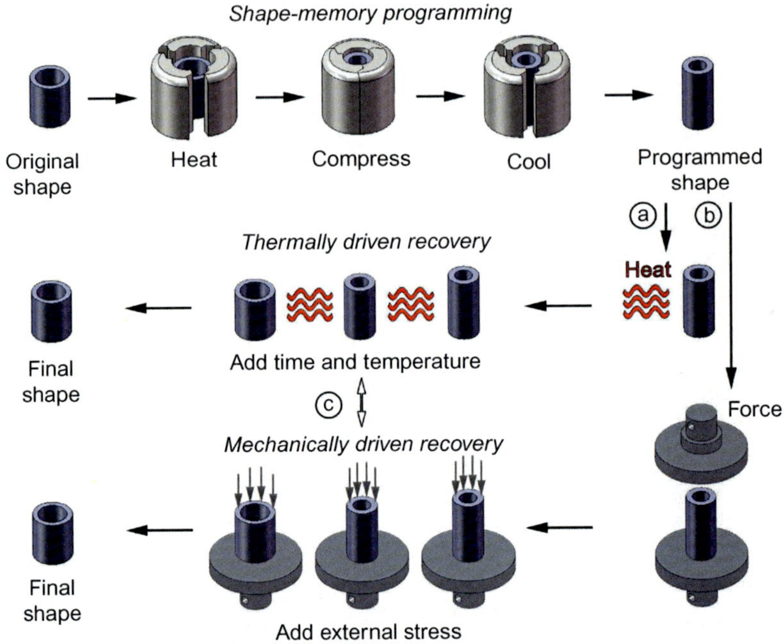

Figure 2.1 (a) Thermal activation is used to drive SMP from programmed shape to final shape. (b) Mechanical activation is used to drive SMP from programmed shape to final shape. (c) A combination of mechanical force and temperature can be used for activation. Adapted from Yakacki et al. (2011). Permission obtained from Elsevier.

a polymer may actually enhance its mechanical properties (toughness, failure strain) depending upon the location of its T_g in relation to the testing temperature. An initially glassy polymer may absorb water, thus making it more ductile and increasing its failure strain and toughness. The extent of these shifts in mechanical properties is highly dependent upon the immersion time, hydrophilicity, and type of water molecule and can be used to tailor the mechanical properties for long-term biomedical applications (Safranski et al., 2013).

The shape-memory effect in polymers is based on changes in entropic elasticity of the polymer system. At the macroscopic level, the SMP is programmed into a temporary shape and then ideally recovers back to its original shape. At the macromolecular level, the SMP's chains are initially in a low-energy state when the SMP is in its original shape. Cross-links, chemical or physical, serve to memorize and fix the original shape. When the SMP is programmed (heated and deformed), the polymer chains are strained to a high-energy state, with cooling below T_a locking in this high-energy state. The polymer chains would prefer to return to the original low-energy shape, but this does not occur due to vitrification or crystallization. During recovery, the applied thermal energy removes the polymer from its vitrified or crystallized state, which allows for movement of the polymer chains back to their low-energy state. The SMP returns from its temporary shape to its original shape, acting as an entropic spring (Lendlein and Kelch, 2002; Liu et al., 2007). Recently, mechanically activating an SMP has been demonstrated, where mechanical force (rather than temperature) assists in driving the polymer from its temporary shape (high energy) to its original shape (low energy) (Figure 2.1) (Yakacki et al., 2011). This allows for rapid activation of the polymer from the temporary shape to the original shape. Either thermal or mechanically assisted recovery (or a combination of both) is possible for SMPs, allowing for further options when using in biomedical devices.

Following a previous classification scheme (Liu et al., 2007), SMPs are often divided into four classes: (a) chemically cross-linked glassy thermosets, (b) chemically cross-linked semicrystalline rubbers, (c) physically cross-linked thermoplastics, and (d) physically cross-linked block copolymers (Figure 2.2). Class I SMPs are chemically cross-linked thermoset networks, such as chemically cross-linked methacrylates, thiol-ene-acrylates, and epoxies, that activate due to a glass transition

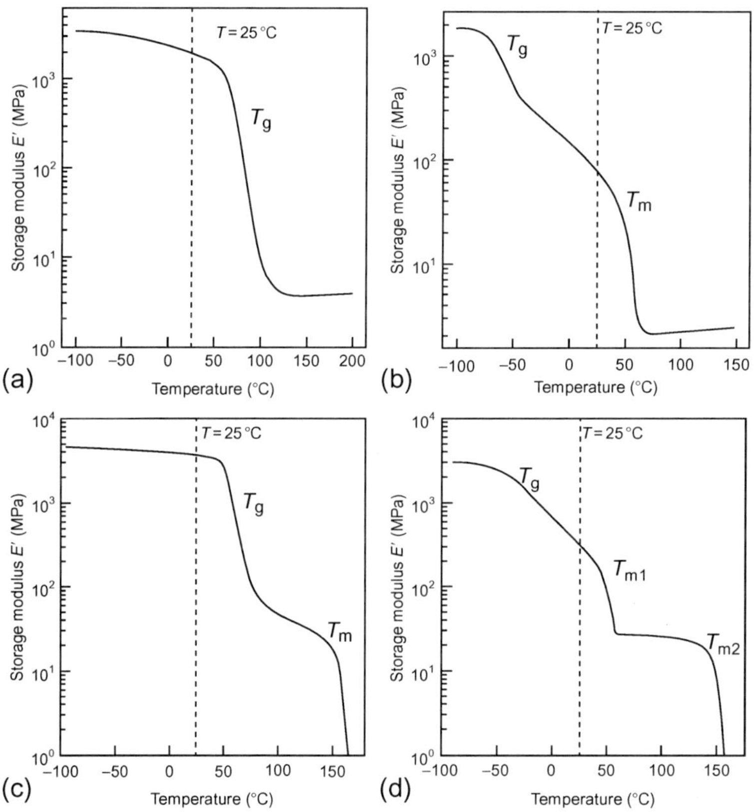

Figure 2.2 Classification scheme of SMPs with different activation mechanisms: (a) chemically cross-linked glassy thermosets, (b) chemically cross-linked semicrystalline rubbers, (c) physically cross-linked thermoplastics, and (d) physically cross-linked block copolymers.
Reproduced from Liu et al. (2007), with permission from The Royal Society of Chemistry.

(Safranski and Gall, 2008; Nair et al., 2010; Ware et al., 2012b; Di Prima et al., 2007). Class II SMPs are chemically cross-linked thermoset networks that activate due to a melting transition. Examples of Class II SMPs include polycaprolactone (PCL)-methacrylates and polycyclooctene (Lendlein et al., 2005b; Liu et al., 2002). Class III SMPs are physically cross-linked thermoplastics (copolymers or blends) that activate due to a glass transition, such as POSS-PN copolymers or PLA-PVA blends (Jeon et al., 2000; Liu and Mather, 2003). Class IV SMPs are physically cross-linked thermoplastics (multi-block copolymers) that activate due to a melt transition of the soft segment and consist mostly of multi-block polyurethanes, such as BDO-PCL diol-MDI-based polyurethanes (Kim et al., 1998; Li et al., 1996). Due to the wide variety of SMP systems, designing biomedical devices from these polymers is not limited to a specific chemistry, so other issues like hydrophilicity and biocompatibility can be addressed.

A number of thermo-mechanical properties are used to define the performance of SMPs. These properties are dictated by the chemical and physical structure of the polymer with inherent trade-offs existing for each polymer system. First, the T_a, as dictated by T_g or T_m, controls the rate and extent of shape recovery and is dependent upon the chemical structure and molecular weight of the polymer. As the T_a increases above the surrounding environmental test temperature, the rate and extent of shape recovery decreases. Second, the cross-linking density, chemical or physical, directly controls the recovery force, such that greater the cross-linking density, the higher the recovery force; however, this can also dictate the rate and amount of shape recovery at low cross-linking densities. The failure strain is dependent upon the cross-linking density, chemical structure, and environmental testing temperature. The higher the failure strain, the higher the amount of shape change possible for a given SMP. Since the failure strain is temperature dependent, the temperature to program the SMP from the original shape to the temporary shape may have an optimal value. Often overlooked, the failure strain or strain capacity of the SMP is critical in determining how much shape change the material can go through. Failure strains have reached over 800% for some SMPs, which would allow for very large shape changes (Voit et al., 2010).

The two most widely used equations for SMPs are the total strain recovery rate equation and the strain fixity rate equation (Lendlein and Kelch, 2002). The total strain recovery rate, R_r, or how much shape recovery occurs compared to original shape, is calculated using Equation (2.1), where ε_p is the residual strain after heating and ε_m is the maximum strain during programming for N cycles. The strain fixity rate, R_f, or how well a SMP stays packaged in its temporary shape is calculated using Equation (2.2), where ε_m is the maximum strain during programming, and ε_u is the strain after cooling and unloading for N cycles (Figure 2.3).

$$R_r = \frac{\varepsilon_m - \varepsilon_p(N)}{\varepsilon_m} \times 100 \tag{2.1}$$

$$R_f = \frac{\varepsilon_u(N)}{\varepsilon_m} \times 100 \tag{2.2}$$

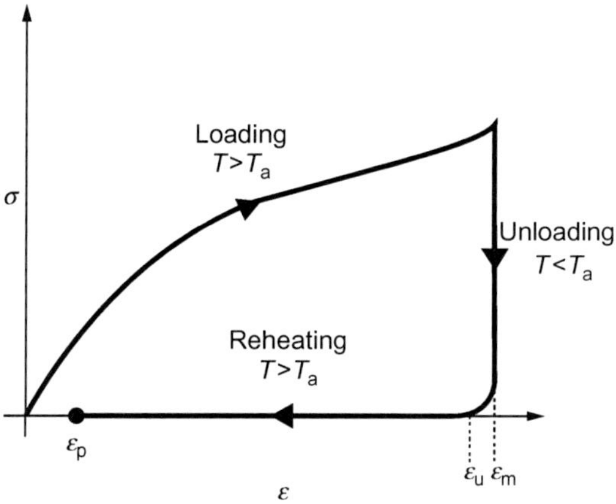

Figure 2.3 Schematic of shape-memory cycle on stress–strain diagram. Adapted from Lendlein and Kelch (2002), with permission obtained from Wiley.

Dynamic mechanical analysis (DMA), differential scanning calorimetry, and mechanical testing are the dominant characterization methods used to determine the thermomechanical properties and performance characteristics of SMPs. SMPs are often characterized under two ideal conditions: (1) free-strain recovery under isothermal conditions or at a fixed heating rate and (2) fixed-strain recovery conditions under isothermal conditions or at a fixed heating rate. Free-strain recovery occurs when no bias load is applied to the SMP; thus, it is able to freely recover its stored strain. Free-strain recovery measures the amount of shape recovery when no strain is held on the SMP during recovery. Fixed-strain recovery occurs when a high bias load is applied to the SMP, thus it cannot move and its strain is fixed. Fixed-strain recovery measures the amount of recovery force (rather than strain), since the strain is fixed during recovery of the SMP (Figure 2.4). Recovery can be assessed using a variety of testing approaches. Tension or compression tests in mechanical load frames or in a DMA offer more quantitative analysis rather than bending tests that only measure angles of recovery. Free-strain and fixed-strain tests show the two extreme cases of SMP

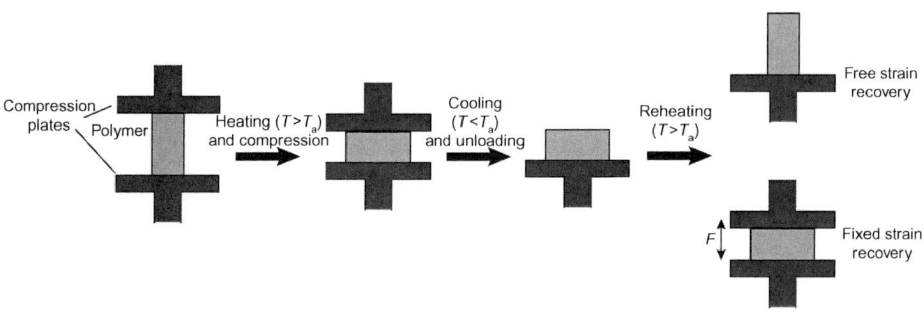

Figure 2.4 Schematic of mechanical characterization of free-strain and fixed-strain recovery. Free-strain recovery occurs when the SMP is not constrained and the material recovers with no bias force against it. Fixed-strain recovery occurs when the SMP is fully constrained and the material exerts a force during recovery.

deployment. In real applications, SMPs often have some bias load against them and are deployed under partial-strain conditions; thus, deployment with varying bias forces should be taken into account (Lakhera et al., 2012a). While these two tests are idealized for the laboratory setting, they provide insight into the clinical scenario when deploying SMPs *in vivo*.

The use of SMPs in biomedical applications has long been a focus in the "smart" materials community. SMPs hold great promise, especially for minimally invasive surgery, where a device could be implanted in one shape and then activated *in vivo* into a second shape that serves a functional purpose. Other biomedical applications may include using SMPs to apply forces *in vivo* to secure tissues together or to expand and act as a scaffold. To date, SMPs have mainly been applied in the field of orthopedic and cardiovascular devices.

This chapter will review the mechanical properties of SMPs, especially focusing on the thermo-mechanical properties (T_a, failure strain, shape recovery, shape fixity, and recovery forces) (Table 2.1) of SMPs that are undergoing development for biomedical

Table 2.1 Shape-memory properties of SMPs

Type of SMP	T_a (°C)	Modulus (MPa)	Shape recovery (%)	Shape fixity (%)	Strain (%)	References
(Meth)acrylate	–29 to 112	0.5–128.5	100	>99	~800	Yakacki et al. (2008a), Safranski and Gall (2008), Li et al. (1996), Lakhera et al. (2012a), and Gall et al. (2005)
Semicrystalline degradable	16 to 60	2.4–71	92–99	92–97	~550	Lendlein et al. (2001, 2005b), Liu et al. (2002), and Feldkamp and Rousseau (2011)
Polyurethane	40 to 92	1.3–7	84–100	96–99	~271	Tobushi et al. (1996), Hearon et al. (2011), and Baer et al. (2006)

applications. The chapter will focus on methacrylate SMPs, semicrystalline degradable SMPs, and polyurethane SMPs. While many different polymer chemistries are under academic investigation for SMP biomedical devices, these three classes represent the SMPs that have undergone the most clinical development. The mechanical properties of clinically used and preclinical SMP devices will be detailed as well as future SMP biomedical applications.

2.2 Mechanical properties of shape-memory polymers (SMPs)

2.2.1 Methacrylate SMPs

Methacrylate and acrylate-based SMPs are some of the more widely studied chemically cross-linked SMPs for biomedical applications that undergo a shape change via T_g (Yakacki et al., 2007, 2008a,b,c; Ware et al., 2012a; Smith et al., 2009, 2011; Safranski et al., 2013; Safranski and Gall, 2008; Voit et al., 2010; Lakhera et al., 2012a,b; Gall et al., 2005; Nguyen et al., 2010; Yakacki and Gall, 2010; Choi et al., 2006, 2012; Ortega et al., 2012; Choi and Lendlein, 2007; Song et al., 2010). SMP epoxy systems also fall into this category, but are mostly being developed for non-biomedical applications and are thus reviewed elsewhere (Di Prima et al., 2007; Xie and Rousseau, 2009; Feldkamp and Rousseau, 2011). Other SMPs are being developed from thiol-ene and thiol-acrylate systems (Nair et al., 2010; Ware et al., 2012b). Several research groups have studied the thermo-mechanical properties of (meth)acrylate-based SMPs; however, some of the most extensive studies have been performed by Gall et al.

Initial studies focused on a model SMP system of poly(ethylene glycol) dimethacrylate (PEGDMA) and tert-butyl acrylate for use in cardiovascular applications (Gall et al., 2005; Yakacki et al., 2007). These SMPs demonstrated 100% strain recovery up to 80% strain for programming. Programming temperatures above and below T_g were evaluated, and recovery was shown to occur at a lower temperature when a programming temperature below T_g was used. Isothermal free-strain recovery tests showed an increase in recovery as temperature increased or decreasing programming temperature (Gall et al., 2005). These properties allow for activation of a SMP with a T_g above body temperature to activate at physiological conditions.

Further investigation and tailoring of the SMP's chemical structure yielded SMPs with similar T_g and varying cross-linking density with T_g from 50 to 55 °C and rubbery moduli from 1.5 to 11.5 MPa (Yakacki et al., 2007). As cross-linker concentration increases for SMPs with equivalent T_g, the recovery time decreases from 300 to 30 s, and all networks reached 100% shape recovery. In this system, the increased cross-linker concentration acts as a driving force for complete shape recovery. For SMPs with equivalent cross-linker concentration, SMPs with lower T_g started to recover before SMPs with higher T_g. Within this study, prototype stents were also produced and their shape-memory deployment demonstrated at physiological conditions (Yakacki et al., 2007).

In another study, the T_g and rubbery modulus of a model SMP based on PEGDMA and methyl methacrylate (MMA) could be independently tailored from 56 to 92 °C and 9.3 to 23.0 MPa by controlling the molecular weight of PEGDMA and MMA concentration (Yakacki et al., 2008a). In particular, it was found that the T_g controls the free-strain recovery while the cross-linking density is not a direct factor. This is in opposition to the previous work, where cross-linking density contributed to the free-strain recovery response. However, there seems to be a diminishing effect of cross-linking density on free-strain recovery. Once the cross-linking density reaches a certain threshold, T_g becomes the dominant factor in controlling free-strain recovery. For SMPs with equivalent T_g, cross-linking density (measured via rubbery modulus) directly controls the amount of recovery stress exerted under fixed-strain conditions, as the recovery stress is directly proportional to the rubbery modulus. For SMPs with equivalent cross-linking density and varying T_g, the recovery stress is equivalent; thus T_g does not control the recovery stress (Yakacki et al., 2008a; Figure 2.5).

These initial investigations explored the fundamental relationships between T_g, cross-linking density, shape recovery, and recovery stress. In order to optimize SMPs for biomedical applications, further studies explored other fundamental relationships between T_g, cross-linking density, chemical structure, and failure strain in order to maximize shape change and offer further tailorability. For example, chemically cross-linked SMPs that have T_g as the T_a display a peak in their failure strain as a function of temperature, typically near the onset of T_g, as defined by DMA. The peak failure strain increases as the cross-linking density decreases (Yakacki et al., 2008c). By significantly decreasing the cross-linking density and tailoring the T_g, up to 800% strain recovery has been demonstrated (Voit et al., 2010). This peak's temperature position is independent of cross-linking density and will shift as the T_g of the SMP changes (Safranski and Gall, 2008). Similarly, a peak in toughness also occurs for these SMPs within a temperature range near the onset of T_g (Smith et al., 2009, 2011). As a result, the optimal programming temperature for most of these SMPs is not above T_g, but either at T_g or its onset. This allows for maximization of shape change and limits material damage.

The methacrylate SMPs offer a wide variety of T_g values from −29 to 112 °C and rubbery modulus from 2.8 to 129.5 MPa, where their thermo-mechanical properties in relation to their failure strain has been explored (Safranski and Gall, 2008). At a low rubbery modulus ($E < 10$ MPa), the chemical structure plays a role in the failure strain capacity; however, at high rubbery modulus ($E > 10$ MPa), the cross-linking density dominates over the chemical structure's influence on the failure strain capacity (Figure 2.6). This emphasizes that a wide variety of monomers are possible for methacrylate networks and chemical structure can play a significant role in the thermo-mechanical properties and performance.

In order to apply these SMPs to actual biomedical devices, the effect of different sterilization methods and the effect of long-term storage on the thermo-mechanical properties must also be considered (Yakacki et al., 2008b; Ortega et al., 2012). In one study, six different sterilization techniques (steam, ethylene oxide, low

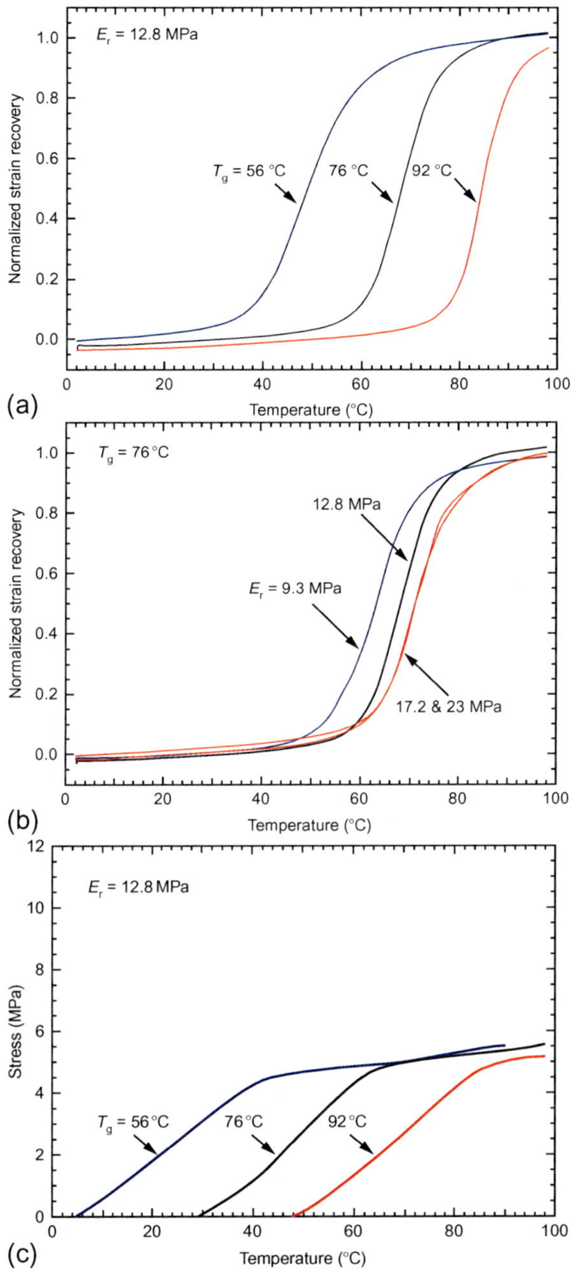

Figure 2.5 (a) Free-strain recovery as a function of temperature for varying glass transition. (b) Free-strain recovery as a function of temperature for varying rubbery modulus. (c) Fixed-strain recovery as a function of temperature for varying glass transition.

(Continued)

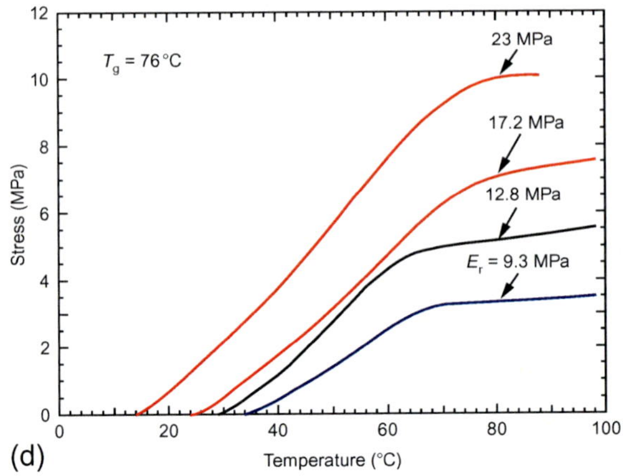

Figure 2.5 Continued. (d) Fixed-strain recovery as a function of temperature for varying rubbery modulus.
Adapted from Yakacki et al. (2008a) with permission from Wiley.

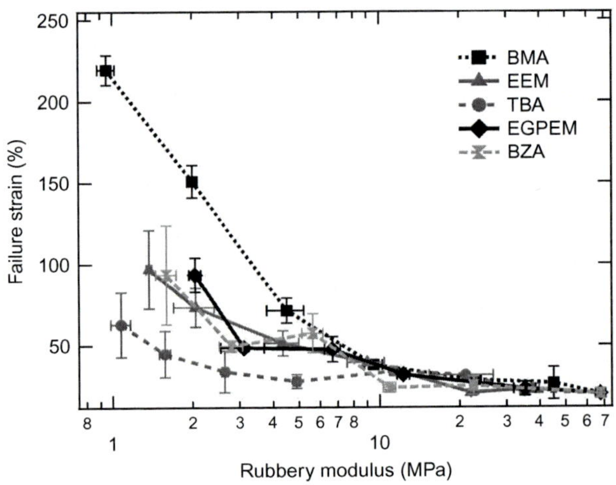

Figure 2.6 Failure strain as a function of rubbery modulus for five series of chemically cross-linked methacrylate networks composed of mixtures of PEGDMA and benzyl methacrylate (BMA), or ethoxy ethyl methacrylate (EEM), or tert-butyl acrylate (TBA), or ethylene glycol phenyl ether methacrylate (EGPEM), or benzyl acrylate (BZA). Failure strain was measured from tensile testing each network at its respective T_g.
Adapted from Safranski and Gall (2008), with permission from Elsevier.

temperature plasma, e-beam radiation, gamma radiation, and nitrogen dioxide) were used on the methacrylate SMPs. Low-temperature plasma altered the surface oxidation, thus negatively affecting the biocompatibility of the SMP. Gamma radiation decreased the T_g and increased the rubbery modulus by a statistically significant amount, but practical performance was not evaluated under altered conditions. The other sterilization methods did not significantly alter the thermo-mechanical properties. Methacrylate SMPs were programmed and stored for over 1 year at 20 °C. SMPs exhibited full shape recovery under free-strain conditions. The T_a increased by up to 9 °C and the rate of recovery increased by up to 9 × due to physical aging. Storage and aging of SMPs would allow for faster activation *in vivo* if the increase in T_a did not negatively affect recovery.

These model SMP systems made from chemically cross-linked methacrylates have established many of the fundamental relationships between chemical structure, cross-linking density, T_g, and SMP performance, such as free-strain recovery, fixed-strain recovery, and overall shape-change due to their highly tailorable chemical structure.

2.2.2 Semicrystalline degradable chemically cross-linked SMPs

PCL-based SMPs are another system being studied for use in biomedical applications. These are chemically cross-linked networks, either photopolymerized or thermally cross-linked, but use a crystalline segment and a T_m to switch from the original shape to the temporary shape (Lendlein et al., 2001, 2005b; Kelch et al., 2007).

Initially, PCL diols of varying molecular weight were methacrylated and subsequently photo-cross-linked to produce semicrystalline cross-linked networks. The T_m ranged from 32 to 50 °C as the molecular weight of the PCL diol increased from 1500 to 10,000 g/mol. The mechanical properties were well characterized with elastic moduli at room temperature ranging from 2.4 to 71 MPa and failure strains from 16.1% to 290%, producing very durable SMPs. The failure strain at 70 °C above T_a ranged from 24% to 210% as molecular weight increased, thus decreasing cross-linking density. The free-strain recovery ranged from 92% to 97% and shape fixity varied from 92% to 97% over five thermo-mechanical cycles (Lendlein et al., 2005b).

A second system of PCL dimethacrylates were mixed with a varying amount of butyl acrylate, forming a co-network of a semicrystalline degradable cross-linker and a nondegradable monomer. T_m decreased from 51 to 45 °C as amount of butyl acrylate increased. Failure strain ranged from 12% to 550% depending upon the molecular weight of the cross-linker and the amount of co-monomer. Modulus decreased and failure strain increased as the amount of butyl acrylate increased due to a decrease in cross-linking density. The total strain recovery remained high (93–98%) as butyl acrylate concentration increased, suggesting no influence on recovery properties; however, at high concentrations of butyl acrylate (70%), the strain fixity decreased to 82%, suggesting high concentrations of monomer disrupt the crystallinity and the ability to hold a temporary shape (Lendlein et al., 2001).

In a similar SMP system consisting of a semicrystalline oligo[(ε-hydroxycaproate)-co-glycolate] dimethacrylate or its co-network with butyl acrylate, the T_a could be varied from 18 to 52 °C by changing glycolate content. Some SMPs were able to show near complete strain recovery and shape fixity near 94%. Failure strain ranged from 120% to 360% as the molecular weight of the cross-linker increased. Degradation rate could be controlled by adjusting amorphous monomer content in the cross-linkers. Select networks showed activation near 35–36 °C, making them suitable for biomedical applications (Kelch et al., 2007). However, many of these networks have not undergone the fixed-strain testing to characterize recovery stress and are not intended for biomedical applications that experience high mechanical forces.

In another SMP system, polycyclooctene was cross-linked with small concentrations of peroxide and displayed rapid free-strain recovery in less than 1 s. As the peroxide concentration increased, the crystallinity decreased from 25.5% to 2.6%, which resulted in poor shape recovery. T_m increased by increasing the amount of the trans-configuration. Also, the T_m decreased from 60.3 to 16.7 °C as peroxide concentration increased (0–10%) (Liu et al., 2002). This system exhibited highly tailorable properties by adjustment of monomer structure and initiator concentration and may see use in biomedical applications, such as dental or orthopedic fields.

With these semicrystalline SMPs, control of crystallinity is key because it not only dictates T_m, but also failure strain and modulus. There is an inherent trade-off between activation, crystallinity, and mechanical performance, where a lower T_a requires a lower molecular weight monomer and often a less crystalline monomer, which sacrifices mechanical properties. Currently, some of these SMPs are being studied in combination with biodegradation for biomedical applications, such as drug release (Wischke et al., 2009, 2010, 2013; Wischke and Lendlein, 2010; Neffe et al., 2009).

2.2.3 Polyurethane SMPs

In the 1990s, much of the research on SMPs originated in Japan, particularly focusing on the shape-memory polyurethanes (Tobushi et al., 1996, 1998; Takahashi et al., 1996). Mitsubishi Heavy Industries subsidiary SMP Technologies, Inc. has been selling thermoplastic and thermoset polyurethane SMPs for several years often using the trade name Diaplex™. While many studies have evaluated SMP polyurethanes, Maitland and Kim have particularly studied these SMPs extensively (Kim et al., 1996, 1998, 2000, 2001; Jeong et al., 2000; Cabanlit et al., 2007; Maitland et al., 2002; Hearon et al., 2011; Baer et al., 2006; Wilson et al., 2007).

Early work on shape-memory polyurethanes by Kim focused on a system of shape-memory polyurethanes based on PCL-soft segment and MDI-BD-hard segments with the molecular weight of the PCL diol ranging from 2000 to 8000 g/mol and the soft segment content ranging from 50% to 90%. The sharpness of the T_a transition increased as the molecular weight and soft segment content increased, which improved the shape-memory behavior. The shape fixity reached near 99% and the shape recovery reached near 85% for SMPs with highest molecular weight of PCL diol (8000 g/mol) and high soft segment content (80%) (Kim et al., 1996).

Initially, Maitland evaluated several Mitsubishi materials in laser activated cardiovascular applications, such as micro-actuators for removing thrombi to treat stroke and releasing embolic coils to treat aneurysms. Activation of the coil could be achieved in 5 s in a simulated environment (Cabanlit et al., 2007; Maitland et al., 2002; Small et al., 2005, 2010; Baer et al., 2007). These evaluations provided successful results that necessitated further examination of the Mitsubishi SMPs as biomedical materials.

In 2006, an independent evaluation of the shape-memory properties of the thermoset and thermoplastic SMP polyurethanes from Mitsubishi was made (Baer et al.,

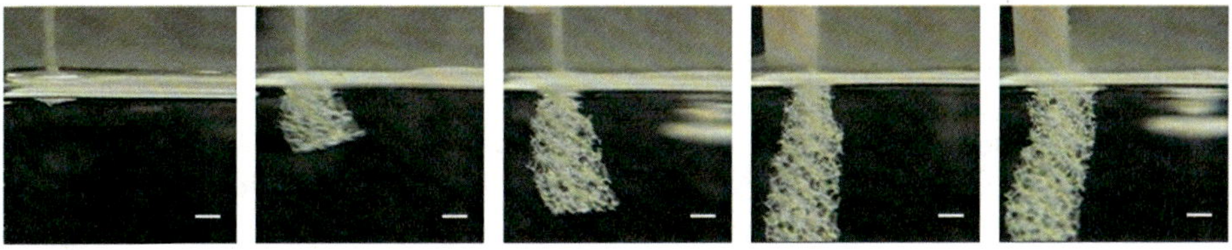

Figure 2.7 Recovery of shape-memory polyurethane foam. Water bath temperature is 80 °C. The approximate time between images is 1 s and scale bar is 2.5 mm. Reproduced from Singhal et al. (2012), with permission from Wiley.

2006). The T_g of the soft segment ranged from 46 to 74 °C via tan delta from DMA and the rubbery modulus ranged from 1.3 to 5.9 MPa. For the SMPs, failure strain was investigated as cure temperature was varied. As the first cure temperature decreased, the failure strain increased from 51% to 95% at 37 °C. However, no clear trend was seen when tested at 80 °C, where the failure strain ranged from 241% to 271%. The free-strain recovery ranged from 84% to 89% and shape fixity ranged from 96% to 99% depending upon amount of strain, cure conditions, and recovery temperature (Baer et al., 2006). Due to sufficient mechanical properties, biological compatibility testing was investigated and found to have excellent biocompatibility for vascular applications (Cabanlit et al., 2007).

Newer polyurethane networks were synthesized from aliphatic monomers with T_g ranging from 40 to 92 °C and modulus from 3 to 7 MPa by varying the chemical structure. After an initial SM cycle, the SMPs have 98–100% recovery (Wilson et al., 2007). These networks set the baseline for producing devices with greater recovery. Using these chemistries, low density SMP polyurethane foams were also created, exhibiting 97–98% shape recovery and up to 70 × volume expansion (Figure 2.7). The foams have a recovery stress near 10 kPa under fixed-strain conditions. With very low density at 0.015 g/cm^3 and favorable biocompatibility, these materials are under further development by Shape Memory Therapeutics, Inc. (Singhal et al., 2012). Polyurethanes have had a long history in biomedical devices, in particular cardiovascular devices. These SMPs, especially as foams, can be tailored to meet a wide variety of biomedical applications.

2.3 Mechanical properties of SMP biomedical devices

2.3.1 *Orthopedic SMP devices*

The promise of SMPs in biomedical applications has yet to be fully realized. However, several technologies have been successfully introduced into the orthopedic marketplace. These include combinations of both mechanical recovery and thermal recovery. In particular, a company called MedShape (Atlanta, GA) has successfully cleared two shape-memory devices through the United States Food and Drug Administration (US FDA) for human use and in products intended for permanent implantation.

The first product cleared through the US FDA utilized a thermoset-acrylic-based co-polymer (referred to as Memori®) with shape-memory behavior in both mechanical and thermal recovery. This product (WedgeLoc™; refer to premarket application #K083792 (MedShape Solutions, 2009a)) serves as a suture anchor in soft-tissue reconstruction procedures such as rotator cuff repair (Figure 2.8; MedShape, 2012a). The pullout strength of a suture anchor is dependent upon its bearing area, where increasing the

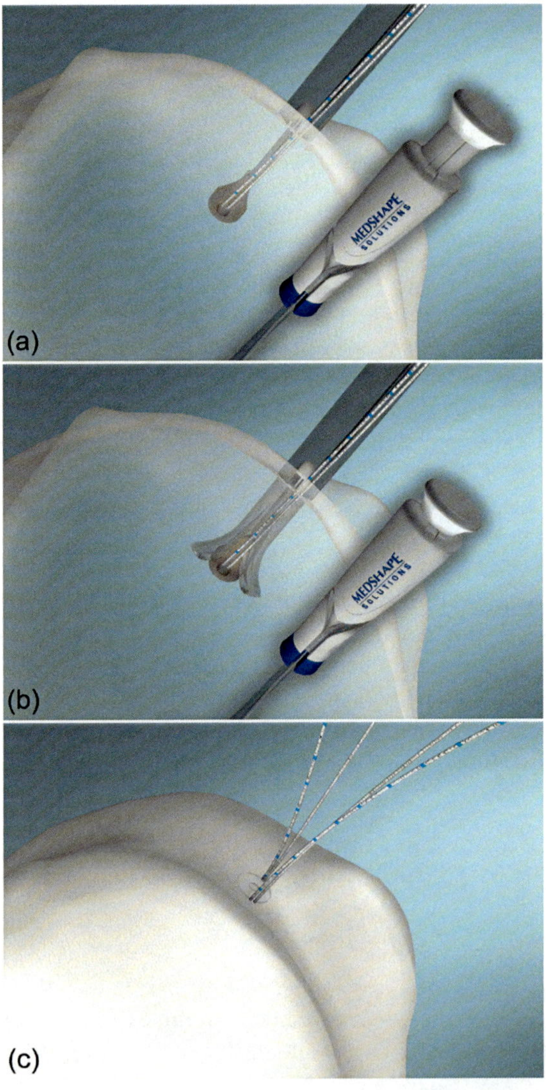

Figure 2.8 (a) WedgeLoc™ driver positioned over site of implantation. (b) Wedgeloc™ implant deployed within bone tunnel. (c) WedgeLoc™ implant with driver removed.

bearing area increases the pullout strength (Yakacki et al., 2009b). By using a SMP, the suture anchor could be implanted in a small profile and then expand in place to increase the bearing area and pullout force. Wedgeloc™ is initially (mechanically) deployed within the cancellous layer of bone to provide initial fixation. However, the material can continue expanding over time due to thermal recovery to accommodate changes to the surrounding bone substrate. The SMP material was tailored to more closely match the modulus of cancellous bone.

This SMP falls under the Class I chemically cross-linked glassy thermosets and utilizes a T_g for shape change at approximately 70 °C, and a rubbery modulus near 11 MPa. At room temperature, Memori® has a Young's modulus near 200 MPa, but begins thermal recovery at body temperature, which can be rapidly accelerated at or over 50 °C. Compressive strain to failure exceeds 50%. The material is exceptionally durable and has shown stability under long-term storage conditions over 40% (compressive) strain for periods of up to 2 years.

A follow-up product was introduced by MedShape using a polymer based on thermoplastic PEEK (polyetheretherketone; referred to as PEEK Altera®) that exhibits shape-memory through mechanical recovery. This product (Morphix®; refer to premarket applications #K092102 and #K92914 (MedShape Solutions, 2009b,c)) also serves as a suture anchor in soft-tissue repair procedures identical to those for the previous WedgeLoc™ product (Figure 2.9). However, the material is exclusively mechanically deployed (without any thermal activation) and intended to bridge both cortical and cancellous layers of bone. Much like the previous device, the additional expansion of the material can be achieved to accommodate changes in surrounding bone. However, this expansion is accomplished via subsequent cyclic loading of the sutures trapped in the bone through the expansion component (referred to as the eyelet). As the anchor is loaded over time and during rehab, the loading itself provides the additional mechanical impetus required to further deploy the shape-memory implant. This PEEK-based polymer system utilizes a mechanical recovery for shape change and has a Young's modulus approaching 3 GPa at body temperature. The material has proven to be exceptionally durable, with storage stability for periods of up to 4 years.

As a result of the success of the mechanically activated SMP *in vivo*, MedShape has launched additional orthopedic devices utilizing its unique properties, including the ExoShape® Soft Tissue Fastener. This device is deployed within bone in conjunction with autologous or autogenous soft-tissue grafts, locking the soft tissue into the bone itself. The implant is provided to the clinician in its low-profile state and mechanically deployed once positioned with the soft tissue for repair in the bone (MedShape, 2012b, 2013a). Traditionally, soft-tissue fixation utilizes screw-based devices that may twist and damage soft-tissue grafts during insertion. The shape-memory behavior allows for easier insertion and expansion of the device without twisting of the soft-tissue graft. MedShape has leveraged the behavior of this SMP material into a wide variety of temporary geometries to accommodate many different clinical applications. Two independent product lines are based on this approach and have been successfully used clinically as early as January 2011 (ExoShape® (Figures 2.10 and 2.11); refer to premarket applications #K101808 and #K111471 (MedShape Solutions, 2010, 2011),

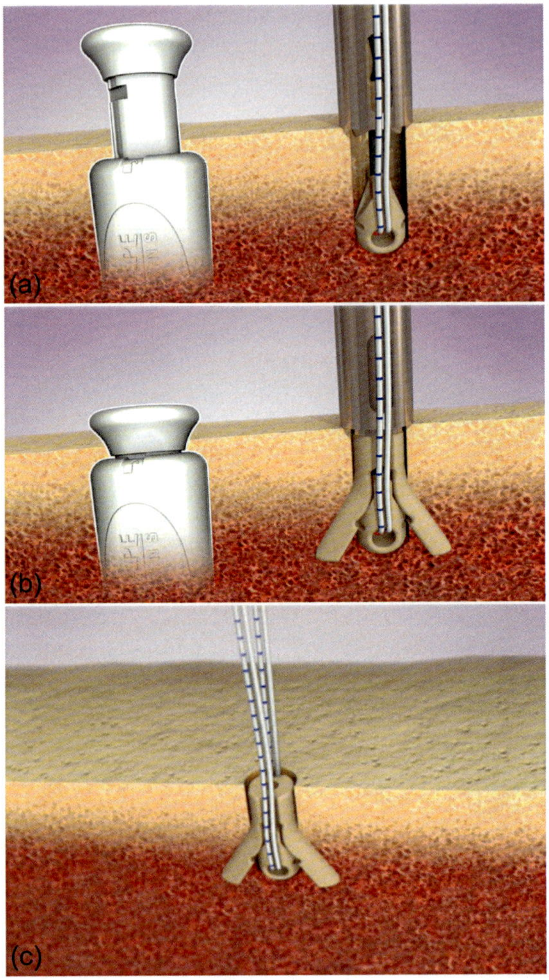

Figure 2.9 (a) Morphix® driver positioned over site of implantation. (b) Morphix® implant deployed within bone tunnel. (c) Morphix® implant with driver removed.

Figure 2.10 ExoShape® device in programmed temporary shape (left) and deployed shape (right).

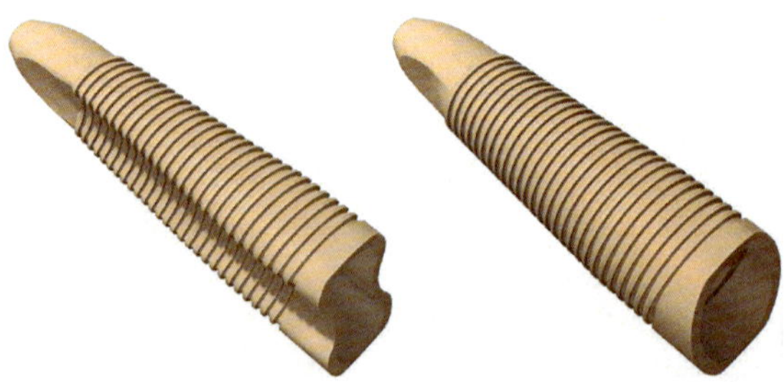

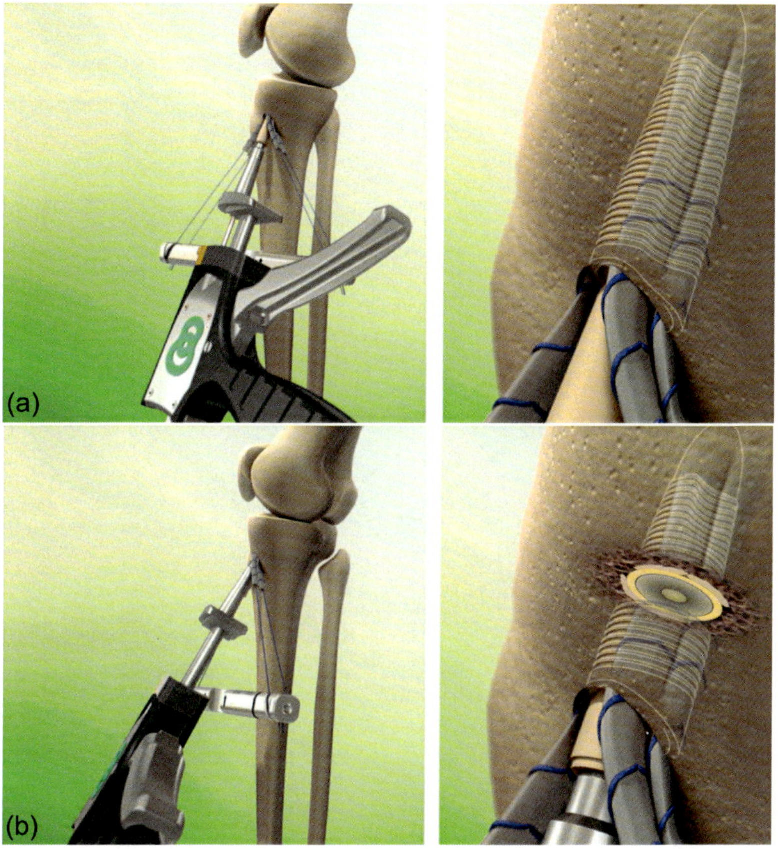

Figure 2.11 (a) ExoShape® implant as inserted into bone tunnel with soft tissue. (b) ExoShape® implant deploying into bone tunnel with soft tissue (section view showing implant expansion and soft-tissue compression).

and Eclipse™ (Figure 2.12); refer to premarket application #K123350 (MedShape, 2013b)). In benchtop testing, the ExoShape® device has exhibited average pullout strengths of 1233 N and 1254 N of bovine extensor tendon from synthetic bone and porcine bone, respectively (Smith et al., 2012). Due to its radial expansion, the device exerts an average resultant normal force of 1780 N, which has been shown to promote high pullout strength. Though the number of SMP medical devices approved for human use in orthopedics remains limited, their successful commercialization continues to provide evidence of the promise for these types of biomaterials in a wider variety of applications.

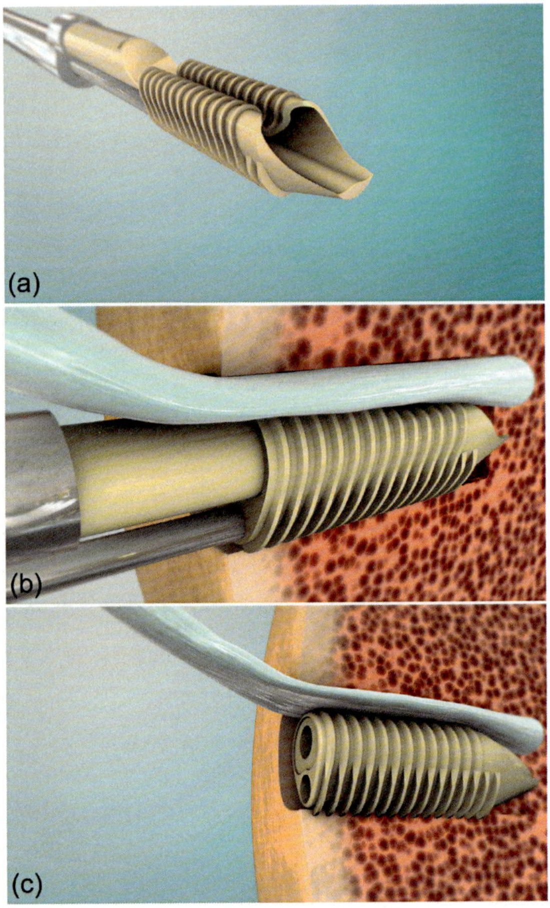

Figure 2.12 (a) Eclipse™ implant in pre-deployed (programmed) state and loaded on driver. (b) Eclipse™ implant as inserted into bone tunnel with soft tissue. (c) Eclipse™ implant deployed in bone tunnel with soft tissue and driver removed.

2.3.2 Cardiovascular SMP devices

Cardiovascular medicine was the first arena to see the successful utilization of shape-memory materials. These were primarily shape-memory metal devices based on nickel titanium alloys (refer to NiTiNOL), and had very simple geometries. Early devices based on these materials included kink-resistant guide wires, which utilized the pseudoelastic properties of the alloy (strain-induced martensite), and vena cava filters (refer to Simon NitiNOL Vena Cava Filter) that utilized the thermal activation properties (austenite transformation) to allow for deployment upon exposure to body temperature. Later, self-deploying stents (refer to Symphony® stent, originally Nitinol Medical Technologies later acquired by Boston Scientific Corporation, and Memotherm® stent, originally Angiomed later acquired by C.R. Bard) also saw extensive use of these alloys in their various modalities. Though a significant amount of research (both pre-clinical and clinical) has been conducted on SMP cardiovascular devices, no devices to date have successfully utilized SMP in a commercial cardiovascular application.

A significant amount of research has been undertaken to evaluate the application of shape-memory biomaterials in cardiovascular devices. In most cases, this research has focused on their use in the construction of stents or stent grafts (Small et al., 2010). The primary benefits of this approach include reduction in complexity for stent delivery, closer matching of the native modulus of the vessel, and the opportunity to eliminate the use of metals that may not be compatible with magnetic resonance imaging. Research conducted by Shandas and Gall focused on the use of thermoset-acrylic-based co-polymers similar to those successfully utilized in orthopedic applications (Gall et al., 2005; Yakacki et al., 2007).

Alternatively, a variety of thermoplastic-based polymers have been evaluated in stent applications. These have primarily been focused on the use of polyurethane-based SMPs (Colombo and Karvouni, 2000). In particular, shape-memory biodegradable polymers have been of recent interest in that they combine the advantages of low complexity and self-deployment with bioresorption. As early as 2000, Tamai et al. (2000) reported the use of a biodegradable shape-memory stent in humans. The stent utilized the thermal recovery properties of PLLA to deploy a cardiovascular stent via a heated balloon (injected with sterile contrast media/saline mixture at 70 °C to initiate the shape recovery, followed by mechanical expansion using balloon dilatation). The stent was reported to be capable of continued expansion over a 3-month time period at body temperature and in response to physiological remodeling of the target vessel. Recently, 10-year post-operative follow-up was reported with results equivalent to bare metal stents (Nishio et al., 2012). The Ikagi-Tamai (shape-memory) bioresorbable stent received approval for human use in peripheral vascular applications in 2007 (CE Mark via European Union only; no FDA approval reported to date).

Additional research into SMP stents has proven promising, including incorporation of drug-eluting characteristics (Wache et al., 2003) and the use of braided structures to achieve higher strain capacity and durability (Kim et al., 2010). Thermoplastic polyurethanes (TPUs) have also been utilized in stent research with mixed results (Baer et al., 2007). However, none of these approaches has seen commercial or clinical use.

In addition to stents, several other cardiovascular related SMP technologies have been under development. mNEMOSCIENCE (Aachen, Germany) developed a SMP primarily intended to serve as a self-tightening suture material (Lendlein and Langer, 2002). The initial intent was for treatment of patent foramen ovale, a congenital condition that involves a septal defect between chambers of the heart. They also targeted the use of their material to assist in femoral artery access closure (sealing of the puncture made in the femoral artery during intravascular procedures). This technology was licensed to Aporo Biomedical (Sausalito, CA). To date, this technology has not seen commercial use in either application.

Aneurysms have also seen treatments under development that utilize SMP technologies. These have primarily been in foam, including TPU (Small et al., 2010) and polymers based on poly-vinyl-alcohol (PVA) (Tadavarthy et al., 1975). Early prototypes of TPU-based shape-memory foams showed success by Maitland (Shape Memory Therapeutics, Inc.) when delivered via an intravascular approach and then activated via laser (Maitland et al., 2007; Singhal et al., 2012). This group has also researched early activation by using water uptake to decrease T_g down to 12–40 °C from 64 to 80 °C with an activation rate ranging from 2 min to 24 h (Singhal et al., 2013). Since the SMP foam cannot be seen via X-ray, 4 vol.% tungsten particulate filler was loaded into the shape-memory polyurethane in order to impart radio-opacity (Rodriguez et al., 2012). *In vitro* models of aneurysms and shape-memory deployment have been studied to predict the stresses produced by the SMP (Hwang et al., 2012), thermal and fluid dynamic changes (Small et al., 2009), and changes in vascular dynamics (Ortega et al., 2007). While significant research has gone into this application of SMP, this medical technology has yet to gain FDA clearance.

Of particular interest has been work on thermally induced phase separation, which provides a higher total shape recovery rate over more classical homogenous foams like those represented by PVA. Successful early adoption of PVA foams as embolic material in the treatment of intracranial aneurysms (Cook Medical, Bloomington, IL) has encouraged the development of SMP versions of the same. The current embolic polymer foam is injected into the aneurysm as small particles in solution. These particles are primarily used to occlude defects such as hypervascular lesions or aterio-venous malformations. They have not seen general use in aneurysm occlusion due to their embolic nature (easily swept downstream and could embolize unintentionally).

However, PVA foam structures of much larger format were developed and evaluated, utilizing shape-memory attributes common with hydration, as early as 1975 (Tadavarthy et al., 1975). Though not commonly attributed to shape memory, the act of compressing open-cell foam structures under temperature and vacuum allowed for the storage of temporary (low-profile) geometries that could recover when exposed to body temperature, and highly aqueous environments. The act of shape recovery using hydration *in vivo* allowed for a more controlled embolization of vascular aneurysms while encouraging the formation of localized thrombus and preventing unintended embolization. Though some clinical investigation use was reported for this approach, no commercial use has followed.

2.4 Future of SMPs in biomedical applications

The future of SMPs in biomedical applications is promising. Both thermal and mechanical recovery has been successfully utilized for soft-tissue repair. In addition, some of these materials have been evaluated in a variety of new applications, including soft tissue reinforcement fabrics, bone staples, meniscal repair darts, and immobilization casts. In addition, evaluation of shape-memory composites have been reported. These include the integration of hydroxyapatite (HA) into poly(*rac*-lactide), which is a thermoplastic biodegradable aliphatic polyester (Madbouly and Lendlein, 2010).

The introduction of HA is intended to produce a bioactive composite that promotes osteointegration as part of the bioabsorption of the polymer construct. There are many possible applications for these materials in bioprosthetic heart valves and ophthalmic implants, including for the treatments of presbyopia and glaucoma.

2.5 Conclusions

The mechanical properties of SMPs are highly dependent upon their chemical and physical structure. Inherent trade-offs exist in the mechanical properties in each SMP system, and precise tailoring of mechanical properties is possible by fine-tuning the chemical structure and the thermo-mechanical programming. Most SMPs today have nearly 100% shape recovery under some conditions in the laboratory. However optimization of the remaining mechanical properties for each individual biomedical application remains challenging. To undertake the production of a biomedical device, the designer must fully understand the mechanical properties of the SMP because the material and the device design are intrinsically connected to one another. The methacrylate, semicrystalline, and polyurethane systems represent the most developed SMPs and have been successfully applied in orthopedic and cardiovascular applications. The ability of these materials to accommodate physiological remodeling, as well as their MRI compatibility and potential for bioresorption, make them an ideal choice in many other medical applications. It is highly likely that this decade will see the utilization of these specialty materials in a greater number of biomedical devices than in any previous decade. As more medical technologies leverage these advantages, their use will become widespread.

References

Baer, G., et al., 2006. Shape-memory behavior of thermally stimulated polyurethane for medical applications. J. Appl. Polym. Sci. 103 (6), 3882–3892.

Baer, G.M., et al., 2007. Fabrication and in vitro deployment of a laser-activated shape memory polymer vascular stent. Biomed. Eng. Online 6, 43.

Bar-Cohen, Y. (Ed.), 2004. Electroactive Polymer (EAP) Actuators as Artificial Muscles: Reality, Potential, and Challenges, second ed. SPIE Press, Bellingham, Washington.

Behl, M., Razzaq, M.Y., Lendlein, A., 2010. Multifunctional shape-memory polymers. Adv. Mater. 22 (31), 3388–3410.

Cabanlit, M., et al., 2007. Polyurethane shape-memory polymers demonstrate functional biocompatibility in vitro. Macromol. Biosci. 7 (1), 48–55.

Choi, N.-y., Lendlein, A., 2007. Degradable shape-memory polymer networks from oligo [(L-lactide)-ran-glycolide]dimethacrylates. Soft Matter 3 (7), 901–909.

Choi, N.Y., Kelch, S., Lendlein, A., 2006. Synthesis, shape-memory functionality and hydrolytical degradation studies on polymer networks from poly(rac-lactide)-b-poly(propylene oxide)-b-poly(rac-lactide) dimethacrylates. Adv. Eng. Mater. 8 (5), 439–445.

Choi, J., et al., 2012. Effect of physical aging on the shape-memory behavior of amorphous networks. Polymer 53 (12), 2453–2464.

Chung, T., Romo-Uribe, A., Mather, P.T., 2007. Two-way reversible shape memory in a semi-crystalline network. Macromolecules 41 (1), 184–192.

Colombo, A., Karvouni, E., 2000. Biodegradable stents: "fulfilling the mission and stepping away". Circulation 102 (4), 371–373.

Di Prima, M., et al., 2007. Thermo-mechanical behavior of epoxy shape memory polymer foams. Smart Mater. Struct. 16 (6), 2330.

Feldkamp, D.M., Rousseau, I.A., 2011. Effect of chemical composition on the deformability of shape-memory epoxies. Macromol. Mater. Eng. 296 (12), 1128–1141.

Gall, K., et al., 2005. Thermomechanics of the shape memory effect in polymers for biomedical applications. J. Biomed. Mater. Res. A 73 (3), 339–348.

He, C., Kim, S.W., Lee, D.S., 2008. In situ gelling stimuli-sensitive block copolymer hydrogels for drug delivery. J. Control. Release 127 (3), 189–207.

Hearon, K., et al., 2011. Post-polymerization crosslinked polyurethane shape-memory polymers. J. Appl. Polym. Sci. 121 (1), 144–153.

Hwang, W., et al., 2012. Estimation of aneurysm wall stresses created by treatment with a shape memory polymer foam device. Biomech. Model. Mechanobiol. 11 (5), 715–729.

Jeon, H.G., Mather, P.T., Haddad, T.S., 2000. Shape memory and nanostructure in poly (norbornyl-POSS) copolymers. Polym. Int. 49 (5), 453–457.

Jeong, H., Lee, S., Kim, B., 2000. Shape memory polyurethane containing amorphous reversible phase. J. Mater. Sci. 35 (7), 1579–1583.

Kelch, S., et al., 2007. Shape-memory polymer networks from oligo[(epsilon-hydroxycaproate)-co-glycolate]dimethacrylates and butyl acrylate with adjustable hydrolytic degradation rate. Biomacromolecules 8 (3), 1018–1027.

Kim, B.K., Lee, S.Y., Xu, M., 1996. Polyurethanes having shape memory effects. Polymer 37 (26), 5781–5793.

Kim, B.K., et al., 1998. Polyurethane ionomers having shape memory effects. Polymer 39 (13), 2803–2808.

Kim, B.K., et al., 2000. Shape-memory behavior of segmented polyurethanes with an amorphous reversible phase: the effect of block length and content. J. Polym. Sci. B Polym. Phys. 38 (20), 2652–2657.

Kim, B.K., et al., 2001. Shape memory behavior of amorphous polyurethanes. J. Macromol. Sci. B 40 (6), 1179–1191.

Kim, J., Kang, T., Yu, W., 2010. Simulation of mechanical behavior of temperature-responsive braided stents made of shape memory polyurethanes. J. Biomech. 43, 632–643.

Lakhera, N., et al., 2012a. Partially constrained recovery of (meth)acrylate shape-memory polymer networks. J. Appl. Polym. Sci. 126 (1), 72–82.

Lakhera, N., et al., 2012b. Biodegradable thermoset shape-memory polymer developed from poly(β-amino ester) networks. J. Polym. Sci. B Polym. Phys. 50 (11), 777–789.

Lendlein, A., Kelch, S., 2002. Shape-memory polymers. Angew. Chem. Int. Ed. Engl. 41 (12), 2035–2057.

Lendlein, A., Kelch, S., 2005. Shape-memory polymers as stimuli-sensitive implant materials. Clin. Hemorheol. Microcirc. 32 (2), 105–116.

Lendlein, A., Langer, R., 2002. Biodegradable, elastic shape-memory polymers for potential biomedical applications. Science 296 (5573), 1673–1676.

Lendlein, A., Schmidt, A.M., Langer, R., 2001. AB-polymer networks based on oligo(epsilon-caprolactone) segments showing shape-memory properties. Proc. Natl. Acad. Sci. U. S. A. 98 (3), 842–847.

Lendlein, A., et al., 2005a. Light-induced shape-memory polymers. Nature 434 (7035), 879–882.

Lendlein, A., et al., 2005b. Shape-memory polymer networks from oligo(ϵ-caprolactone) dimethacrylates. J. Polym. Sci. A Polym. Chem. 43 (7), 1369–1381.
Li, F., et al., 1996. Crystallinity and morphology of segmented polyurethanes with different soft-segment length. J. Appl. Polym. Sci. 62 (4), 631–638.
Liu, C., Mather, P.T., 2003. In: Proceedings of the Annual Technical Conference—Society of Plastic Engineers. Society of Plastic Engineers, Brookfield, CT.
Liu, C., et al., 2002. Chemically cross-linked polycyclooctene: synthesis, characterization, and shape memory behavior. Macromolecules 35 (27), 9868–9874.
Liu, C., Qin, H., Mather, P.T., 2007. Review of progress in shape-memory polymers. J. Mater. Chem. 17 (16), 1543–1558.
Luo, X., Mather, P.T., 2010. Triple-shape polymeric composites (TSPCs). Adv. Funct. Mater. 20 (16), 2649–2656.
Madbouly, S., Lendlein, A., 2010. Shape-memory polymer composites. In: Lendlein, A. (Ed.), Shape-Memory Polymers. Springer, Berlin, Heidelberg, pp. 41–95.
Maitland, D.J., et al., 2002. Photothermal properties of shape memory polymer micro-actuators for treating stroke. Lasers Surg. Med. 30 (1), 1–11.
Maitland, D.J., et al., 2007. Prototype laser-activated shape memory polymer foam device for embolic treatment of aneurysms. J. Biomed. Opt. 12 (3), 030504.
MedShape Solutions, 2009a. 510(k) Summary, K083792. U.S. Food and Drug Administration.
MedShape Solutions, 2009b. Special 510(k) Summary, K091202. U.S. Food and Drug Administration.
MedShape Solutions, 2009c. Special 510(k) Summary, K092914. U.S. Food and Drug Administration.
MedShape Solutions, 2010. 510(k) Summary, K101808. U.S. Food and Drug Administration.
MedShape Solutions, 2011. Special 510(k) Summary, K111471. U.S. Food and Drug Administration.
MedShape, Inc., 2012a. Morphix product sheet, MK-10014. Available from: http://www.medshape.com/images/product-sheets/MK-10014-01%20Product%20Brochure%20Morphix.pdf.
MedShape, Inc., 2012b. ExoShape product sheet, MK-10042. Available from: http://www.medshape.com/images/product-sheets/exoshape_product_brochure.pdf.
MedShape, Inc., 2013a. Eclipse product sheet, MK-10095. Available from: http://www.medshape.com/images/product-sheets/eclipse_product_brochure.pdf.
MedShape, Inc., 2013b. 510(k) Summary, K123350. U.S. Food and Drug Administration.
Mohr, R., et al., 2006. Initiation of shape-memory effect by inductive heating of magnetic nanoparticles in thermoplastic polymers. Proc. Natl. Acad. Sci. U. S. A. 103 (10), 3540–3545.
Nair, D.P., et al., 2010. Photopolymerized thiol-ene systems as shape memory polymers. Polymer 51 (19), 4383–4389.
Neffe, A.T., et al., 2009. Polymer networks combining controlled drug release, biodegradation, and shape memory capability. Adv. Mater. 21 (32–33), 3394–3398.
Nguyen, T.D., et al., 2010. Modeling the relaxation mechanisms of amorphous shape memory polymers. Adv. Mater. 22 (31), 3411–3423.
Nishio, S., et al., 2012. Long-term (>10 years) clinical outcomes of first-in-human biodegradable poly-L-lactic acid coronary stents: Igaki-Tamai stents. Circulation 125 (19), 2343–2353.
Ortega, J., et al., 2007. Vascular dynamics of a shape memory polymer foam aneurysm treatment technique. Ann. Biomed. Eng. 35 (11), 1870–1884.
Ortega, A.M., et al., 2012. Effect of crosslinking and long-term storage on the shape-memory behavior of (meth)acrylate-based shape-memory polymers. Soft Matter 8 (28), 7381–7392.

Pierce, B.F., et al., 2011. Demonstrating the influence of water on shape-memory polymer networks based on poly[(rac-lactide)-co-glycolide] segments in vitro. Int. J. Artif. Organs 34 (2), 172–179.

Qin, H., Mather, P.T., 2008. Combined one-way and two-way shape memory in a glass-forming nematic network. Macromolecules 42 (1), 273–280.

Qiu, Y., Park, K., 2001. Environment-sensitive hydrogels for drug delivery. Adv. Drug Deliv. Rev. 53 (3), 321–339.

Rodriguez, J.N., et al., 2012. Opacification of shape memory polymer foam designed for treatment of intracranial aneurysms. Ann. Biomed. Eng. 40 (4), 883–897.

Safranski, D.L., Gall, K., 2008. Effect of chemical structure and crosslinking density on the thermo-mechanical properties and toughness of (meth)acrylate shape memory polymer networks. Polymer 49 (20), 4446–4455.

Safranski, D.L., Smith, K.E., Gall, K., 2013. Mechanical requirements of shape-memory polymers in biomedical devices. Polym. Rev. 53 (1), 76–91.

Singhal, P., et al., 2012. Ultra low density and highly crosslinked biocompatible shape memory polyurethane foams. J. Polym. Sci. B Polym. Phys. 50, 724–737.

Singhal, P., et al., 2013. Controlling the actuation rate of low-density shape-memory polymer foams in water. Macromol. Chem. Phys. 214, 1204–1214.

Small IV., W., et al., 2005. Laser-activated shape memory polymer intravascular thrombectomy device. Opt. Express 13 (20), 8204–8213.

Small, W.t., et al., 2009. Magnetic resonance flow velocity and temperature mapping of a shape memory polymer foam device. Biomed. Eng. Online 8, 42.

Small, W.t., et al., 2010. Biomedical applications of thermally activated shape memory polymers. J. Mater. Chem. 20 (18), 3356–3366.

Smith, K.E., et al., 2009. The effect of the glass transition temperature on the toughness of photopolymerizable (meth)acrylate networks under physiological conditions. Polymer (Guildf) 50 (21), 5112–5123.

Smith, K.E., et al., 2011. Long-term toughness of photopolymerizable (meth)acrylate networks in aqueous environments. Acta Biomater. 7 (2), 558–567.

Smith, K.E., et al., 2012. Anterior cruciate ligament fixation: is radial force a predictor of the pullout strength of soft-tissue interference devices? Knee 19 (6), 786–792.

Song, L., et al., 2010. Tailored (meth)acrylate shape-memory polymer networks for ophthalmic applications. Macromol. Biosci. 10 (10), 1194–1202.

Tadavarthy, S., Moller, J., Amplatz, K., 1975. Polyvinyl alcohol (Ivalon)—a new embolic material. Am. J. Roentgenol. 125, 609–616.

Takahashi, T., Hayashi, N., Hayashi, S., 1996. Structure and properties of shape-memory polyurethane block copolymers. J. Appl. Polym. Sci. 60 (7), 1061–1069.

Tamai, H., et al., 2000. Initial and 6-month results of biodegradable poly-L-lactic acid coronary stents in humans. Circulation 102 (4), 399–404.

Tobushi, H., et al., 1996. Thermomechanical properties in a thin film of shape memory polymer of polyurethane series. Smart Mater. Struct. 5, 483–491.

Tobushi, H., et al., 1998. Shape fixity and shape recovery in a film of shape memory polymer of polyurethane series. J. Intell. Mater. Syst. Struct. 9 (2), 127–136.

Voit, W., et al., 2010. High-strain shape-memory polymers. Adv. Funct. Mater. 20 (1), 162–171.

Wache, M., et al., 2003. Development of a polymer stent with shape memory effect as a drug delivery system. J. Mater. Sci. Mater. Med. 14, 109–112.

Ware, T., et al., 2012a. Triple-shape memory polymers based on self-complementary hydrogen bonding. Macromolecules 45 (2), 1062–1069.

Ware, T., et al., 2012b. Three-dimensional flexible electronics enabled by shape memory polymer substrates for responsive neural interfaces. Macromol. Mater. Eng. 297 (12), 1193–1202.
Wilson, T., et al., 2007. Shape memory polymers based on uniform aliphatic urethane networks. J. Appl. Polym. Sci. 106 (1), 540–551.
Wischke, C., Lendlein, A., 2010. Shape-memory polymers as drug carriers—a multifunctional system. Pharm. Res. 27 (4), 527–529.
Wischke, C., et al., 2009. Evaluation of a degradable shape-memory polymer network as matrix for controlled drug release. J. Control. Release 138 (3), 243–250.
Wischke, C., et al., 2010. Comparing techniques for drug loading of shape-memory polymer networks—effect on their functionalities. Eur. J. Pharm. Sci. 41 (1), 136–147.
Wischke, C., Behl, M., Lendlein, A., 2013. Drug-releasing shape-memory polymers—the role of morphology, processing effects, and matrix degradation. Expert Opin. Drug Deliv. 10, 1193–1205.
Xie, T., 2010. Tunable polymer multi-shape memory effect. Nature 464 (7286), 267–270.
Xie, T., Rousseau, I.A., 2009. Facile tailoring of thermal transition temperatures of epoxy shape memory polymers. Polymer 50 (8), 1852–1856.
Yakacki, C., Gall, K., 2010. Shape-memory polymers for biomedical applications. In: Lendlein, A. (Ed.), Shape-Memory Polymers. Springer, Berlin, Heidelberg, pp. 147–175.
Yakacki, C.M., et al., 2007. Unconstrained recovery characterization of shape-memory polymer networks for cardiovascular applications. Biomaterials 28 (14), 2255–2263.
Yakacki, C.M., et al., 2008a. Strong, tailored, biocompatible shape-memory polymer networks. Adv. Funct. Mater. 18 (16), 2428–2435.
Yakacki, C.M., et al., 2008b. Cytotoxicity and thermomechanical behavior of biomedical shape-memory polymer networks post-sterilization. Biomed. Mater. 3 (1), 015010.
Yakacki, C.M., et al., 2008c. Deformation limits in shape-memory polymers. Adv. Eng. Mater. 10 (1–2), 112–119.
Yakacki, C.M., et al., 2009a. Shape-memory polymer networks with Fe_3O_4 nanoparticles for remote activation. J. Appl. Polym. Sci. 112 (5), 3166–3176.
Yakacki, C.M., et al., 2009b. Bearing area: a new indication for suture anchor pullout strength? J. Orthop. Res. 27 (8), 1048–1054.
Yakacki, C.M., et al., 2011. Impact of shape-memory programming on mechanically-driven recovery in polymers. Polymer 52 (21), 4947–4954.
Yang, B., et al., 2004. On the effects of moisture in a polyurethane shape memory polymer. Smart Mater. Struct. 13 (1), 191.
Yang, B., et al., 2005. Effects of moisture on the glass transition temperature of polyurethane shape memory polymer filled with nano-carbon powder. Eur. Polym. J. 41 (5), 1123–1128.
Yang, B., et al., 2006. Effects of moisture on the thermomechanical properties of a polyurethane shape memory polymer. Polymer 47 (4), 1348–1356.
Yu, Y.J., et al., 2011. The effect of moisture absorption on the physical properties of polyurethane shape memory polymer foams. Smart Mater. Struct. 20 (8), 085010.

Characterization of shape-memory polymers for biomedical applications

3

K. Dyamenahalli, A. Famili, R. Shandas
University of Colorado, Aurora, CO, USA

3.1 Introduction

Potential uses of shape-memory polymers (SMPs) and their composites in the medical field are numerous and include endovascular devices, such as stents and embolic coils, intra-abdominal patch repair of inguinal hernias or pelvic organ prolapse, intra-ocular lenses, and drug delivery devices. The goal of this chapter is to familiarize the reader with modern laboratory tools available to study properties of SMPs in view of their proposed function. While some of the techniques described herein can be generalized to the characterization of traditional polymers or SMPs designed for industrial uses, most were selected specifically for their relevance to SMPs intended for biomedical applications. In such roles, the utility of SMPs is most often found in the mechanical properties they display following a thermal transition, typically occurring near body temperature. Primary among these properties are the glass transition temperature, glassy and rubbery moduli, strain-recovery and fixity rates, and recovery stress. That said, this chapter encompasses a much wider range of techniques, from microstructural characterization to measurement of oxidative stability and surface fouling. In addition to discussing theoretical concepts and practical considerations associated with each SMP characterization technique, we attempt to lead the reader through the process of identifying the most relevant properties to evaluate and the comparative advantages of each technique, in an application-specific manner. Accordingly, we begin with a series of Tables 3.1–3.5, which score the ability of various material characterization techniques to evaluate SMP properties. Guidance for further reading, a listing of important ASTM and ISO reference standards, and additional resources have also been provided.

3.2 Structural and chemical characterization

Extensive structural and chemical characterization is necessary to understand the nature of SMPs and predict their behavior. While a precise composition is typically targeted at the start of any synthesis procedure, it must be verified experimentally

Shape Memory Polymers for Biomedical Applications. http://dx.doi.org/10.1016/B978-0-85709-698-2.00003-9

Table 3.1 Techniques for structural and chemical analysis

	UV–vis spectroscopy	FTIR spectroscopy	GPC	WAXD	NMR spectroscopy	MS
Molecular weight and polydispersity	–	–	**	–	*	**
Functional groups	*	**	–	–	**	–
Chemical composition	*	**	–	–	**	*
Chain conformations	–	*	*	**	**	–
Transitions	–	**	–	–	**	–
Residual monomers	**	**	–	–	**	**
End groups	*	**	–	–	**	*
Degree of crystallinity	–	–	–	**	*	–

**, strong technique for acquiring this information; *, weak technique for acquiring this information; –, technique inadequate for acquiring this information; UV–vis, ultraviolet–visible; FTIR, Fourier transform infrared; GPC, gel permeation chromatography; WAXD, wide-angle X-ray diffraction; NMR, nuclear magnetic resonance; MS, mass spectrometry.

Table 3.2 Techniques for mechanical and thermo-mechanical analysis

	Tensometry	DMA	DSC	TGA	Rheology
Isothermal elastic deformation properties	**	*	–	–	–
Flexural and shear moduli	*	**	–	–	**
Complex, storage and loss moduli	–	**	–	–	–
Shape recovery parameters	–	**	–	–	–
Creep and stress relaxation	**	**	–	–	–
Thermal decomposition behavior	–	–	*	**	–
T_g and T_m	–	**	**	*	–
Sub-T_g thermal transitions	–	**	*	*	–
Viscosity	–	**	**	–	**

**, strong technique for acquiring this information; *, weak technique for acquiring this information; –, technique inadequate for acquiring this information; DMA, dynamic mechanical analysis; DSC, differential scanning calorimetry; TGA, thermogravimetric analysis.

Table 3.3 **Techniques for analysis of surface properties**

	AFM	Contact angle measurements	XPS	TOF-SIMS
Surface chemistry	**	*	**	**
Surface wetting and free energy	–	**	–	–
Surface functionalization	**	–	**	**
Surface topology	**	*	–	–
Surface mechanical properties	**	–	–	–

**, strong technique for acquiring this information; *, weak technique for acquiring this information; –, technique inadequate for acquiring this information; AFM, atomic force microscopy; XPS, X-ray photoelectron spectroscopy; TOF-SIMS, time-of-flight secondary ion mass spectrometry.

using multiple specific methods. The combined output of these analyses provides insight into the chemical structure of the synthesized SMP, with each providing insight into one or more desired polymer properties, as outlined in Table 3.1.

3.2.1 *Ultraviolet–visible spectroscopy*

Ultraviolet–visible (UV–vis) spectroscopy is a technique most commonly applied to quantitative measurement of solutions, specifically for determining concentrations of known solutes. However, its application to solid-state samples can also provide valuable insights. Some of the key advantages of UV–vis spectroscopy are its relative ease of use, cost-effectiveness, and sampling speed. Hence, it can be a good starting point for proof-of-concept work or to guide early experimentation.

The physical principles underlying this method are straightforward, making the instrumentation simple and robust. Light of known wavelength and intensity is directed at the sample and its final intensity, after passing through, is measured by a detector. By comparing the incident radiation (I_0) and the transmitted radiation (I), the amount of light absorbed by the sample at that particular wavelength can be easily calculated. Using the Beer–Lambert law, this absorption can be used to measure concentrations of known solutes:

$$A = \log_{10}\left(\frac{I_0}{I}\right) = \varepsilon \cdot c \cdot L$$

In this equation, A is absorbance, ε is the molar absorbtivity (L mol^{-1} cm^{-1}), c is the concentration of the dissolved solute (mol L^{-1}), and L is the path length (cm). UV–vis spectroscopy is relatively weak at identifying compounds; it is much more useful in quantitative assessments. In SMP characterization, UV–vis spectroscopy is an especially effective method for measuring basic optical characteristics of a sample

Table 3.4 Techniques for optical/imaging properties

	SEM	TEM	Phantom-based X-ray imaging	Phantom-based MR imaging	UV–vis spectroscopy	FTIR spectroscopy	Ellipsometry
Near-visible absorbance/ transmittance spectra	–	–	–	–	**	**	–
Refraction, aberration, and birefringence	–	–	–	–	–	–	**
Radio-opacity	–	–	**	–	–	–	–
MR signal and artifacts	–	–	–	**	–	–	–
Porosity, density, and free space	*	**	–	–	–	–	–

**, strong technique for acquiring this information; *, weak technique for acquiring this information; –, technique inadequate for acquiring this information; SEM, scanning electron microscopy; TEM, transmission electron microscopy; UV–vis, ultraviolet–visible; FTIR, Fourier transform infrared.

Table 3.5 **Techniques for biocompatibility analysis**

	In vitro cytotoxicity	*In vitro* functional testing	*In vivo* sensitization	*In vivo* irritation	*In vivo* functional testing
Material stability	*	*	*	*	**
Cytotoxicity	**	*	**	**	*
Pyrogenicity	–	–	**	**	*
Cellular functional response	–	**	–	–	*
Physiological functional response	–	–	–	–	**
Protein adsorption	–	**	–	–	**

**, strong technique for acquiring this information; *, weak technique for acquiring this information.

and the concentrations of its known extractables or degradation products. Optical characteristics measured in the solid phase will be of particular interest for ocular device applications, where UV-blocking properties must be characterized and quantified and optical clarity in the visible region is critical (Song et al., 2010). In addition, knowledge of the absorption spectrum is important for light-activated SMP systems, depending on the wavelength of light in question (Wilson et al., 2007). Extraction studies, used to quantify the ability of unreacted monomers or other additives (e.g., plasticizers or stabilizers) to diffuse out of the SMP network, often employ UV–vis spectroscopy to measure the concentration of these compounds in the extraction medium. However, more sensitive methods, such as high-performance liquid chromatography (HPLC), can also be used (Haider and Karlsson, 1999).

3.2.2 *Fourier transform infrared spectroscopy*

Fourier transform infrared spectroscopy (FTIR) is an invaluable analytical tool, especially when assessing bond conversion during polymerization. Like UV–vis spectroscopy, FTIR relies on transmission of radiation through a sample. However, moving from the UV and visible to the infrared regions of the electromagnetic spectrum allows for detection of molecular vibrational states, which provides information on chemical structure and bonding.

For a molecule to absorb energy in the infrared energy range, it must possess a mode of vibration that causes a shift in dipole moment. This dipole moment can be caused either by permanent dipoles, which occur when two atoms in a molecule have significantly different electronegativity, or asymmetrical stretching or bending in a molecule that has no permanent dipole. The constituent atoms responsible for dipole moments will influence the energy required to vibrate or stretch these bonds, allowing IR absorption peaks to be linked with chemical structure. These spectra act as fingerprints for particular types of bonding, allowing for their identification and relative quantification.

In SMP applications, FTIR can provide a vast array of data. In addition to information about general bonding and structure within the polymer network, FTIR can identify and quantify functional groups. This is particularly advantageous when functional groups are either involved in the shape-memory transition or are to be used for subsequent tethering/modification of the polymer, such as with a biomacromolecule. Perhaps the most valuable function of FTIR is its ability to monitor polymerization-specific parameters, such as degree of conversion. By tracking the evolution of absorbance peaks associated with functional groups formed or consumed during polymerization (e.g., vinyl groups), the polymerization process can be tracked in real time. Reactions can be optimized by measuring conversion as a function of time, temperature, initiator concentration, and other parameters (Moraes et al., 2008).

For many polymer systems, attenuated total reflectance FTIR (ATR-FTIR) can be used to extend FTIR analytical principles to polymers in solution or to isolate surface properties of bulk polymers. For example, it may be used to assess the effects of storage or sterilization methods on SMP surface chemistry, including oxidation and other degradation processes. Additionally, ATR-FTIR analysis can be used to identify protein surface adsorption, with the additional benefit of providing structural information about the protein after adsorption. Conveniently, most modern FTIR spectrometers can be converted simply by mounting an ATR accessory to the sample compartment. In the ATR accessory, infrared light passes through a crystal element having a refractive index greater than that of the sample, so that it reflects at least once off the sample surface and produces an evanescent wave that typically penetrates between 0.5 and 2 μm into the sample. The beam is collected by a detector as it exits the crystal. This scheme is shown in Figure 3.1.

3.2.3 Gel permeation chromatography

Gel permeation chromatography (GPC) is by far the most common choice in polymer characterization for the evaluation of molecular weight (MW) and polydispersity index (PDI), which measures the distribution or heterogeneity in molecular mass in a polymer sample. Both are critical parameters; most mechanical properties vary considerably with MW, and PDI plays a key part in determining the sharpness of thermal transitions.

GPC is based on the principles of size-exclusion chromatography, by which polymers are separated based on their hydrodynamic radius, as illustrated in Figure 3.2. A column is packed with microporous polystyrene beads with carefully controlled pore sizing. As the polymer solution permeates the column, molecules will either pass primarily through interstitial spaces (for molecules too large to enter the pores)

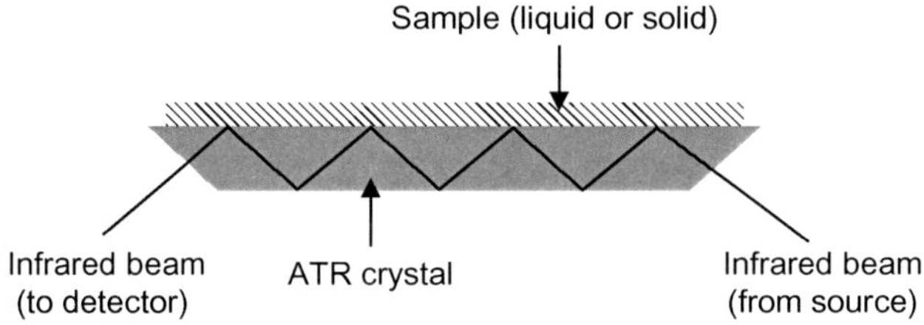

Figure 3.1 Multiple-reflection, attenuated total reflectance (ATR) system for use with FTIR spectrometers. In the ATR accessory, infrared light passes through a crystal element having a refractive index greater than that of the sample, so that it reflects at least once off the sample surface and produces an evanescent wave that typically penetrates between 0.5 and 2 μm into the sample. The beam is collected by a detector as it exits the crystal.

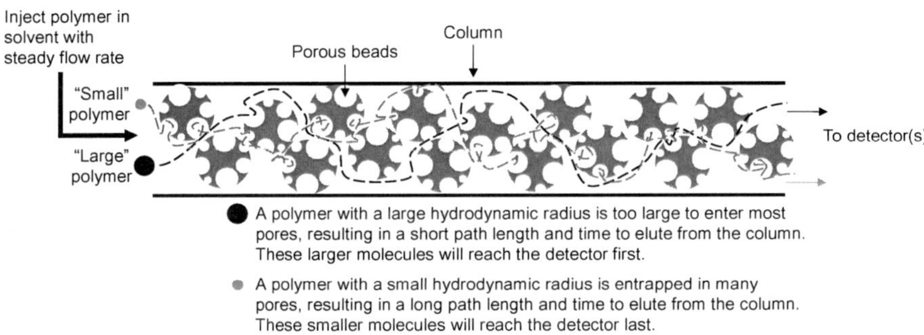

Figure 3.2 In size-exclusion chromatography, the principle underlying gel permeation chromatography, polymers in a solvent are pumped through a column packed with microporous beads. Larger molecules are unable to enter the majority of pores and therefore pass through the column relatively rapidly. Smaller molecules are able to enter many more pores and must travel a greater distance, resulting in slower passage through the column. This elution profile is measured by detectors at the outlet of the column.

and elute rapidly from the column, or will be transported into and between the beads (for molecules small enough to enter the pores), eluting slowly due to the increased path length. The amount of polymer exiting the column as a function of time is measured by an appropriate detector, generally some combination of refractive index, viscosity, and/or light scattering (Odian, 2004).

The application of GPC to SMP systems composed of linear or branched polymers is readily understandable. Given the variety of these systems that are formed from the co-polymerization of homo-polymers, GPC plays a critical role in characterizing both the homo-polymers and the resulting co-polymer. That said, many SMP applications use cross-linked systems, and the utility of GPC may not be as apparent. GPC is still an important tool in characterizing these polymers, especially when measuring the MW and PDI of the pre-cursors used in their synthesis (Nagahama et al., 2009). For instance, a recent study using a semi-crystalline PCL-based SMP found that the MW of PCL segments could be used to control the shape-memory behavior of the network, in particular the strain-recovery rate, due to its dependence on cross-link density (Paderni et al., 2012).

3.2.4 Nuclear magnetic resonance spectroscopy

Understanding nuclear magnetic resonance (NMR) spectroscopy theory requires a complex discussion with more space than can be allotted here. Since theoretical and mechanistic discussions are not the focus of this chapter, readers are instead directed to a number of other works with thorough discussions in this regard (Sanders and Hunter, 1993; Keeler, 2010; Jacobsen, 2007). We provide brief details below.

Given the insolubility of most SMP systems, solid-state NMR is generally more valuable for NMR characterization than the liquid-state alternative. From these studies, information regarding chemical composition, network architecture, cross-link density, degree of conversion, and, most importantly, shape-memory transitions can be garnered at the molecular level. As first reported by Lendlein and colleagues (Bertmer et al., 2005), in a covalently cross-linked system, the shape-memory effect is characterized by way of double-quantum excitation, which reflects the strength of dipolar coupling in the network. When elongated and fixed in the temporary state, segments between cross-linking points are stretched and partially aligned, resulting in greater dipolar coupling. After recovering the permanent shape, this alignment is lost and dipolar coupling in the network is reduced. The shift in the excitation time associated with maximum double-quantum coherence reflects this change in the network and correlates strongly with the shape-memory effect. Shape-memory reversibility can also be characterized by monitoring this effect before deformation and again after recovery of the permanent shape.

3.2.5 Wide-angle X-ray diffraction

Entirely crystalline polymers are rarely encountered; most polymeric systems display characteristics of both crystalline and amorphous solids. This balance between crystalline and amorphous domains in the polymer architecture underlies the shape-memory effect in several classes of SMPs and thus represents an important property to characterize.

When an incident X-ray interacts with a material in a wide-angle X-ray diffraction (WAXD) instrument, the electrons begin to oscillate at the same frequency as the incoming beam. If the atoms have no regular arrangement (i.e., in entirely amorphous materials), the oscillations of the electrons will destructively interfere with one another, and little to no energy leaves the system. However, if there is a regular arrangement of atoms (i.e., crystalline domains), constructive interference will result in X-ray beams leaving the sample in well-defined directions. When studying a polymeric sample, the amorphous regions produce very broad peaks in the diffraction spectrum and crystalline regions produce sharp peaks. The crystallinity in the sample can be calculated by comparing the area under the curves in these regions, resulting in a measure of mass fraction crystallinity.

WAXD has been broadly applied to the characterization of SMP materials, often times coupled with DSC measurements for a more complete picture of crystallinity. For example, Coughlin et al. used WAXD measurements to characterize the effect of cross-linking on polycyclooctene (PCO) and the resultant impact on shape-memory behavior (Liu et al., 2002). They noted a monotonic decrease in the degree of crystallinity with increased cross-linking, explained by the constraining of crystal growth by cross-linking points. For the PCO system, they also concluded that the rate and extent of strain recovery both increase with the decreasing degree of crystallinity. This mechanistic understanding gives them the ability to tailor these parameters to the given application, improving the flexibility of their system.

WAXD can determine precise crystal structures in SMP samples, aiding the understanding of shape-memory effects in systems where crystallinity is involved in shape recovery and storage. However, its application is somewhat limited by the relative difficulty in translating data to a structural determination.

3.3 Mechanical and thermo-mechanical characterization

As noted earlier, the utility of SMPs intended for biomedical device applications is most often judged by the mechanical properties they display about thermal transition. Accordingly, this section encompasses some of the most ubiquitous and useful techniques for SMP characterization, including tensile/compression testing, dynamic mechanical analysis (DMA), differential scanning calorimetry (DSC), thermogravimetric analysis (TGA), and rheology.

3.3.1 Mechanical tensile and compression testing

Tension/tensile and compression testing are fundamental to materials science and comprise some of the simplest methods available to characterize the mechanical properties of polymers. Perhaps the most basic of these is the uniaxial tensile test, in which a sample is subjected to a fixed strain rate, along a single axis, until failure. The applied force and extension are measured and recorded simultaneously at regular intervals; the results take the form of a stress–strain curve. Important parameters derived from this curve include ultimate tensile strength (peak stress), Young's modulus (the slope of the initial linear portion), Poisson's ratio, elongation at yield (typically expressed as % of original strain), and elongation at failure. Typical material tensile systems operate at a single temperature throughout each test, with control provided by insulated chambers connected to recirculating water baths or furnaces. When testing SMPs, it is critical to take thermal transition temperatures into account and test samples at the temperature(s) seen in the end-application.

While uniaxial testing is sufficient for isotropic samples, anisotropic samples (e.g., polymer composites in which the discontinuous phase or additive takes the form of fibers), require the use of biaxial systems. There are three main types of biaxial tensile testing: (1) *planar biaxial tests*, in which two forces of independent origin are introduced along two primary axes; (2) *bursting tests*, in which a disc-shaped specimen is clamped along its edge and inflated by a gas or fluid until it bursts; and (3) *cylinder tests*, which require a hollow, cylindrical sample that is subjected to internal pressure and axial tension.

Compression tests generate similar results, but the moduli determined in compression may be higher than those found in tension if the material exhibits anisotropy. In general, however, compression testing is used for materials that cannot withstand tensile loading, such as gels and extremely hydrophilic polymers. Additionally, in some cases, polymers may fail in a brittle manner under tension, while exhibiting significant ductility under compression. These differences may reflect variations in the applied stress fields during testing, but are more often due to variations in molecular and small-scale responses inherent to the polymer specimen (Nielsen and Landel, 1994).

3.3.2 Dynamic mechanical analysis

DMA or dynamic mechanical analysis is a powerful and commonly used tool to study the viscoelastic behavior of polymers. In simple terms, it involves measuring a material's response to an oscillating stress. The phase lag between the applied stress and measured strain reflects the material's tendency to flow (viscosity), while the sample recovery reflects the material's stiffness (modulus). Unlike traditional tensile testing, however, DMA provides a modulus value for each cycle of the sinusoidal stress, allowing the investigator to sweep across a range of temperatures and frequencies or shear rates. Temperature and frequency sweeps are the most common operational modes for DMA. It is also important to note that the modulus obtained in DMA may be different from the Young's modulus obtained from the linear region of a classical stress–strain curve. DMA provides complex, elastic/storage, and imaginary/loss moduli (E^*, E', and E'', respectively). The elastic modulus reveals the material's ability to store and return energy, while the loss modulus reveals its propensity for viscous energy loss. Along with moduli and viscosity, DMA can measure thermal transitions in polymers, including the glass transition temperature (T_g), which separates the glassy and rubbery regimes of semi-crystalline polymers and is critical in the characterization of SMPs. In a typical plot of storage modulus versus temperature, sub-T_g transitions, which reflect molecular vibrations on the order of bond bending and stretching and side-group motion, can also often be seen. They are less prominent than the T_g, since they are associated with comparatively small changes in modulus. Figure 3.3 illustrates these transitions and describes some of the important parameters measured by DMA. It also shows how DMA data can be used to calculate free strain-recovery and fixity rates and recovery stress.

DMA instrumentation consists of sample clamps, which secure the test sample; a linear drive motor, which provides load for the applied force; a displacement sensor; and a temperature-controlled chamber (furnace and liquid nitrogen line). Sample and clamp geometry are highly dependent on the desired testing mode.

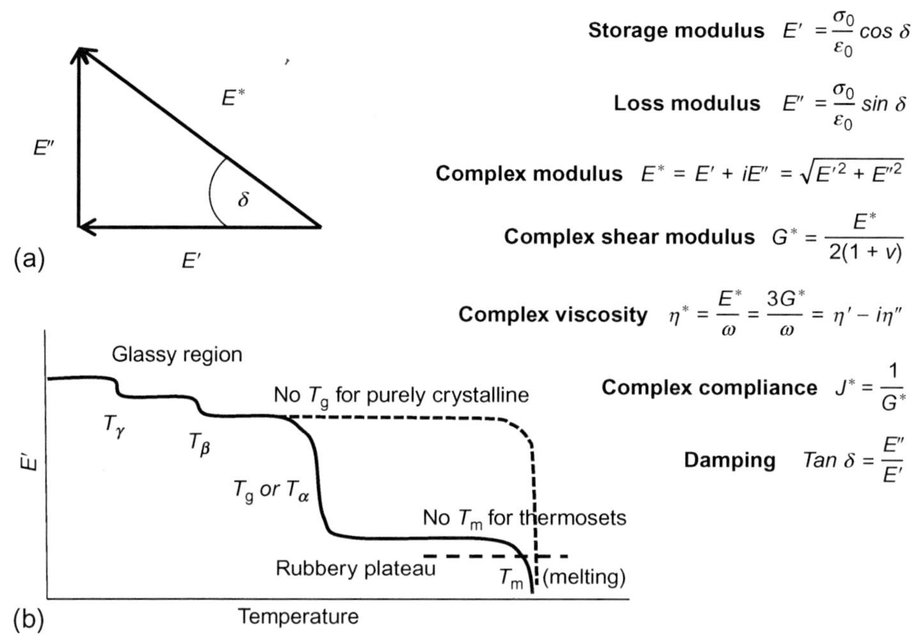

Figure 3.3 (a) The amplitude of the DMA signal and phase angle are used to calculate the tan δ, storage and loss moduli, viscosity, and other important material properties. Phase lag between stress and strain (δ), frequency (ω), stress (σ), strain (ε). (b) Prototypical DMA temperature scan of a polymer, showing decrease in storage modulus as temperature increases due to increased molecular motion (bond bending and stretching, side chain motion, etc.) and free volume.

3.3.3 *Differential scanning calorimetry*

The changes in physical and chemical properties underlying temperature- or time-dependent polymer transitions are accompanied by changes in enthalpy. As its name suggests, DSC can measure these changes in heat flow in an experimental sample in reference to a known sample. The observed thermal transitions are very useful for assessing uniformity between batches of the same material or determining the thermal properties of new materials. DSC can measure glass transitions, melting and boiling points, crystallization time and temperature, crystallinity percentage, heats of fusion and other reactions, reaction kinetics, specific heat, oxidative/thermal stability, rate and degree of polymerization, and sample purity. That said, DSC is not ideally suited to assess all these properties, and other techniques may be superior. For instance, observed thermal transitions in an unknown polymer can be compared to those of common polymers in published reference databases, but they do not uniquely identify composition. FTIR is far more effective for determining polymer composition. Similarly, melting points, which reflect MW and thermal processing history, are

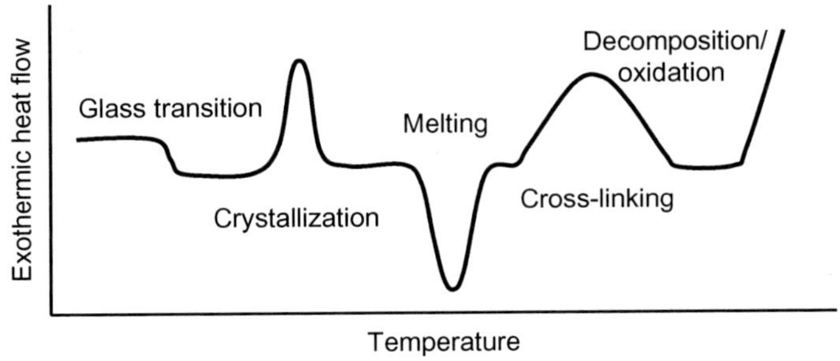

Figure 3.4 Typical DSC curve of cross-linked polymer showing thermal transitions.

sometimes available from standard compilations, and DSC can reveal polymer degradation if the measured melting point is lower than expected. However, structural/chemical decomposition is best measured using TGA. DSC is comparatively useful for measuring melting temperature (T_m) and T_g, but sub-T_g thermal transitions are usually too weak or broad to be detected by DSC and require DMA. A typical DSC curve of heat flow as a function of temperature is shown in Figure 3.4. More recently, investigators have used DSC to measure thermal conductivity in polymers (Hu et al., 2007) and to predict drug solubility in polymers with the fox equation (Haddadin et al., 2009).

There are several variants of DSC, but differential thermal analysis, in which temperature and temperature differences are measured in association with time- and temperature-dependent material transitions, is the most common. In differential photocalorimetry, the sample is exposed to UV–vis radiation. When running a DSC experiment, investigators must optimize both sample and instrument parameters. Polymer samples should be as thin as possible and cover as much of the plate as possible. Just as with DMA, careful control of heating and cooling rates is critical. Figure 3.5 displays a simplified DSC instrument schematic.

3.3.4 Thermogravimetric analysis

TGA measures the rate and amount of mass change in a material as a function of temperature or time in a controlled atmosphere. It can determine selected characteristics of materials that exhibit mass loss or gain as a result of decomposition, oxidation, dehydration, or loss of other volatile components. These characteristics include composition (of multi-component polymer systems), thermal and oxidative stability, decomposition kinetics, and moisture or volatile component content.

TGA instruments rely on precise measurements of three variables: temperature, temperature change, and mass change. Accordingly, they consist of a precise balance and a programmable furnace that allows for either a constant heating rate (more common) or variable heating, in order to achieve a constant mass loss rate (useful for studying specific reaction kinetics). The experimental material sample is placed on a balance pan inside the furnace. If a reference sample is used, it must be placed

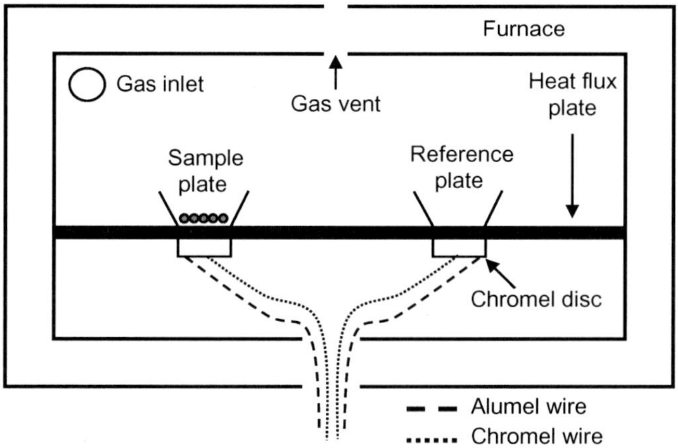

Figure 3.5 DSC instrument schematic. Alumel wire measures sample temperature (T). Chromel wire measures ΔT.

on a separate balance in a different chamber. The furnace chamber also allows the atmosphere surrounding the sample to be purged with an inert gas, such as nitrogen or helium, to prevent oxidation. As the sample is heated, its components decompose and the weight percentage corresponding to each resulting mass change can be measured. Some modern TGA instruments, which use quartz crystal microbalances, can measure mass changes on the order of micrograms (versus milligrams for conventional TGA). For structure determination, thermogravimetric analyzers can be coupled to an FTIR or mass spectrometer, and temperatures of up to 2000 °C may be used for gas phase analysis.

3.3.5 Rheology

The field of rheology is concerned with the viscoelastic behavior of matter, particularly its tendency to flow and respond plastically to an applied force, rather than elastically. Viscoelasticity can be related directly to the configuration of individual polymer molecules, network junctions, and entanglements, all of which can change in response to an applied force. Local rearrangements occur much more rapidly than larger segmental motions, so the stress response is relatively long and continuous. This effect is lessened in low MW polymers, which display near-Newtonian behavior (viscosity independent of applied shear stress), due to a lack of significant entanglements and the absence of chain stretching, rotation, or other relaxation processes. High MW polymers exhibit *shear thinning*, in which viscosity decreases as a function of the shear rate.

Rheometers are most often used to study liquids, but soft solids, such as polymers, are also routinely studied. As such, they can be used to monitor polymerization, like FTIR, and gel formation by measuring associated changes in viscosity. More generally, rheology enables the translation of measured force, pressure, torque, and angular velocity, into stress and strain. These can, in turn, be used to calculate other

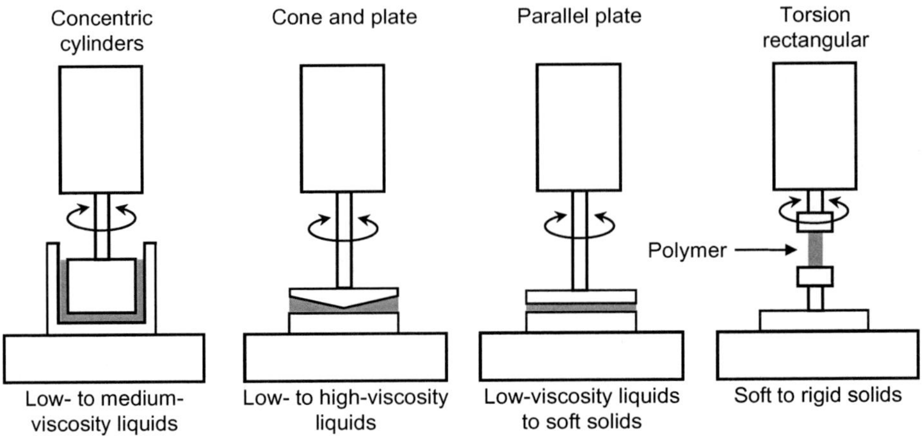

Figure 3.6 Sample geometry and viscosity govern the selection of rheology fixtures.

rheological properties. A typical set-up establishes contact between the sample and two surfaces (*slip surfaces*), at least one of which is attached to a drive motor. Characterization of both steady and oscillatory shear properties can be made. Several fixture geometries have been developed to accommodate different sample geometries and viscosities. The four most common geometries are shown in Figure 3.6.

Concentric cylinders are best for very low viscosity systems, including polymer suspensions in solvents or colloidal mixtures that are prone to settling. Note that for systems with extremely low viscosities, the contact area should be maximized so that an adequate force is seen at the transducer. The cone and plate is a particularly versatile set-up for characterization in the non-linear viscoelastic region and is the most common fixture used in rheology. It has the benefits of constant shear rate along the flow axis and low sample volume, but is quite sensitive to plate separation and cone angle (typically $\sim 1°$). It can be used with suspensions or emulsions, but the suspended particles must be no larger than one-tenth the truncation gap. In addition, care should be taken to avoid shear heating. Parallel plate fixtures are simple to use with respect to sample preparation and loading. They are appropriate for samples ranging from low-viscosity liquids to soft solids, but produce non-uniform velocity fields requiring complex integration over the sample diameter. For both the cone and plate and parallel plate fixtures, instabilities in the shear field can cause ejections of the fluid at high rates. The last fixture shown in Figure 3.6 is adequate for solid samples; however, most instruments are inaccurate at high strains.

3.4 Surface characterization

The success or failure of polymers employed in biomedical device applications is often determined by their surface properties. It is well known that protein surface fouling and cell attachment/function are highly dependent on surface patterning in polymers. The term "surface" can be defined qualitatively as the zone where the structure and composition differ from that of the bulk material, as influenced by the interface between that material and the surrounding medium (i.e., air, water, blood, etc.). In the case of polymers, this zone can be significantly deeper than other materials, extending anywhere from 10 to 100 nm from the interface. Because of the heightened reactivity of this interfacial zone and its critical role in determining the response of biological systems to the material, its chemical makeup and structure must be thoroughly understood.

3.4.1 Atomic force microscopy

On a basic level, it is desirable to understand the morphology of a material's surface on a scale relevant to biological systems. Atomic force microscopy (AFM) accomplishes this task by providing a map of surface topography with nanoscale resolution. In fact, modern AFM instruments often have sub-nanometer resolution. They essentially consist of a sharp tip/probe mounted to a cantilever. When the tip is brought in close proximity with a surface, forces of interaction between the tip and surface result in a deflection of the cantilever. This deflection is registered through changes in voltage (when piezoelectric elements are incorporated into the cantilever), laser beam deflection, or optical interferometry. Interaction forces include the mechanical contact force, van der Waals forces, capillary forces, electrostatic forces, chemical bonding, and magnetic forces, among others.

AFM has advanced greatly since its commercial introduction in the late 1980s, resulting in the application of *scanning probe microscopy* to provide an array of surface information including surface potential, thermal conductivity, chemical interaction strength, and biorecognition of specific biomolecules. Together, these variants can provide an impressively complete collection of the nature of a polymer's surface. In an SMP system, measurements of surface variations can be used to infer morphology and molecular structure of different regions in the network, including the existence and evolution of crystallites (Saywer et al., 2008). However, AFM does have several disadvantages, many of which are specific to soft materials like SMPs. For instance, the area and depth of an AFM scan is limited, meaning it is unlikely that the entire surface of a sample could be imaged. Instead, a small section must be selected to represent the entire surface. In addition, soft materials can be influenced by the small forces applied by the cantilever tip, causing sampling artifacts. However, such concerns have been minimized by the recent application of real-time correction algorithms such as feature-oriented scanning.

3.4.2 Contact angle measurements

A drop of water sitting on a surface can be a surprisingly powerful tool in characterizing interfacial energies. Determining the angle formed between the surface and droplet is a balance between the cohesive force attracting the water molecules to each other and the adhesive force, which is driven by attraction between water molecules

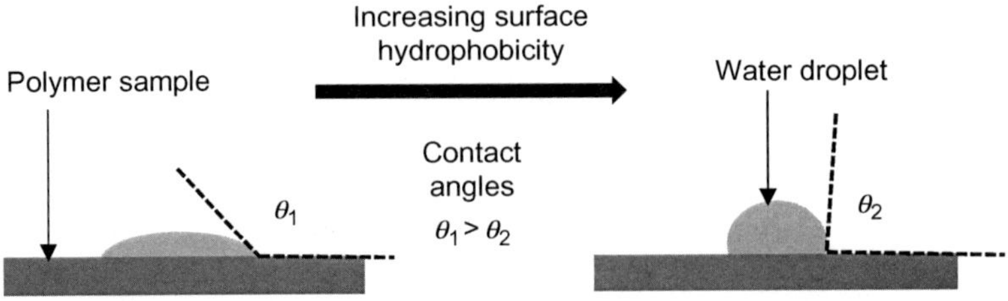

Figure 3.7 Contact angle is dependent on the forces of interaction among molecules of the liquid droplet and between those of the liquid droplet, solid sample surface, and air. It reflects the contribution of polar, dispersive, and other forces to the total surface free energy and can predict a material's interactions with cells, proteins, and small molecules.

and the molecules comprising the surface of the material. For instance, a polar, hydrophilic surface will form a greater angle of contact with a water droplet than a non-polar, hydrophobic surface (Figure 3.7). Surface free energy, which is correlated with contact angle, has been shown to be a very useful and easily obtained parameter that hints to that material's performance in a biological system. For example, Iwata and Arima showed that adhesion of human umbilical vein endothelial cells and HeLA cells onto self-assembled monolayers of alkanethiols was strongly dependent on the wettability of the surface, as determined by contact angle measurements (Arima and Iwata, 2007). Surface free energy can be partitioned into individual components, each of which represents a contribution from a specific type of interfacial interaction. The primary interaction forces include London dispersion forces, polar forces, hydrogen bonding, induction, and acid–base interactions. There are several methods to calculate surface free energy and its components, depending on the material being studied; readers are referred to excellent reviews on the subject, such as the work by Żenkiewicz (2007). Note that liquids other than water are often used when estimating non-polar contributions to surface energy. Additionally, readers should keep in mind that contact angle measurements are notoriously sensitive, with slight differences in sample preparation capable of significantly altering experimental results. Concerns include surface roughness, surface and liquid purity, and absorption of the liquid into the polymer. The sessile drop experiment is the most sensitive to these factors, but more sophisticated instruments exist that instead measure advancing and receding contact angles or perform capillary-based measurements, which improve accuracy and repeatability.

3.4.3 X-ray photoelectron spectroscopy

Based on the photoelectric effect, X-ray photoelectron spectroscopy (XPS) involves focusing X-rays onto a sample and subsequently detecting the kinetic energy and number of electrons that are ejected. Interaction of X-ray photons with atoms at the surface of the material cause inner shell electrons to be liberated. Since the energies of the incident X-ray photons are known, the *binding energy* of the liberated electrons can be calculated based on their kinetic energy. Binding energies simply represent the difference in energy between the neutral and ionized atoms. They are characteristic of the atoms from which the electrons were liberated and their environment, allowing determination of the atomic percentages of the chemical elements present at the surface of the material and their chemical and electronic states. Since only electrons near the surface of the material are ejected with enough kinetic energy to escape the sample, XPS limits the information returned about the sample to the region within 1–12 nm of the surface.

Compared with many other surface characterization techniques (e.g., SEM), the lack of sample preparation and non-destructive nature of the analysis are major advantages of XPS. Due to the surface localization and sensitivity of XPS, its application to SMP characterization can provide valuable information about surface composition, contamination and oxidation state, and characterization of surface modifications. For example, after immobilization of a biomolecule on the surface of a SMP device, XPS could be used to (a) confirm covalent linking of the molecule to the SMP surface; (b) provide a stoichiometric analysis of biomolecule content; and (c) permit an estimation of the thickness of the surface brush. XPS likely provides the most expansive set of information of any surface characterization technique relevant to SMPs; however, the rarity and high cost of XPS instruments and the reliance on experienced operators limit its utility.

If more detailed surface characterization is required than can be provided by XPS, time-of-flight secondary ion mass spectrometry (TOF-SIMS) analysis may be used. This technique can provide not only the mass spectra of the top one to two atomic layers of the material, but also detailed surface maps and depth profiles. While TOF-SIMS is not as common as XPS in organic applications, its use in SMP applications may increase as composite materials, incorporating inorganic fillers, are more heavily investigated.

3.5 Imaging-based characterization

3.5.1 Electron microscopy

Transmission and scanning electron microscopy (TEM and SEM) have long been used for structural characterization of polymers. In lieu of light and optical glass lenses, electron microscopes employ electrons (having a much lower wavelength) and electromagnetic lenses, allowing them to resolve structures well under 1 nm. When deciding whether to use TEM or SEM, one must consider material processing restrictions as well as the desired resolution. Table 3.6 summarizes these considerations. With either modality, the user must balance image quality, contrast, and radiation damage, as with all soft materials.

Table 3.6 Comparison of transmission and scanning electron microscopy

	TEM	SEM
Sample preparation	Ultrathin section	Thick, conductive
Peak resolution	~0.5 Å	~0.5 nm
Beam intensity/voltage	High (~100 keV)	Low–medium
Final image	Interior (2D)	Surface or interior via fracture (3D)

3.5.2 Transmission electron microscopy

Like biological specimens, synthetic polymers consist primarily of low atomic number elements, whose elastic interactions with high-energy electrons are fairly weak. There is almost no absorption of electrons directed at samples thin enough for TEM. Generating contrast in polymer TEM can thus be difficult. However, inelastic interactions can be strong. This allows for powerful spectroscopic techniques, but can also lead to radiation damage, a constraint that affects polymers far more than inorganic samples (Libera and Egerton, 2010). Radiation damage is a particular concern with TEM, as it employs high voltages to accelerate the electrons (40–400 keV). Even so, several well-established techniques can be used to image polymers, including bright- and dark-field imaging, high-resolution imaging (to investigate molecular-level structures in crystalline polymer solids), electron diffraction, and analytical microscopy.

SMPs inherently contain spatial variations in density, crystallinity, and crystal orientation, and it is often important to characterize the distribution and size of crystalline and amorphous regions. As illustrated in Figure 3.8, crystallinity generates Bragg diffraction. In dark-field imaging, the aperture of the objective lens is set to block the primary beam and allow scattered electrons to pass. This produces an image containing bright crystallites and dark amorphous surroundings. Amorphous regions do not exhibit appreciable spatial variations in density, leading to forward scattering. However, they can still produce variations in the energy or phase of incident electrons, providing additional sources of contrast (electron energy-loss spectroscopy and phase contrast, respectively). Figure 3.7 illustrates the difference between amplitude and phase contrast. Composite SMPs containing heavy elements are straightforward to image using standard TEM. They produce significant Rutherford scattering, in which electrons are scattered at high angles and can be blocked by an objective aperture to generate image contrast, with the heavy discontinuous phase appearing dark. Modern and comprehensive works have been published covering contrast mechanisms, resolution, and specimen preparation in polymer TEM (Michler, 2008; Saywer et al., 2008). Special attention should be paid to positive and negative staining methods; for instance, compounds containing double bonds can be selectively stained with osmium tetroxide (OsO_4). It is often used to stain one phase of block copolymers, revealing their microstructure.

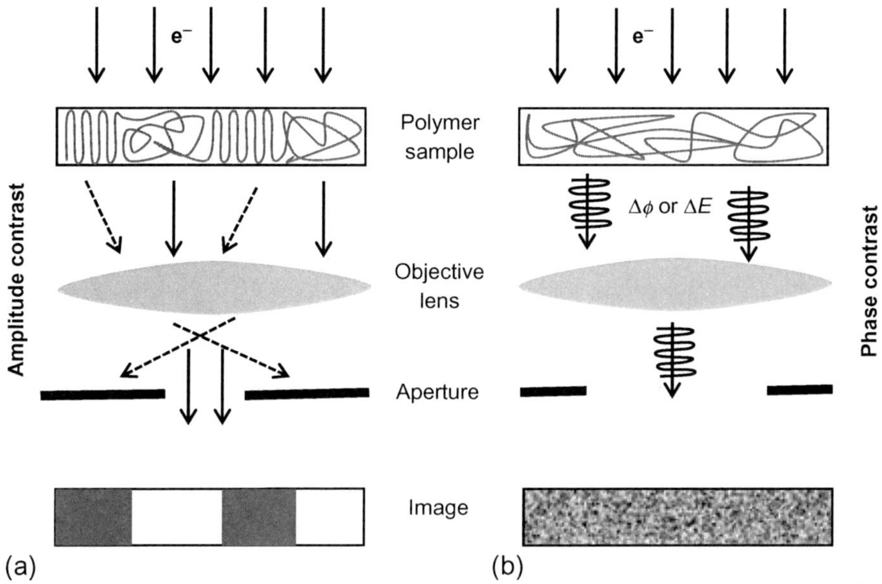

Figure 3.8 (a) Amplitude contrast in polymer TEM arises when an objective aperture is used to selectively block electrons scattered at high angles from crystalline segments. (b) Variation in the phase or energy of electrons departing the sample can provide contrast within largely amorphous polymers having only minor spatial variations in density.

3.5.3 Scanning electron microscopy

SEM is generally used to examine the surface topography of polymers, though internal structures can be imaged by introducing fractures. The image resolution of SEM is typically an order of magnitude poorer than TEM, but it has excellent depth of field, allowing it to produce accurate representations of a polymer's three-dimensional shape. In addition, since SEM does not rely on transmission, samples up to several centimeters in size can be imaged.

Image contrast in SEM can be generated through several mechanisms. *Surface-tilt contrast* arises due to the angle between the incident electron beam and the sample surface, which makes the surface features normal to the beam appear darkest. *Shadow* and *diffusion contrast* causes edges and protrusions on the surface to appear bright. *Material contrast* results from spatial variations in the sample's secondary emission rate, which depends primarily on the constituent atoms.

Sample preparation for SEM is generally much simpler than for TEM. The sample is simply placed in the specimen holder with an electroconductive adhesive. However, with polymers and other insulating specimens, care must be taken to prevent surface charging from the incident electron beam, as this can create severe imaging artifacts. Ultra-thin heavy metal coatings such as gold, platinum, or their palladium alloys are often applied to prevent surface charging, though it is sometimes adequate to simply reduce the accelerating voltage.

3.5.4 Phantom-based medical imaging

When characterizing SMPs for biomedical device applications, it is often necessary to assess signal and artifacts generated from radiography and magnetic resonance-based imaging modalities. These modalities, which include digital X-ray, fluoroscopy, computed tomography (CT), and magnetic resonance imaging (MRI), are often used to confirm proper device placement in the body. Initial assessment is most often performed in artificial *imaging phantoms*, which are designed to simulate the imaging characteristics of the target organ or delivery site (e.g., vascular compartment, brain parenchyma etc.). Due to the abundance of water in the body, the simplest phantoms often consist of an acrylic polymer (or equivalent) container filled with water or saline, in which the specimen of interest is suspended. However, more purposeful phantoms can be constructed, as discussed below. General considerations when designing imaging phantoms for X-ray and MRI imaging are shown in Figure 3.9.

3.5.5 Digital X-ray, CT, and fluoroscopy

Polymers are made primarily of low atomic number elements, including carbon, hydrogen, oxygen, and nitrogen, which are poor attenuators of photons. Developing radio-opaque SMPs typically requires the addition of heavy-element fillers (Salamone, 1996; Moszner and Salz, 2001). For instance, barium sulfate, zirconium oxide, and tantalum have been used in the orthopedic field for bone cement (Behl et al., 2010; Bohner, 2010; Lye et al., 2009); tantalum-filled SMPs have been evaluated as embolic coil materials (Heaton, 2004); and iodinated monomers have been incorporated into denture base resins (Davy et al., 1997). Methods also exist for *a priori* design of radiographic phantoms having specific elemental compositions and physical densities (Lam, 1981), but it is most often sufficient to use normal saline (0.90% w/v NaCl) as the scattering medium.

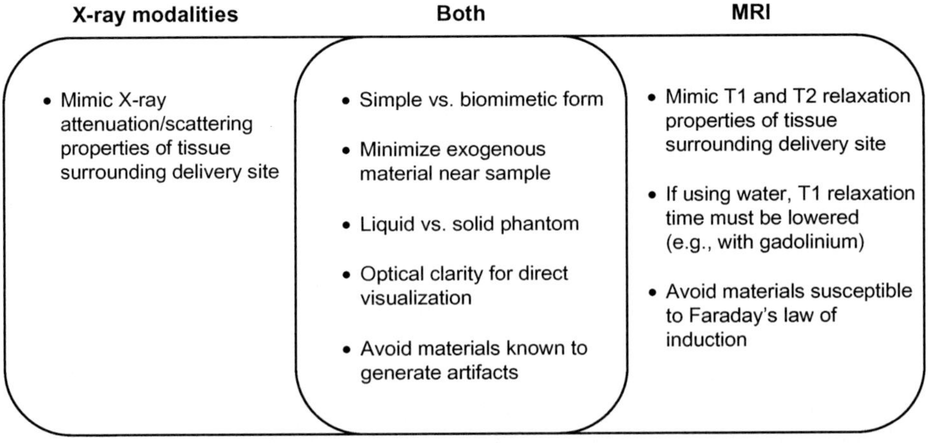

Figure 3.9 Design considerations for imaging phantoms intended to assess SMP biomedical devices.

3.5.6 Magnetic resonance imaging

The goal of a MRI phantom is to surround the specimen of interest in an artificial environment that mirrors the T1 and T2 relaxation properties and conductivity of tissue surrounding the putative device delivery site. Since MRI signal arises primarily from the relaxation of oriented protons found in water molecules, a simple MRI phantom can be designed using water. However, a paramagnetic contrast agent such as gadolinium must be added (at approximately 5–10 mmol) to reduce the T1 relaxation time to useable levels. It is often useful to study the geometry and properties of accreditation phantoms used to validate clinical scanners. For instance, the American College of Radiology accreditation phantom uses a solution of 10 mmol nickel chloride and 45 mmol sodium chloride to simulate biological conductivity and includes a contrast vial containing 20 mmol nickel chloride and 15 mmol sodium chloride, allowing for a difference in the T1 and T2 relaxation times. Due to the strong magnetic fields used in MRI, care must be taken not to include ferromagnetic materials or conductive materials susceptible to torque or current generation through Faraday's law of induction.

3.6 Biological testing

Given the immense variety and complexity of biological responses to foreign bodies, characterizing the response of biological systems to implanted materials can be a daunting task. Because of this, the field has strived to standardize test procedures to ensure repeatability of experiments and facilitate direct comparisons between materials. However, these efforts have only been moderately successful; wide variation still exists. Section 3.9 includes standards for biological testing, many of which provide detailed experimental protocols. Determining which protocol is appropriate for a given material will depend heavily on the nature of the material and the clinical application for which it is designed.

3.6.1 In vitro *testing*

Cell- or tissue-culture based testing can be used to gather a variety of information on how certain biological systems, in a controlled environment, will react to a material. For a typical SMP application, three major categories of testing are used: cytotoxicity testing, functional testing, and hemocompatibility testing. Cytotoxicity testing is one of the most crucial steps in characterizing a SMP for biomedical applications and should be performed as early as realistically possible in the material development process. While it does not provide a complete picture, *in vitro* testing can still provide valuable insight that can guide subsequent product development.

The purpose of *in vitro* cytotoxicity testing is to determine whether exposure to a material, or substances extracted from that material, is toxic at the cellular level. However, because toxicity involves multiple mechanisms, there are various methods by which its effects can be assessed, either quantitatively (cell count or cellular morphology) or qualitatively (metabolic activity, membrane integrity, necrosis, or apoptosis). In addition, there are three methods by which cells can be exposed to the material of interest: direct contact, agar diffusion or extraction. In direct contact tests, cells are grown to approximately 80% confluence in a culture dish and, concomitant with a change in the culture medium, a coupon of the sample material is placed in the culture dish. After a period of incubation, the sample is removed and the cells are fixed and histochemically stained for microscopy analysis. In the agar diffusion test, cells are grown to near-confluence in a culture dish and the medium is replaced with fresh medium containing 2% agar and a vital stain. After the agar solidifies, the sample material is placed on top of the agar gel and the plate is incubated, after which live cells can be identified. In the extraction test, a sample of the material is incubated in medium for a period of time, after which the material is removed and the medium is added to nearly confluent cells. This test is the most flexible assay that can be used for quantitative assessment of cytotoxicity, allowing evaluation of specific toxicity mechanisms. However, the direct contact and agar diffusion tests may be considered better analogues to the clinical implementation of a device.

In vitro testing can also be used to measure functional responses at the cellular level. These tests take characterization beyond the simple question of toxicity and attempt to determine how cells will functionally respond to implantation of the sample material, whether such a response is desirable or not. This level of testing is especially important for polymers that are bio-functionalized, or otherwise modified with the intention of eliciting a specific cellular/physiological response. For example, in an application where tissue ingrowth into a SMP network is crucial, functional testing might entail seeding cells with a sample of the SMP, followed by electron microscopy and histological analysis of sample cross-sections to determine the extent of cellular penetration (Marra et al., 1999). While *in vitro* functional testing can provide a rapid and inexpensive means of optimizing polymer parameters, only *in vivo* testing can give a complete picture of how the material will behave after implantation.

Hemocompatibility testing is a critical step for devices that will come into contact with blood. As blood is a complex system, materials can interact with it in a variety of ways, many of which can be deleterious to the clinical application. Several tests are outlined by ISO 10993-4 as first steps in establishing the hemocompatibility of a material. These tests are designed to assess the potential for a material to cause adverse effects upon contact with blood, whether at the site of the device itself or downstream of it. Accordingly, the expected mode of interaction between the material and blood must be established first. The aforementioned ISO standard breaks this into three categories: external communicating device—blood path indirect (a device that contacts the blood path at one point as a conduit into the vascular system); external communicating device-circulating blood (a device that contacts circulating blood); and implant device (a device principally contacting blood). Based on the category, several Level 1 (primary) and Level 2 (optional) tests are outlined to evaluate potential adverse interactions. Primarily, these tests assess responses related to thrombosis, coagulation, platelets, hematology, and immunology. While some of these assessments can be performed by *in vitro* tests (e.g., immunological testing), most require *in vivo* or *ex vivo* work. Based on the results of the Level 1 tests, Level 2 testing may be required if specific interactions need additional investigation.

3.6.2 In vivo *testing*

While useful for modeling biological systems, *in vitro* testing cannot begin to duplicate all the complexities of a living system. As such, *in vivo* testing is a necessary step in the development of any biomaterial. *In vivo* assessments are meant to ensure a) that a given material is not harmful to the patient and b) that it performs its intended role. As with *in vitro* studies, several organizations have published standardized protocols to be followed when performing *in vivo* experimentation. The reader is directed to Section 3.9 for these references.

The appropriate *in vivo* testing protocol to be implemented will depend on the specific application of the SMP device, including the duration and mode of contact. Contact duration is specified as limited ($\leq$24 h), prolonged (between 24 h and 30 days), or permanent ($\geq$30 days), and the modes of contact are categorized as surface device, external communicating device, or implant device. While a multitude of testing regimens exist depending on the combination of duration and mode of contact, three tests are generally recommended by ISO 10993 for all medical devices and will be briefly described here: cytotoxicity (as described in Section 3.6.1), sensitization, and irritation. Sensitization studies highlight immunologic mechanisms influencing host reactions to an implanted device, with an emphasis on local over-systemic responses. Sensitization studies may be performed using individual chemicals used to synthesize the test material (to isolate specific responses), the entire material itself, or extracts from the material. Typical test methods include the guinea pig maximization test, the closed patch test and the murine lymph node assay. Irritation studies estimate the potential for an implanted material to cause dermal irritation, generally by applying the material or its extracts to a dermal, mucosal, or ocular surface of young adult albino rabbits. For devices that will be externally communicating or have internal contact, intradermal injections of material extracts are recommended. In a typical SMP application, where extracts will likely contain hydrophilic and lipophilic components, it is important to include testing with solvents for both classes of chemicals. For devices that will have only external communication with intact or abraded skin, the test material or its extractions should be applied directly to both skin types. In both of these testing methods, extended exposure ($\geq$4 h) is followed by grading for erythema or eschar formation, edema, or other observed reactions. Repeated exposure studies may also be necessary.

3.7 Example applications

In this section, we will approach three distinct SMP biomedical device applications from the perspective of an investigator. Each case study will lead the reader through the process of identifying important application-specific material properties and the techniques useful in characterizing them.

Case study 1: SMP vascular stent

Vascular stents are mesh tubes used to keep blood vessels open following the repair of a stenosis secondary to a pathological biological process. For instance, atherosclerotic lesions in the coronary arteries of the heart, which restrict blood flow to the myocardium, can be treated by balloon dilation (angioplasty) of the constricted region followed by placement of a stent to maintain patency in the long term. Stents are typically made of metals, with or without a polymer coating designed for elution of anti-fibrotic drugs and prevention of encapsulation. However, fully polymeric stents have gained FDA approval and SMPs appear to be well suited for percutaneous vascular devices, as they can recover a complex 3D conformation after prolonged storage in a catheter under deformation.

Comparison of a group of candidate SMPs for vascular stent applications would require extensive testing. First, the mechanical and thermo-mechanical properties would have to be assessed. Simple uniaxial tensile testing in a temperature-controlled chamber would determine whether the SMP stent could withstand typical peak stresses seen during device deployment or retraction. It would also be important to determine how the SMP stent transitions from room to body temperature. While DSC could accurately determine thermal transition temperatures, DMA may be more appropriate, since it can also provide the modulus and recovery stress over that same range. Recovery stress may be particularly important as this would help to determine whether the deployed device exerts sufficient force on the arterial wall to maintain patency following angioplasty.

Compositional and structural characterization is a ubiquitous requirement in polymeric biomaterial development and includes analysis of MW and weight distribution, the degree of branching and crystallinity, and component concentrations. However, it has unique importance when designing materials intended for delivery to the vascular compartment. FDA guidelines require materials in contact with blood to undergo testing for cytotoxicity (*in vitro*), hemolysis, complement activation, cell adhesion, protein adsorption, thrombogenicity (whole-blood clotting time, platelet, and fibrinogen turnover, etc.), and pyrogenicity, among others. Particular attention should be paid to chemical composition and leaching, which reflect the monomeric composition, impurities introduced by the fabrication process, and the degree of conversion. Variables such as protein and cell adsorption can be tested directly using human serum proteins or whole blood. However, candidate polymers can be pre-screened for their tendency to interact with proteins or cells using contact angle measurements. It is well known that hydrophilic/ionic surfaces tend to increase cell adhesion, while protein fouling can be driven by hydrophobic interactions between the substrate and protein core or ionic interactions.

Case study 2: growth factor-modified neurovascular SMP device

A SMP device has been designed for a neurovascular application, in which the device is meant to promote neuronal regeneration at the site of implantation. To promote regeneration, the device has been surface-modified with neuronal growth factors.

As a first step, the raw material itself should be tested for *in vitro* biocompatibility, followed by testing of the material after surface modification. To confirm immobilization of the growth factor on the device's surface and to determine the amount of growth factor tethered to the surface, solid-state NMR, AFM, or XPS could be used, with NMR or AFM providing a quicker analysis but XPS providing better accuracy (Charbonneau et al., 2012). Functional *in vitro* studies should follow demonstrating the potential of the device to promote neuronal outgrowth and the added benefit of the immobilized growth factors. These studies should also identify the optimal concentration of tethered growth factor for maximized response. For example, primary hippocampal neurons isolated from rats could be cultured on surfaces of the SMP material itself, modified SMP, and poly-L-lysine coated surfaces (positive control) (Tu et al., 2011). After a period of incubation, cells would undergo morphological assessment in addition to neurofilament antibody staining to qualitatively assess neurite outgrowth.

Testing of shape-memory and mechanical properties would follow traditional characterization methods, including DMA or DSC for thermo-mechanical testing and solid-state NMR and FTIR for chemical characterization. In this case, chemical characterization might focus on ensuring the presence of functional groups amenable to immobilization of the growth factor on the surface of the material.

Case study 3: subcutaneous SMP drug delivery device

In this case study, a SMP device has been developed with the intention of being administered subcutaneously, in a minimally invasive fashion. Once implanted, the device will deploy to its permanent shape, opening up macro-scale "pores" through which a drug will diffuse. The device will be loaded with enough of the drug to sustain several months of delivery at therapeutic levels.

Besides universal characterization steps, including thermo-mechanical testing and chemical characterization, biocompatibility testing and examinations of the kinetics of drug release and incorporation will be pivotal for this device. Cytotoxicity testing should begin with *in vitro* exposure of a relevant cell line (e.g., L929, fibroblasts isolated from the subcutaneous tissue of mice) to extractions from the material, as outlined in ISO 10993, followed by an MTT assay to determine whether metabolic activity is affected. Finding no cytotoxic effects, biocompatibility testing should move to *in vivo* studies for sensitization and irritation with the protocol extending at least 8 weeks. This 8-week timeframe will allow for evaluation of (a) the onset and intensity of acute inflammation; (b) the time required for acute inflammation to subside; and (c) any indication of chronic inflammation, which generally takes about 8 weeks to present.

The combination device/drug side of the system will also need careful examination to ensure the mechanisms and kinetics of drug release are thoroughly understood. Considerations include drug stability, kinetics of drug release from the system, uniformity of drug distribution, and the physical state of the drug within the network (crystalline or solid dispersion). The first two considerations are best assessed by *in vitro* release testing, in which the device is placed in a release medium (e.g.,

PBS, pH 7.4) at physiologically relevant conditions and samples of the release medium are taken periodically. HPLC, mass spectrometry (MS), or UV–vis spectroscopy can be used to determine the amount of drug released at a given time and the fraction of that drug that is pharmaceutically active. Drug stability is especially critical for delivery of large-molecule drugs, such as proteins or peptides; however, more sensitive methods such as ELISA are generally needed to make these assessments. Drug distribution and physical state can be assessed by XPS or AFM if it can be assumed that conditions at the surface are indicative of the entire network. Otherwise, more advanced techniques such as confocal Raman spectroscopy may be employed (Breitenbach et al., 1999; Balss et al., 2008).

3.8 Future trends and conclusions

Shape-memory behavior in polymers intended for biomedical applications has been studied extensively since the 1970s. However, advances in existing characterization techniques and development of new methods will continue into the foreseeable future. Adoption of new methods has been driven in part by the emergence of functionalized SMPs, including nanocomposites and surface-modified SMPs coated with bio-antigens/receptors. With these new materials, the study of interfaces (between the continuous and discontinuous phases of a composite or immobilized surface biomolecules and foreign surfaces) takes center stage. Accordingly, surface analysis techniques like XPS, which determine the identity and oxidation state of elements within 10 nm of a material's surface, are being seen more commonly in the literature. Another interesting trend is the combination of existing analytical instruments. For instance, simultaneous thermal analysis (STA) is the application of DSC and TGA to a sample in a single instrument. This is possible because the environmental conditions of the test (atmospheric composition, gas flow rate, heating rate, etc.) are identical for both signals. The results are often enhanced further by coupling the STA machine to an FTIR instrument or mass spectrometer. Advances in imaging techniques, such as dynamic *in situ* TEM (DTEM), may also provide important data on the micro-structural changes in SMPs during thermal transitions. DTEM allows for real-time atomic-level observations of changes in materials in response to external stimuli, such as heat, stress, light, or electromagnetic fields. It undoubtedly augments an investigator's ability to study the fundamental processes occurring during SMP device synthesis and use.

Computational modeling and simulation may also play a key role in the future of SMP characterization, particularly in initial feasibility and proof-of-concept studies. Commercial software packages such as SolidWorks® and ANSYS® are routinely used to model the deformation and internal stresses expected in biomaterials, once deployed in the body, and could one day be used to model more complex behavior. For instance, an investigator could conceivably simulate the trans-catheter delivery of a SMP stent into a coronary artery and predict the likelihood of stent displacement, vessel rupture, or the time to complete encapsulation. Such simulations would require information about the device geometry, mechanical properties of the SMP and vessel wall, arterial blood flow, and even protein/cell adsorption kinetics. Clearly, computational simulations are also well suited for evaluation of drug release from SMPs and may provide a rapid means of testing the effects of polymer composition, MW, and other variables on drug release kinetics.

This chapter provided an overview of characterization methods relevant to the development and implementation of SMP biomaterials, with an emphasis on human medical device applications. The task of assembling a comprehensive material description is now more automated, faster, and more accurate than it has ever been. Even so, the investigator must always bear in mind that the identification of important material properties and the methods best suited to evaluate them are highly application-specific and that SMP validation should be a constant process of feedback and refinement, rather than a single event.

3.9 Sources of further information

- ISO 10993: Biological Evaluation of Medical Devices.
- Test Methods for Biological Safety Evaluation of Medical Devices, Assessment of Medical Device, Notice 36 (Pharmaceutical and Food Safety Bureau, Ministry of Health, Labour and Welfare, Japan).
- USP <87>: Biological Reactivity Tests *In Vivo*.
- USP <88>: Biological Reactivity Tests *In Vitro*.
- ASTM F748-06: Standard Practice for Selecting Generic Biological Test Methods for Materials and Devices.
- ASTM D3418/ISO 11357: Transition Temperatures and Enthalpies of Fusion and Crystallization of Polymers by Differential Scanning Calorimetry.
- ASTM D4065: Dynamic Mechanical Properties.
- ASTM D638/ISO 527: Tensile Properties of Plastics.
- ASTM D695/ISO 604: Compressive Properties of Rigid Plastics.
- Menard, K.P., 1999. Dynamic Mechanical Analysis: A Practical Introduction, Boca Raton, FL: CRC Press.

References

Arima, Y., Iwata, H., 2007. Effect of wettability and surface functional groups on protein adsorption and cell adhesion using well-defined mixed self-assembled monolayers. Biomaterials 28 (20), 3074–3082. Available at: http://www.ncbi.nlm.nih.gov/pubmed/17428532.

Balss, K.M., et al., 2008. Quantitative spatial distribution of sirolimus and polymers in drug-eluting stents using confocal Raman microscopy. J. Biomed. Mater. Res. A 85 (1), 258–270. Available at: http://www.ncbi.nlm.nih.gov/pubmed/17876804.

Behl, M., Razzaq, M.Y., Lendlein, A., 2010. Multifunctional shape-memory polymers. Adv. Mater. (Deerfield Beach, FL) 22 (31), 3388–3410, Available at: http://www.ncbi.nlm.nih.gov/pubmed/20574951 (accessed 04.08.11).

Bertmer, M., et al., 2005. Biodegradable shape-memory polymer networks: characterization with solid-state NMR. Macromolecules 38 (9), 3793–3799. Available at: http://pubs.acs.org/doi/abs/10.1021/ma0501489.

Bohner, M., 2010. Design of ceramic-based cements and putties for bone graft substitution. Eur. Cell. Mater. 20, 1–12. Available at: http://www.ncbi.nlm.nih.gov/pubmed/20574942.

Breitenbach, J., Schrof, W., Neumann, J., 1999. Confocal Raman-spectroscopy: analytical approach to solid dispersions and mapping of drugs. Pharm. Res. 16 (7), 1109–1113. Available at: http://www.springerlink.com/index/j915203714138461.pdf.

Charbonneau, C., et al., 2012. Chondroitin sulfate and epidermal growth factor immobilization after plasma polymerization: a versatile anti-apoptotic coating to promote healing around stent grafts. Macromol. Biosci. 12 (6), 812–821. Available at: http://www.ncbi.nlm.nih.gov/pubmed/22457238.

Davy, K.W., Anseau, M.R., Berry, C., 1997. Iodinated methacrylate copolymers as X-ray opaque denture base acrylics. J. Dent. 25 (6), 499–505. Available at: http://www.ncbi.nlm.nih.gov/pubmed/9604581.

Haddadin, R., et al., 2009. Estimation of drug solubility in polymers via differential scanning calorimetry and utilization of the fox equation. Pharm. Dev. Technol. 14 (1), 18–26, Available at: http://www.ncbi.nlm.nih.gov/pubmed/18825543 (accessed 16.02.13).

Haider, N., Karlsson, S., 1999. A rapid ultrasonic extraction technique to identify and quantify additives in poly(ethylene). Analyst 124 (5), 797–800. Available at: http://xlink.rsc.org/?DOI=a809025d.

Heaton, B., 2004. A Shape Memory Polymer for Intracranial Aneurysm Coils: An Investigation of Mechanical and Radiographic Properties of a Tantalum-Filled Shape Memory Polymer Composite. Georgia Institute of Technology, Atlanta.

Hu, M., Yu, D., Wei, J., 2007. Thermal conductivity determination of small polymer samples by differential scanning calorimetry. Polym. Test. 26 (3), 333–337, Available at: http://linkinghub.elsevier.com/retrieve/pii/S0142941806002145 (accessed 12.02.13).

Jacobsen, N.E., 2007. NMR Spectroscopy Explained: Simplified Theory, Applications and Examples for Organic Chemistry and Structural Biology. Wiley-Interscience, Hoboken, NJ.

Keeler, J., 2010. Understanding NMR Spectroscopy, second ed. John Wiley & Sons, Inc., Chichester, UK.

Lam, G.K.Y., 1981. Systematic method of formulating liquid phantoms with a given elemental composition and density. Med. Phys. 8 (6), 894–896.

Libera, M.R., Egerton, R.F., 2010. Advances in the transmission electron microscopy of polymers. Polym. Rev. 50 (3), 321–339, Available at: http://www.tandfonline.com/doi/abs/10.1080/15583724.2010.493256 (accessed 20.11.12).

Liu, C., et al., 2002. Chemically cross-linked polycyclooctene: synthesis, characterization, and shape memory behavior. Macromolecules 35 (27), 9868–9874. Available at: http://pubs.acs.org/doi/abs/10.1021/ma021141j.

Lye, K.W., et al., 2009. Bone cements and their potential use in a mandibular endoprosthesis. Tissue Eng. B Rev. 15 (4), 485–496. Available at: http://www.pubmedcentral.nih.gov/articlerender.fcgi?artid=3113466&tool=pmcentrez&rendertype=abstract.

Marra, K.G., et al., 1999. In vitro analysis of biodegradable polymer blend/hydroxyapatite composites for bone tissue engineering. J. Biomed. Mater. Res. 47 (3), 324–335. Available at: http://www.ncbi.nlm.nih.gov/pubmed/10487883.

Michler, G.H., 2008. Electron Microscopy of Polymers. Springer-Verlag, Leipzig.

Moraes, L.G.P., et al., 2008. Infrared spectroscopy: a tool for determination of the degree of conversion in dental composites. J. Appl. Oral Sci. 16 (2), 145–149. Available at: http://www.scielo.br/scielo.php?script=sci_arttext&pid=S1678-77572008000200012&lng=en&nrm=iso&tlng=en.

Moszner, N., Salz, U., 2001. New developments of polymeric dental composites. Prog. Polym. Sci. 26 (1), 535–576.

Nagahama, K., et al., 2009. Biodegradable shape-memory polymers exhibiting sharp thermal transitions and controlled drug release. Biomacromolecules 10 (7), 1789–1794.

Nielsen, L.E., Landel, R.F., 1994. Mechanical Properties of Polymers and Composites, second ed. Marcel Dekker, Inc., New York.

Odian, G., 2004. Principles of Polymerization. John Wiley & Sons, Inc., Hoboken.

Paderni, K., et al., 2012. Shape-memory polymer networks from sol–gel cross-linked alkoxysilane-terminated poly(ε-caprolactone). J. Mater. Sci. 47 (10), 4354–4362. Available at: http://www.springerlink.com/index/10.1007/s10853-012-6289-2.

Salamone, J., 1996. Radiopaque polymers. In: Polymeric Materials Encyclopedia: Q-S, CRC Press, Boca Raton, FL, pp. 7346–7350.

Sanders, J.K.M., Hunter, B.K., 1993. Modern NMR Spectroscopy: A Guide for Chemists, second ed. Oxford University Press, Oxford, UK.

Saywer, L.C., Grubb, D.T., Meyers, G.F., 2008. Polymer Microscopy, third ed. Springer, New York.

Song, L., et al., 2010. In vitro evaluation of chemically cross-linked shape-memory acrylate–methacrylate copolymer networks as ocular implants. J. Phys. Chem. B 114 (21), 7172–7178. Available at: http://www.ncbi.nlm.nih.gov/pubmed/20462221.

Tu, Q., et al., 2011. The effect of acetylcholine-like biomimetic polymers on neuronal growth. Biomaterials 32 (12), 3253–3264. Available at: http://www.ncbi.nlm.nih.gov/pubmed/21303719.

Wilson, T.S., et al., 2007. Shape memory polymers based on uniform aliphatic urethane networks. J. Appl. Polym. Sci. 106 (1), 540–551. Available at: http://doi.wiley.com/10.1002/app.26593.

Żenkiewicz, M., 2007. Methods for the calculation of surface free energy of solids. J. Achiev. Mater. Manuf. Eng. 24 (1), 137–145.

Mechanical testing of shape-memory polymers for biomedical applications

4

H. Tobushi[1], *R. Matsui*[1], *K. Takeda*[1], *S. Hayashi*[2]
[1]Aichi Institute of Technology, Toyota, Japan; [2]SMP Technologies Inc., Tokyo, Japan

4.1 Introduction

The polyurethane shape-memory polymer (SMP) has high-performance and mechanical properties and has therefore been used practically in various fields (Takahashi et al., 1996; Ito et al., 1996; Huang et al., 2012; Tobushi et al., 2013; Otsuka and Wayman, 1998). In biomedical applications, the following mechanical properties are necessary: high flexibility and rigidity, strength, elongation, durability of cyclic deformation, and long-term use. The mechanical properties of SMPs depend on stress, strain, temperature, time, and their hysteresis. In order to evaluate the properties, mechanical testing for each property is performed. In the present chapter, tests for basic mechanical properties, tensile deformation, creep and stress relaxation, shape fixity and shape recovery, shape fixity and shape recovery of foam, recovery stress, and secondary shape forming will be explained. Future trends will be also introduced.

4.2 Testing for basic mechanical properties

Flexibility and rigidity are of primary importance for SMP elements in biomedical applications and are prescribed by the elastic modulus of the materials. The elastic modulus of SMPs differs significantly at temperatures above and below the glass transition temperature T_g. The elastic modulus is high at temperatures below T_g and low at temperatures above T_g. The shape fixity and shape recovery of SMPs are used based on the dependence of elastic modulus on temperature.

Elastic modulus is high at temperatures below T_g due to the elastic energy of crystal and amorphous phases and low at temperatures above T_g due to elastic entropy based on micro-Brownian motion of amorphous phase. The dynamic response of viscoelastic materials can be evaluated using harmonic mechanical loading with small amplitudes. The strain will be out of phase, phase lag, with the applied stress. The elastic portion of the material will store energy, whereas the viscous part dissipates energy. This is expressed as storage elastic modulus E' and loss modulus E''. They are related by the loss tangent defined as $\tan \delta = E''/E'$. The dependence of storage

Shape Memory Polymers for Biomedical Applications. http://dx.doi.org/10.1016/B978-0-85709-698-2.00004-0

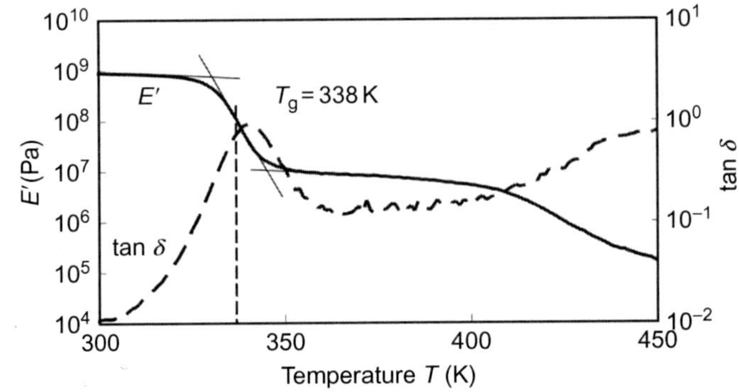

Figure 4.1 Dynamic mechanical properties of polyurethane shape-memory polymer.

elastic modulus E' and loss tangent tan δ on temperature for polyurethane SMP obtained by the dynamic mechanical test is shown in Figure 4.1. The elastic modulus E' is high at low temperature, decreases markedly in the glass transition region, and is low at high temperature. The elastic modulus E' at low temperature is larger than that at high temperature by about 100 times. The value of tan δ in the vicinity of the glass transition temperature T_g is about 1, showing the superior property of energy dissipation in this region.

In the case of SMP foam, the dynamic mechanical test is performed under compression. SMP is composed of soft and hard segments. The micro-Brownian motion of soft segments of SMP is active above T_g. Therefore, elastic modulus is low above T_g, and correspondingly, SMP deforms easily, and the original shape is recovered during unloading. The micro-Brownian motion of soft segments is frozen below T_g. Therefore, the elastic modulus is high below T_g, and SMP is hard to deform.

4.3 Testing for tensile deformation

In order to evaluate the shape fixity and shape recovery, the stress–strain relationship of SMP is necessary. The deformation property of SMP is visco-elastic and depends markedly on temperature T. The stress–strain relationship of visco-elastic material depends on strain rate $d\varepsilon/dt$. The most basic test to evaluate the deformation properties of the material is the tension test. As mentioned above, the deformation property of SMP depends markedly on both temperature and strain rate. The tension test, therefore, is carried out at various temperatures and strain rates. The test temperature is designated at the glass transition temperature T_g, above T_g and below T_g. The elastic modulus, yield stress, and work-hardening coefficient differ at temperatures at T_g, above T_g and below T_g.

Based on the basic mechanical properties of SMP, if the SMP element deformed above T_g is cooled down to below T_g, the deformed shape is fixed. This property is called shape fixity. In the state below T_g, since the SMP element is hard, it can carry a large load. Following this cooling process, if the shape-fixed SMP element is heated up to above T_g, it regains its original shape. This property is called shape recovery. As mentioned above, the SMP element changes shape when heated and retains its new shape when cooled. If the material is then reheated, it remembers its original shape and returns to it. These phenomena are the basic mechanism of shape fixity and shape recovery of the SMP element.

The stress–strain curves of the material are obtained by the tension test under various strain rates $d\varepsilon/dt$ at various temperatures T. At temperatures above T_g, deformation resistance is low and strain is recovered during unloading. At low temperature, deformation resistance is high and residual strain appears after unloading if it is loaded over the yield point. At all temperatures, deformation resistance increases in proportion to strain rate $d\varepsilon/dt$.

4.4 Testing for creep and stress relaxation

In applications of SMPs, if the SMP element is subjected to constant tightening force or pressure, the amount of deformation must be kept constant during the period of use. In a similar manner, if the SMP element is subjected to constant tightening or fixing displacement, the amount of force must be kept constant during the period of use. In general, the visco-elastic phenomena appear in polymers. If the visco-elastic properties appear in the SMP elements, the displacement under constant force may change, or the force under constant displacement may change. These behaviors are evaluated by creep or stress relaxation, respectively. The properties of creep and stress relaxation depend on stress, strain, temperature, and time (Tobushi et al., 1996a).

4.4.1 Creep test

In the creep test, the applied stress is kept constant, and the change in strain with the lapse of time is observed. The creep strain increases gradually under constant stress. The creep strain is large at temperatures above T_g and small at temperatures below T_g. The creep test is therefore performed at various temperatures above and below T_g. The temperature in the chamber is controlled to keep it constant during the test.

In the case of SMP foam, the creep test is performed in compression.

In the case of observing the short-term property, the test is carried out by the tension or compression test machine. In the case of observing the long-term property, the test is carried out by giving a constant dead weight in the temperature-controlled chamber. In the test, the displacement is automatically recorded.

In the creep test, at first, the change in strain under constant stress σ_0 is recorded with the lapse of time. The creep strain is observed until the prescribed time t_1. At t_1, the stress σ_0 is removed. The free stress state is held after t_1 and the behavior of strain is observed. The strain decreases gradually, that is, creep recovery appears.

In the case of cyclic creep test, these loading and unloading processes are repeated, as shown in Figure 4.2.

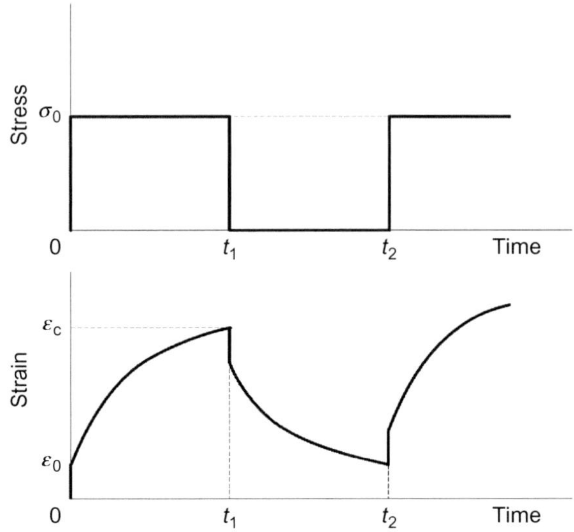

Figure 4.2 Creep and creep recovery test.

4.4.2 Stress relaxation test

In the stress relaxation test, the applied strain is kept constant and the change in stress with the lapse of time is observed. The stress decreases gradually under constant strain. The stress relaxation is large at temperatures above T_g and small at temperatures below T_g. The stress relaxation test is therefore performed at various temperatures above and below T_g. The temperature in the chamber is controlled to keep it constant during the test.

In the case of SMP foam, the stress relaxation test is performed in compression.

In the case of observing the short-term property, the test is carried out by the tension or compression test machine. In the case of observing the long-term property, the test is carried out by using a constant displacement device in the temperature-controlled chamber. In the test, the stress relaxation is automatically recorded.

In the stress relaxation test, at first, the change in stress under constant strain ε_0 is recorded with the lapse of time. The stress relaxation is observed until the prescribed time t_1. In the case of cyclic stress relaxation test, the stress σ_0, which is the same as in the initial stage, is obtained by applying the strain ε_1 at t_1, and the behavior of stress is observed after t_1. In the cyclic test, these loading processes are repeated, as shown in Figure 4.3.

4.5 Testing for shape fixity and shape recovery

In order to evaluate the shape fixity and shape recovery of SMP, the thermo-mechanical test with loading–unloading and heating–cooling is performed (Tobushi et al., 1996a,b).

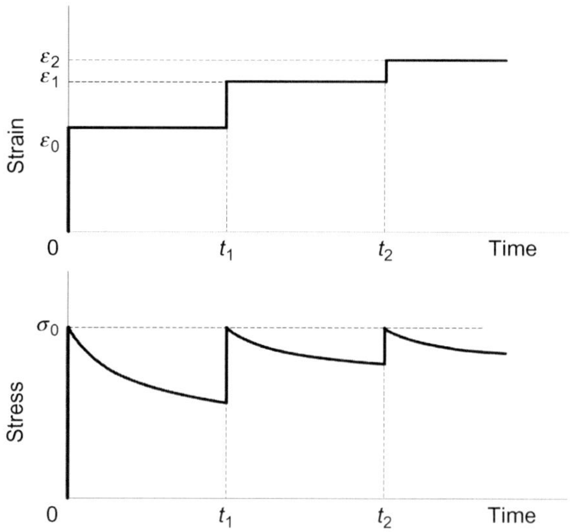

Figure 4.3 Stress relaxation test.

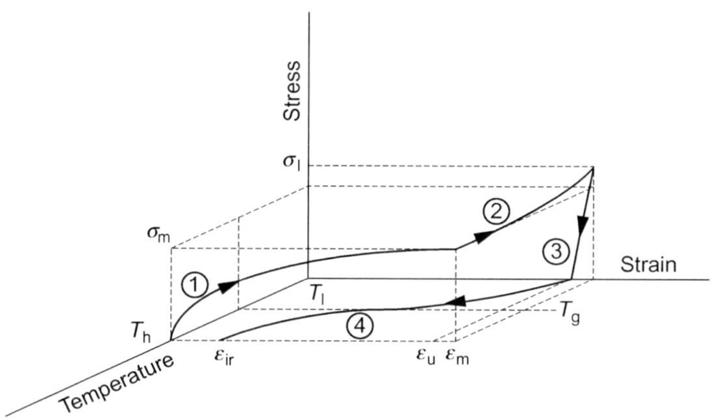

Figure 4.4 Three-dimensional stress–strain–temperature diagram showing the loading path in the thermo-mechanical test for shape fixity and shape recovery.

The three-dimensional stress–strain–temperature diagram in the thermo-mechanical test for shape fixity and shape recovery is shown in Figure 4.4. The maximum strain ε_m is applied at high temperature T_h in process ①. Maintaining ε_m constant, the specimen is cooled to T_l in process ②. The specimen is unloaded at T_l in process ③, and the strain ε_u appears at the unloading finish point. It is heated from T_l to T_h under no-load condition in process ④, and the irrecoverable strain ε_{ir} remains at the heating finish point. T_h is above T_g, and T_l is below T_g.

The stress–strain curve showing the shape fixity and shape recovery in the thermo-mechanical loading test at $\varepsilon_m = 9\%$ for the polyurethane SMP is shown in Figure 4.5.

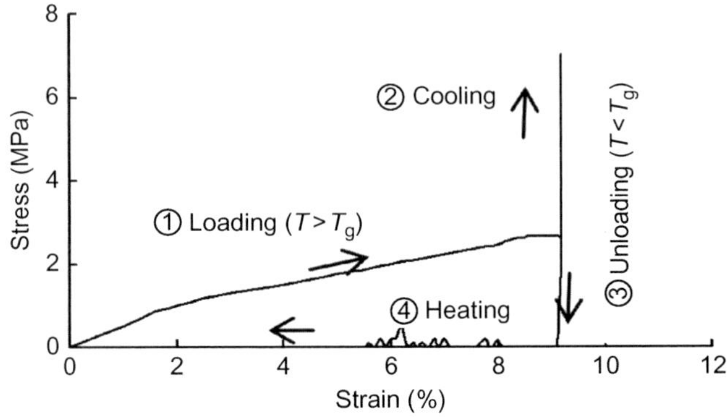

Figure 4.5 Stress–strain relationship in the thermo-mechanical test for shape fixity and shape recovery.

SMP is deformed easily under low stress at high temperature $T > T_g$, curve ①. If it is cooled down to a low temperature $T < T_g$ by keeping the maximum strain ε_m constant ②, stress increases due to the thermal contraction. This stress is larger than the loading stress by about three times. If it is thereafter unloaded at low temperature from this state ③, residual strain ε_u is almost same as the maximum strain ε_m due to high elastic modulus. This property is called the sharp fixity. Since both elastic modulus and yield stress are high in this state at low temperature, it can carry a large load in the elastic range. If it is heated to high temperature $T > T_g$ under no load ④, from the unloaded state at low temperature, strain decreases to ε_{ir} and the original shape is recovered. This property is called the shape recovery.

Note that the stress–strain curve, shape fixity, and shape recovery depend on strain rate in ①, cooling rate in ②, and heating rate in ④.

The ratio of shape fixity R_f and ratio of shape recovery R_r are defined by the following equations,

$$R_f = \frac{\varepsilon_u}{\varepsilon_m} \times 100 \tag{4.1}$$

$$R_r = \frac{\varepsilon_m - \varepsilon_{ir}}{\varepsilon_m} \times 100 \tag{4.2}$$

where ε_u and ε_{ir} represent the strain that appeared at the termination point of unloading below T_g ③ and the irrecoverable strain by heating up to above T_g under no-load condition ④, respectively.

Since recovery strain is large during unloading in the case of loading and unloading at low temperature, the use of the shape fixity in applications is important to correctly evaluate the amount of spring back in SMP elements.

4.6 Testing for shape fixity and shape recovery of foam

The three-dimensional stress–strain–temperature diagram in the thermo-mechanical test for shape fixity and shape recovery of foam is shown in Figure 4.6 (Tobushi et al., 2001, 2003). At first, ① maximum compressive strain $-\varepsilon_m$ is applied at high temperature T_h above T_g. ② Maintaining $-\varepsilon_m$, the specimen is cooled down to low temperature T_l below T_g. Note that stress is reduced to zero at this stage ②. ③ It is held at T_l under no-load condition for time t_l. ④ It is heated up to T_h above T_g under no-load condition. ⑤ It is held at T_h for time t_h. Note that the stress–strain curve in ① depends on strain rate and temperature. The shape fixity and shape recovery depend on cooling rate in ②, the heating temperature, the holding strain and the holding time in ③, and heating rate in ④. Thermo-mechanical paths ①–⑤ are repeated in the cyclic test.

The ratio of shape fixity R_f and ratio of shape recovery R_r are defined by Equations (4.1) and (4.2), in which $-\varepsilon_u$ and $-\varepsilon_{ir}$ represent the compressive strain obtained after holding no-load condition below T_g and the compressive strain obtained after heating up to above T_g under no-load condition, that is, irrecoverable strain, respectively.

4.7 Testing for recovery stress

If SMP is heated by keeping the maximum strain constant, stress increases during heating; that is, recovery stress appears by heating (Tobushi et al., 2003).

The three-dimensional stress–strain–temperature diagram in the recovery stress test is shown in Figure 4.7. As shown in Figure 4.7, the initial loading paths ①–③ are the same as those in the thermo-mechanical tests for shape fixity and shape recovery. In the process ④, no-load condition is maintained at low temperature T_l below T_g for time t_l. In process ⑤, the specimen is heated from T_l to high temperature T_h by keeping constant strain. In process ⑥, it is unloaded at T_h.

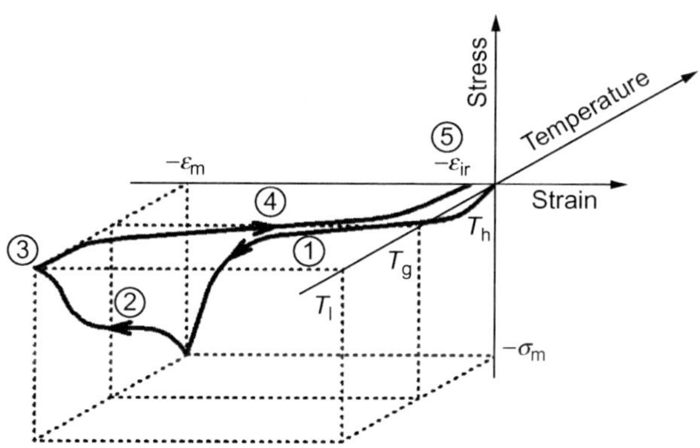

Figure 4.6 Three-dimensional stress–strain–temperature diagram showing the loading path in the thermo-mechanical compression test for shape fixity and shape recovery of SMP foam.

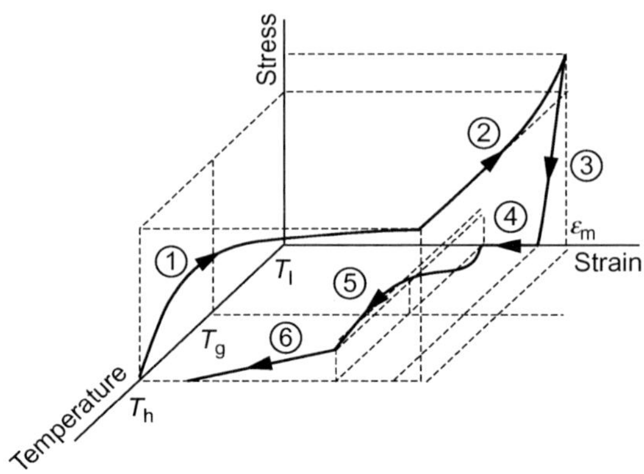

Figure 4.7 Three-dimensional stress–strain–temperature diagram showing the loading path in the recovery stress test.

In the case of SMP foam, the initial loading paths ①–③ are the same as those in the thermo-mechanical test shown in Figure 4.6. The maximum compressive stress is first applied under constant strain rate $d\varepsilon/dt$ at high temperature T_h, path ①. Keeping the maximum strain ε_m constant, it is cooled down to low temperature T_l ②. The stress-free state is held for time t_l at T_l ④. In the process ⑤, it is heated from T_l to T_h while maintaining the maximum compressive strain constant.

The smaller the strain rate $d\varepsilon/dt$, the larger the compressive strain at the maximum stress point is. This gives a higher recovery stress during the subsequent heating. The reason for this is that the foam becomes denser when loaded more slowly. This gives less relaxation during cooling and thereby a larger recovery stress during heating (Tobushi et al., 2003).

4.8 Testing for secondary shape forming

If the deformed SMP is held at temperatures above T_g for a long time, a large irrecoverable strain by heating appears. This phenomenon can be used to obtain the new shape, different from the original shape. This property is therefore called the secondary shape forming. The secondary shape forming is evaluated by three kinds of tests (Tobushi et al., 2003, 2006, 2008). The tension test is used for the film and sheet, the bending test for the sheet, and the compression test for the foam.

4.8.1 Secondary shape forming test for SMP film and sheet

The secondary shape forming of the SMP film and sheet is investigated by the tension test. In the test, load is applied under a constant strain rate for the maximum strain. The tension test is carried out by the following procedure:

1. Maximum strain ε_m is applied at T_g+20 K.
2. Holding ε_m constant, the specimen is cooled to room temperature. The strain is fixed at this stage and is held thereafter. Therefore, the holding strain ε_h, is equal to ε_m.

3. After cooling, the specimen is heated to the prescribed holding temperature T_h (T_g, $T_g + 10$ K and $T_g + 20$ K) by holding ε_h constant.
4. Strain ε_h is held at T_h for the prescribed holding time t_h (0.5, 1, 2, 3, 4, and 8 h).
5. Load is removed after holding ε_h for t_h.
6. The specimen is heated to $T_g + 30$ K under a no-load condition. Note that residual strain appears in this stage.

4.8.2 Secondary shape forming test for SMP sheet

The secondary shape forming of the SMP sheet is investigated by the following three-point bending tests. In the test, deflection rate dy/dt is 2 mm min^{-1} and maximum deflection y_{max} is 15 mm for a distance between two supports of 40 mm.

1. The maximum deflection y_{max} is applied at $T_g + 20$ K under the deflection rate dy/dt of 2 mm min^{-1}.
2. Holding y_{max} constant, the specimen is cooled to room temperature. The deflection is fixed at this stage and held thereafter. Therefore, the holding deflection y_h is equal to y_{max}.
3. After cooling, the specimen with y_h is heated to the prescribed holding temperature T_h (T_g, $T_g + 10$ K and $T_g + 20$ K).
4. The deflection y_h is held at T_h for the prescribed holding time t_h (0.5, 1, 2, 4, and 8 h).
5. The pushing rod is lifted after holding ε_h, for t_h.
6. The specimen is heated to $T_g + 30$ K under a no-load condition.

4.8.3 Secondary shape forming test for SMP foam

The experimental procedure in the secondary shape forming test for the SMP foam held at various temperatures is schematically shown in Figure 4.8. ① At first, maximum compressive strain $-\varepsilon_m$ is applied at $T_g + 30$ K using the testing machine. ② The specimen is compressed by using two compression plates in order to hold $-\varepsilon_m$

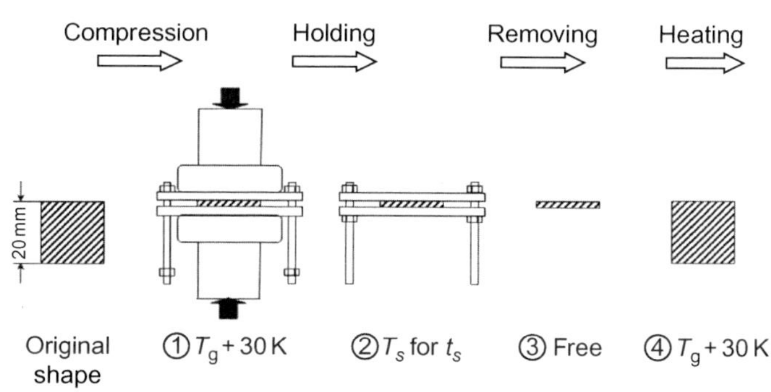

Figure 4.8 Experimental procedure of the secondary-shape-forming test for SMP foam held at various temperatures.

constant, and the compressed shape is held at a certain constant temperature T_s in a furnace. ③ After the prescribed shape-holding time t_s, the specimen is taken out from the furnace and the holding attachment is removed. ④ The shape of the specimen is recovered by heating up to T_g+30 K, and the height of the specimen is measured. By this procedure, residual strain ε_p at T_g+30 K is obtained.

Strain rate $d\varepsilon/dt$ is 10%/min in the loading process to apply $-\varepsilon_m$. Maximum strains ε_m are 50%, 70%, and 90%. In the case of shape holding at high temperature, the shape-holding temperatures T_s are T_g, T_g+30 K and T_g+60 K. The shape-holding times in the furnace t_s are 2, 4, 8, 16, and 24 h. In the case of shape-holding at low temperature, T_s is T_g, T_g-30 K and T_g-60 K, and $t_s=28$ days.

4.9 Future trends

In biomedical applications of SMPs, various additional functions of the material must be further clarified. Subjects to be developed in the future are summarized as follows.

1. The long-term functional property, degradation of the property due to aging, and rupture due to a decrease in strength. These subjects must be tested and clarified.
2. The functional properties may be different between in air and *in vivo* (Ishihara et al., 1998; Nakabayashi and Iwasaki, 2004; Ward et al., 2006, 2007). The functional properties must therefore be tested *in vivo*. The test for the functional properties *in vivo* will be performed in a blood substitute.
3. The gas permeability changes markedly at temperatures above and below T_g in the thin film of the polyurethane SMP. This property can be used in biomedical applications in which it is required as a function of skin. The test for gas permeability of SMPs subjected to stress or strain must be developed.
4. SMP fibers can be used as thread in biomedical applications. A test of the functional properties of SMP fiber must be developed.

References

Huang, W.M., Yang, B., Fu, Y.Q., 2012. Polyurethane Shape Memory Polymers. CRC Press, Florida.

Ishihara, K., Nomura, H., Mihara, T., Kurita, K., Iwasaki, Y., Nakabayashi, N., 1998. Why do phospholipid polymers reduce protein adsorption? J. Biomed. Mater. Res. A 39 (2), 323–330.

Ito, K., Abe, K., Li, H.L., Ujihira, Y., Ishikawa, N., Hayashi, Y., 1996. Variation of free volume size and content of shape memory polymer – polyurethane – upon temperature studied by positron annihilation lifetime techniques and infrared spectroscopy. J. Radioanal. Nucl. Chem. 211 (1), 53–60.

Nakabayashi, N., Iwasaki, Y., 2004. Copolymers of 2-methacryloyloxyethyl phosphorylcholine (MPC) as biomaterials. Biomed. Mater. Eng. 14 (4), 345–354.

Otsuka, K., Wayman, C.W., 1998. Shape Memory Materials. Cambridge University Press, Cambridge, pp. 203–219.

Takahashi, T., Hayashi, N., Hayashi, S., 1996. Structure and properties of shape-memory polyurethane block copolymers. J. Appl. Polym. Sci. 60, 1061–1069.
Tobushi, H., Hara, H., Yamada, E., Hayashi, S., 1996a. Thermomechanical properties in a thin film of shape memory polymer of polyurethane series. Smart Mater. Struct. 5, 483–491.
Tobushi, H., Hayashi, S., Ikai, A., Hara, H., 1996b. Thermomechanical properties of shape memory polymers of polyurethane series and their applications. J. Phys. IV Colloq. C1 6, C1-377–384.
Tobushi, H., Okumura, K., Endo, M., Hayashi, S., 2001. Thermomechanical properties of polyurethane-shape memory polymer foam. J. Intell. Mater. Syst. Struct. 12, 283–287.
Tobushi, H., Shimada, D., Hayashi, S., Endo, M., 2003. Shape fixity and shape recovery of polyurethane shape-memory polymer foams. Proc. Inst. Mech. Eng. L: Mater. Des. Appl. 217, 135–143.
Tobushi, H., Hayashi, S., Hoshio, K., Miwa, N., 2006. Influence of strain-holding conditions on shape recovery and secondary-shape forming in polyurethane-shape memory polymer. Smart Mater. Struct. 15, 1033–1038.
Tobushi, H., Hayashi, S., Hoshio, K., Ejiri, Y., 2008. Shape recovery and irrecoverable strain control in polyurethane shape-memory polymer. Sci. Technol. Adv. Mater. 9, 1–7. http://dx.doi.10.1088/1468-6996/9/1/015009.
Tobushi, H., Matsui, R., Takeda, K., Pieczyska, E.A., 2013. Mechanical Properties of Shape Memory Materials. Nova Science Publishers, New York, pp. 165–234.
Ward, B., Anderson, J., Ebert, M., McVenes, R., Stokes, K., 2006. In vivo biostability of polyether polyurethanes: resistance to metal Ion oxidation. J. Biomed. Mater. Res. A 77 (2), 380–389.
Ward, R., Anderson, J., McVenes, R., Stokes, K., 2007. In vivo biostability of polyether polyurethanes with fluoropolymer and polyethylene oxide surface modifying endgroups; resistance to metal Ion oxidation. J. Biomed. Mater. Res. A 80 (1), 34–44.

Appendix: abbreviations

R_f ratio of shape fixity
R_r ratio of shape recovery
SMP shape-memory polymer
T_g glass transition temperature

Biocompatibility of shape-memory polymers for biomedical applications

5

D.A. Mbeh, R.O. do Nascimento
Laboratory for Innovation and Analysis of Bio-Performance, École Polytechnique, Montréal, QC, Canada

5.1 Introduction

Shape-memory polymers (SMPs) are a category of smart materials with the ability to change shape in response to an environmental stimulus and triggers (e.g., heat, light, magnetic field, chemical, and electricity) (Wei et al., 1998; Metcalfe et al., 2003; El Feninat et al., 2002). Historically, their importance was not recognized until the 1960s, when cross-linked polyethylene (PE) was used for making heat-shrinkable tubes and films (Rainer et al., 1964). More efforts to develop SMPs began in the late 1980s and accelerated in the 1990s. Their shape-changing capacity has enabled SMPs to be used in many applications, such as implants for minimally invasive surgery (Yakacki et al., 2007; Baer et al., 2006), sensors and actuators (Metzger et al., 2002; Small et al., 2005), and heat-shrink tubing and films. The need for these SMPs to be used in a myriad of potential and practical applications including smart medical is well appreciated because of the controversy regarding the biocompatibility of nickel-containing shape-memory alloys (SMAs), their difficult fabrication and/or their cost being significantly higher than those of SMPs (Kim et al., 1996). For example, polymers can be designed to be bioactive, drug eluting (Wache et al., 2003) and/or biodegradable (Lendlein and Langer, 2002) as well as possess shape memory. Contrary to the shape-memory effects in metallic alloys, the effects in polymers are controllable not only by heating but also by exposure to light or through chemical reactions (Irie, 1990).

These materials are to be part of internal medical devices that have intimate contact with tissue and body fluids; therefore, particular attention must be given to the interface between the SMPs and the natural tissue upon implantation. Being synthetic (man made), and thus foreign to the body, these adaptive materials must first satisfy basic criteria such as biofunctionality, biostability, and biocompatibility during implantation. This last element refers to the ability of a biomaterial to perform its desired function with respect to a medical therapy without eliciting any undesirable local or systemic effects in the recipient or beneficiary of that therapy—but rather generating the most appropriate beneficial

Shape Memory Polymers for Biomedical Applications. http://dx.doi.org/10.1016/B978-0-85709-698-2.00005-2

cellular or tissue response in that specific situation and optimizing the clinically relevant performance of that therapy (Williams, 2003).

In this chapter, the general opinion in the literature of the biocompatibility of SMPs, the most conventional techniques for biocompatibility assessment, and the biocompatible coatings of SMPs are reviewed.

5.2 Biocompatibility of shape-memory polymers

In a general context, biocompatibility refers to the ability of a material to perform with an appropriate host response in a specific application (Williams, 2003). Originally, a biocompatible polymer referred to a "plastic" that was tolerated by living organisms; i.e., it did not initiate immune response, control cell adhesion, and/or control water content. It could be an implantable solid-coated surface or an injectable liquid. However, more recent definitions aim to describe the biological mechanism in more detail (Williams, 2008). *In vitro* biocompatibility, or cytotoxicity, is generally evaluated through cell culture systems. *In vivo* experimental, histological, and pathological examination of the peri-implant and host responses—such as immunogenic, carcinogenic, and thrombogenic responses—are also studied. The complexity of these host responses is a result of a series of temporal and spatial processes involving numerous closely interdependent mechanisms of material–tissue interactions. It is these interactions that control the ultimate performance of a material within a biological environment. If we consider the field of biostable materials and permanently implanted devices/implants, the primary goal is minimizing and adjusting material–tissue interactions. The interaction of the living environment and the material should be acceptable and stable for long-term therapies and performances.

Conversely, in the field of biodegradable and bioresorbable polymers, the situation is quite the opposite, with an added dimension of complexity afforded by the degradation and resorption by-products of the implants, which are able to strongly interact with living systems. From this point of view, biocompatibility is a factor that must be considered before biodegradable polymers are selected for their use in medical devices.

Many research groups are pursuing medical applications of SMPs. Two of the earliest reports on biomedical SMP applications also contained some data indicating good biocompatibility (Metcalfe et al., 2003; Lendlein and Langer, 2002). As Lendlein and his collaborators presented in their review in 2010, which included a motivation for the introduction of SMP to biomedical applications, few SMPs are currently commercially available (Lendlein et al., 2010), because their short-, medium-, and long-term biocompatibility must be assessed. Without a supplier of medical-grade SMPs, the burden of establishing biocompatibility currently falls on medical device start-up companies, academic groups, and government laboratories. The first commercially available and biocompatible SMPs are polyurethane (PU) from Mitsubishi Heavy Industries, Ltd. (Nagoya, Japan), now distributed through a subsidiary (DiAPLEX, Ltd.). A significant number of the early published studies have focused on the DiAPLEX materials, documenting good biocompatibility: low cytotoxicity (Fare et al., 2005; De Nardo et al., 2009), low thrombogenicity (Cabanlit et al., 2007), low platelet activation (Fare et al., 2005; Cabanlit et al., 2007), low cytokine activation (Cabanlit et al., 2007), and low *in vivo* inflammatory response (Metcalfe et al., 2003). These results are generally expected from the PU literature (Lamba et al., 1997; Ratner et al., 2004). In addition to the DiAPLEX materials, other published biocompatibility studies on SMPs include poly(L-lactide)-polyurethanes (Small et al., 2010), poly(ε-caprolactone)dimethacrylate (Neuss et al., 2009), and copolymerized methyl methacrylate and poly-(ethylene glycol)dimethacrylate (Yakacki et al., 2008).

Despite some success in biomedical applications, the use of polymers in acceptable permanent implants has yet to be reported, particularly in long-term applications. We must first keep in mind that biocompatibility of biomaterials depends on many parameters (both intrinsic and extrinsic) and that it cannot be easily assessed. In addition, as the expected duration of the implantation is directly related to the material's short- or long-term ability to maintain its stability, biocompatibility must be a priority when selecting biomaterials for specific applications. Ideally, biomaterials used as long-term medical implants must retain their properties and functionality for the remainder of the patient's life.

In general, polymers are well recognized as high-potential biomaterials because of their good biocompatibility; however, we must consider that large-scale industrial production of these polymers is very hard to achieve without additives, and in many cases, the presence of these additives has resulted in biocompatibility problems in long-term implantation. Certain additives, such as plasticizers, stabilizers, catalysts, blowing agents, and, sometimes, pigments, are in fact often used in developing polymeric implants (Singhal et al., 2014). These additives may show toxic effects once in contact with cells, tissues, or organs.

In addition to the presence of additives, the issue of chemical stability is of prime importance and must be carefully considered when designing a SMP that will be suitable for implantation. While some polymers are known to be chemically highly stable upon implantation in humans (i.e., poly-(tetrafluoroethylene), PTFE, and poly(ethyleneterephthalate), PET), others may be more susceptible to chemical degradation because of their intrinsic molecular structure. Indeed, several polymers contain chemical moieties, which may be readily hydrolyzed or oxidized within the aggressive physiological environment of the human body. In other words, the chemical structure of an eventually perfect shape memory polymer should display not only the appropriate mechanical characteristics but also meet the criteria for chemical stability in physiological environment to prevent any failure as biomedical device.

The use of SMP-based implants in hard tissue such as bone has presented the release of particles over time. Bone loss can occur secondary to a biological reaction to particulate debris from implants. It is now widely accepted that this is the principal mechanism responsible for periprosthetic osteolysis. Particulate PE is considered to be the substance causing the most tissue reaction, forming up to 90% of the debris volume (Dattani, 2007). Other particles that have been implicated in development of osteolysis include sub-micron-sized ultra-high-molecular-weight polyethylene (UHMWPE) and polymethylmethacrylate (cement) (Jacobs et al., 2001). These particles most likely exert their effects by either promoting third-body wear of PE, with UHMWPE triggering the cellular response; or they instigate the release of inflammatory mediators, which results in chronic inflammation and tissue damage that erodes the supporting bone with subsequent implant loosening.

In platelet retention experiments, some polymers from the PU family show high thrombogenicity (Lelah et al., 1983). The response of blood to PU surfaces depended on the PU surfaces and on the sequence of PU segments: in fact, the PU segmented copolymers displayed excellent blood compatibility only when the PU soft segment was polytetramethylene oxide, which suggests that a successful application is only possible by selecting the specific PU polymer for a particular application (Cabanlit et al., 2007). The degree of cellular and protein adhesion and the ability to stimulate neutrophils and inflammatory cytokine production are described for two PU-based SMPs, polyesterurethanes (PESU) and thermoset polyetherurethanes (PEU) (Cabanlit et al., 2007). The PESU, which is a thermoplastic SMP, showed higher TNF-α production and a higher potential for macrophage and endothelial activation. And following the implantation of PU-foam-covered implants, some authors observed the presence of toluene diamine (TDA) in the patient's urine (Sepai et al., 1995; Hester et al., 1997). Exposure to TDA released from the coating was known to cause a cancer in animals; for this reason, this type of implant was taken off the market in 1991.

5.3 Biocompatibility assays

In the literature, various studies evaluate the exposition of SMPs to cells through cellular, subcellular, and genetic behavior that can induce cell's death through the disruption of the plasma membrane's integrity, mitochondrial damage, and impairment of the nucleus.

Exposure of the body to SMPs is evaluated to trigger the inflammatory response that will ultimately lead to cell death and tissue damage.

The international standard ISO 10993 (Biological Evaluation of Medical Devices) provides guidelines for biocompatibility testing *in vitro*. According to the standards, testing toxicity of SMPs can be done in direct contact with cells, the so-called cytocompatibility, or cytotoxicity, of their extracts on cells. Extract is obtained according to ASTM F619. In general, no single method can cover the complexity of general toxicity in humans. *In vitro* toxicity testing regimes attempt to measure cytotoxicity, cytocompatibility, cell adhesion, genotoxicity, hemocompatibility, cell proliferation, and a host of other measurable cell parameters.

5.3.1 Cytotoxicity and cytocompatibility

There are a variety of ways to assess cell viability and cytotoxicity of examined compounds or extracts. They include (1) the measurement of mitochondrial activity; (2) the analysis of lactate dehydrogenase (LDH) for the assessment of cell membrane integrity; and (3) the determination of cytokines production as the indicators of cellular pro-inflammatory reaction (Miret et al., 2006). They are mainly performed with immortalized cells (e.g., V79, L929, and 3T3).

5.3.1.1 *Mitochondrial activity*

The monitoring of alterations in mitochondrial activity can be detected with the use of MTT (3-(4,5-dimethylthiazol-2-yl)-2,5-diphenyltetrazolium bromide) and resazurin (7-hydroxy-10-oxidophenoxazin-10-ium-3-one) (Ahmed et al., 1994; Mosmann, 1983).

MTT assay is a commonly used screening method to measure cell viability. It is believed to be based on the reduction of tetrazolium salt (MTT) by mitochondrial succinic dehydrogenases in viable cells, yielding purple formazan crystals that are not soluble in aqueous solutions typical for the cell environment (Mosmann, 1983). The MTT assay was first described by Mosmann (1983) and modified several times by Hansen et al. (1989) and Nielsen and Berg (1985), as Kuzma et al. (2012) have described previously.

Briefly, cells in suspension are seeded in a 96-well microtiter plate and grown in a humidified atmosphere of 5% CO_2 in air at 37 °C. The cells are then exposed to SMP extract. After that, supernatant (which can be used for LDH assay) is carefully removed. MTT solution (5 mg/ml PBS) is added, and the plate is located in optimal atmosphere at 37 °C. The metabolically active cells reduce MTT to blue formazan crystals. After 2 h, MTT-formazan crystals are dissolved overnight in either DMSO or HCl/isopropanol, and absorbance is measured at 570 nm on a multifunctional plate reader and compared with untreated control cells.

Although MTT is economical and widely utilized, it has several disadvantages. It is generally cytotoxic, since the formazan crystals must be solubilized with DMSO or HCl/isopropanol. This procedure kills the cells, allowing only one measurement to be made at a single point in time. Moreover, while MTT reduction only occurs in metabolically active cells, marked changes in metabolic cellular activity can result in significant variabilities in the outcomes, despite the fact that the number of viable cells remains constant (Ventura-Sobrevilla et al., 2011).

There are also other tests: AlamarBlue® assay and PrestoBlue® assay for the cell's metabolism analysis and trypan blue cell-counting assay for cell viability analysis.

5.3.1.2 *Membrane damage*

Cell lysis and membrane damage can be determined by LDH assay. LDH is a stable cytoplasmic enzyme present in all cells. It is rapidly released into the cell culture supernatant when the plasma membrane of cells is damaged. For this reason, the LDH assay is a widely used quantitative test for the toxicity of SMPs. The LDH detection and quantification method is an optical chromophore-based method that is simple, rapid, reliable, and cost-effective and yields reproducible results (Decker and Lohmann-Matthes, 1988; Andre et al., 2004; Vorotnikova et al., 2010).

The assay is a two-step process. In the first step, LDH catalyzes the reduction of NAD+ (nicotinamide adenine dinucleotide) to NADH and H+ by oxidation of lactate to pyruvate. In the second step, the enzyme diaphorase utilizes the newly formed NADH and H+ to catalyze the reduction of a tetrazolium salt to a highly colored formazan salt product.

The above-mentioned supernatant is centrifuged at $500 \times g$ for 10 min and the LDH activity is measured with a standard LDH kit (Sigma, TOX7-1KT). Briefly, aliquots of supernatant and warm reagent are mixed in a 96-well plate; absorbance is recorded using a microplate spectrophotometer system. The LDH measured reflects the quantity released due to cell lysis and cell membrane damage. Thus, when performed correctly, the detectable increase in LDH in growth media used to culture cells directly correlates to the amount of formazan product formed during a specific time period. Therefore, the amount of color formed in the assay is proportional to the number of leaking or lysed cells when the units of LDH per cell for the type of cell have been determined.

5.3.1.3 Cytokines production

Cytokines and other immunologically active molecules are predominantly detected by enzyme-linked immunosorbent assays (ELISA). Enzyme-linked immunosorbent assays are plate-based assays used in the cytotoxicity of SMPs to detect and quantify cytokines such as TNF-α, interleukines (IL-6, 8, 10, etc.) in the co-culture supernatants. In an ELISA, an antigen must be immobilized to a solid surface and then complexed with an antibody that is linked to an enzyme. Detection is accomplished by assessing the conjugated enzyme activity via incubation with a substrate to produce a measureable product. The most crucial element of the detection strategy is a highly specific antibody–antigen interaction.

In general, the culture supernatants are collected after the complete generation of the cytokine to be analyzed. The experiment is conducted according to the manufacturer's test instructions. Conventionally, antigen or antibody is quantified spectrophotometrically by measuring the absorbance of the assay solution in an ELISA plate reader. Disadvantages of conventional ELISA, normally performed in a 96-well microtiter or ELISA plate are: (i) the ELISA plate itself is costly, (ii) the ELISA reader is a bulky, expensive instrument that is not easily available in resource-poor areas, (iii) it requires large volumes of costly reagents and analytes, and (iv) it requires long incubation time (Parween and Nahar, 2013). Therefore, for low-resource settings, it is necessary to have a device or an assay system that is cheap, specific, sensitive, and, most importantly, does not require a costly instrument.

In some cases, to provide more detailed systematic information about the SMP–cell interaction, cell migration and matrix degradation are used. The tightly controlled degradation of the extracellular matrix is mainly dependent on the activity of matrix metalloproteinases (MMPs) and the tissue inhibitors of MMP (Tissue Inhibitor of Metalloproteinase) (Lendlein et al., 2010).

5.3.2 Hemocompatibility

SMPs are used as surgical biodegradable sutures, coronary stents, catheters, or orthodontic applications, where a direct contact with blood occurs. Hemocompatibility has been widely studied, with the intention of establishing a standard for the possible blood–materials interactions. There are so many mechanisms that blood can respond to in an SMP; therefore, the blood compatibility assessment must take into account the fact that if a material will not trigger one response mechanism, it may be highly active in another. Based on the primary process evaluated, hemocompatibility assays can be classified into four categories: blood coagulation, platelets function, hematology, and complement system activation.

5.3.2.1 Blood coagulation

Blood coagulation assay is one of the most frequently used tests to evaluate the hemocompatibility of a biomaterial or a medical device. Blood coagulation is a phenomenon that results from the activation of a clotting factor cascade. The prothrombin time test evaluates the extrinsic and common pathway of coagulation cascade activation; intrinsic and common coagulation pathways are evaluated by measuring the activated partial thromboplastin time; meanwhile, thrombin time examines the thrombin activity or fibrin polymerization.

5.3.2.2 Platelet adhesion

Assessing the hemocompatibility through the response of the platelets consists of the quantification of their number, the evaluation of their structure, and the analysis of platelet factors or components released. The endpoint more frequently evaluated for hemocompatibility of SMPs is platelet adhesion (Zhou et al., 2014; Chan-Chan et al., 2010). The extent of platelet adhesion evaluates the thrombogenic potential of materials. Briefly, platelet-rich plasma (PRP) is prepared by centrifugation (1500 rpm, 15 min) of fresh human whole blood. Fifty microliters of fresh PRP is added to each sample of SMP placed in a 24-well plate and incubated at 37 °C. After washing with 0.9 wt% NaCl aqueous solution (10 min, 3 times), the samples are fixed using 2.5 v% glutaraldehyde solution overnight at 4 °C in the dark. Afterward, the samples are washed again with 0.9 wt% NaCl aqueous solution and subsequently immersed in 30%, 50%, 75%, 90%, 95%, and 100% (v/v) ethanol/water solutions for 10 min each. The morphologies of the platelets on different samples are observed by SEM after drying and sputtering with gold. The amounts of platelets on the samples are determined by counting platelets in six different areas.

5.3.2.3 Hemolysis

Hematology refers to the quantification of cellular and plasma components of the blood. Usually, hematology is evaluated through hemolysis (the release of hemoglobin from totally or partially damaged erythrocytes). *In vitro* hemolysis test is considered a simple and reliable measurement for estimating blood biocompatibility of materials. Hemolysis index is regarded as safe when it is less than 5% (ISO document 10 993-5 1992) (Zhou et al., 2011). To test the hemolysis ratio (HR) of the samples, fresh human whole blood is obtained from healthy donors (Deka et al., 2010). Samples are rinsed with 0.9 wt% NaCl aqueous solution. Every test sample is extracted in 1.5 ml 0.9 wt% NaCl aqueous solution for 30 min at 37 °C. Untreated 0.9 wt% NaCl aqueous solution and distilled water serve as negative and positive controls, respectively. After that, 30 μl diluted whole blood (0.8 ml whole blood is diluted by 1 ml 0.9 wt% NaCl aqueous solution) is added to the samples and incubated for another 60 min. Subsequently, the solutions are centrifuged for 5 min at 3000 rpm. The absorbance of the supernatant is measured at 545 nm.

5.3.2.4 Complement activation

Complement system, a part of the innate system, consists of several plasma proteins, including enzymes and cellular receptors. Once complement activation is initiated, the release of peptide anaphylatoxins (C3a, C4a, and C5a) takes place; these peptides are humoral messengers that bind to specific receptors on neutrophils, monocytes, macrophages, mast cells, and smooth muscle cells and induce, in the end, cell lysis (Monk et al., 2007).

5.3.3 Histocompatibility

An *in vitro* system, considered to be the elementary living system, cannot replicate exactly the biodynamics of the whole human body due to the lack of possible regulation factors (e.g., hormones, nervous system, and immunity) and the lack of biotransformation and excretion pathways for their elimination *in vitro*. Therefore, *in vivo* testing in animal models is necessary prior to human clinical testing. No single animal species represents an ideal general model for the human species. Anatomical, biochemical, physiological, pathological, and/or psychological characteristics must be considered when choosing an animal model (Lendlein et al., 2010; Belanger and Marois, 2001). Guidelines to carry out animal biocompatibility tests are described by the standards organizations of regulatory agencies such as ASTM, ISO, NIH, Food and Drug Administration (FDA), and U.S. and European Pharmacopoeia. *In vivo* tests are used to evaluate physiological effects of the implant and its leachable/soluble/degradation components on local and systemic tissues, tissue response to the implant, and changes in regulator biomolecules. Histologic examination of tissues taken from osteolytic lesions adjacent to both loose and well-fixed implants shows that many types of cells, including macrophages, fibroblasts, osteoclasts, and also some bioactive products, such as enzymes, cytokines, and growth factors, can be found. The inflammatory response of copolymers PCL and PLA after implantation in male wistar rats was studied in detail by Pitt and coworkers (Woodward et al., 1985). In the study realized by Woodruff and his collaborators, inflammatory reactions in bones were less pronounced than in muscles. The investigators do not discuss this observation in great detail, but Woodruff hypothesizes that the pronounced primary inflammatory reaction in muscle might be due to a better vascularization of muscle tissue (Woodruff and Hutmacher, 2010). Until now, inadequate transport between the microvasculature and implanted materials has limited the utility of a variety of biomedical applications, including tissue engineering (Sieminski and Gooch, 2000). The interaction between a biomaterial and surrounding tissue requires sufficient capillary and vessel formation to ensure the transport between the tissue and implanted biomaterials (Binzen et al., 2004) and a sufficient clearance of the biomaterial–tissue interface, for example, from degradation products. Wear particle accumulation at the biomaterial–tissue interface caused concerns regarding the introduction of degradable polymers in medical therapies (Bakker et al., 1990; van Blitterswijk et al., 1991). *In vivo* tissue responses to SMPs and their degradation products can be examined through histological and histomorphometric evaluation.

5.3.3.1 Histological evaluation

Subcutaneous implants and organs are retrieved from the animal sacrificed at predetermined time points, and fixed in a periodate–lysine-paraformaldehyde fixative (Miao and Scutt, 2002) at 4 °C for 1 and 2 days, respectively. The internal organs are grossly inspected at the time of sacrifice for tumor formation. Paraffin sections (5 mm) of the subcutaneous explants are stained for Ki67, a marker for cell proliferation, and with hematoxylin and eosin (H&E). Paraffin sections (5 mm) of the retrieved organs are stained with H&E. All histology slides are blind-assessed by a pathologist. Samples are examined in detail to count the number of lymphocytes, macrophages, mast cells, eosinophils, and neutrophils for each sample at each time point. Other histological evaluations can also be used, such as light microscopy (Zilla et al., 2009).

5.3.3.2 Histomorphometric evaluation

The tissue-covered specimens are retrieved. Samples are fixed in 10% formalin, dehydrated in a graded series of ethanol and embedded in paraffin, after which 6 mm sections are cut in a transversal direction. The sections are cut from at least three arbitrary regions perpendicular to the long axis of the tissue capsule. Paraffin sections are stained with hematoxylin/eosin (HE). All sections are photographed with the Zeiss Imager Z1 together with the AxioCam MRc5 camera, using AxioVision 4.6.3 software (Carl Zeiss Microimaging GmbH, Germany). Histological evaluation on all sections is performed based on the obtained images. For the analyses of HE-stained sections, a refined histomorphometric grading scale is used (Ji et al., 2012). The performed quantitative evaluation of the fibrous capsule in each section is based on four different areas (image size: 678,510 mm^2) of the entire fibrous capsules surrounding the implant (Ji et al., 2012).

5.3.4 Genotoxicity

The study of the genotoxicity of the materials is fundamental to an understanding of the damage that they may cause to the genetic code of their host or other organisms. The similarity showed in the genetic materials of living beings is a powerful tool that can predict similar effects from one species to another (De Lima and Fraceto, 2014). In this respect, available tests that can verify the genotoxic potential of a material, compound, or composite are the *Allium cepa* chromosome aberration test, comet analysis, micronucleus test, and cytogenetic analysis. In this chapter, we focus on the first two methods, providing a brief description of each technique as well as some results of the select literature of SMP.

5.3.4.1 Allium cepa

The presence of pollutants and of potentially toxic products brought about by their degradation induced the World Health Organization (WHO) and the United Nations—through the International Program on Chemical Safety and the United Nations Environment Program (Cabrera and Rodriguez, 1999)—to select *Allium cepa* as a standard test for *in situ* analysis and monitoring of the genotoxicity of materials present in the environment. This technique involves the measurement of chromosomal aberrations caused by chemical agents present in the water and wastewater effluents, among others (De Lima et al., 2010). This technique consist of the exposure of onion roots tips to solutions containing different concentration of the pollutants, a negative control, a medium without any type of contaminants, and a positive control, which is a solution with an agent recognized to cause damage to the DNA. The results obtained with the pollutants should be compared with the control. The study includes at least three concentrations of each pollutant. The *Allium cepa* test could present aberrations of the chromosomes at different phases of cellular division. In this type of test, the polymer as well as the monomer should be studied.

In this test, the proportion of damaged cells is calculated by the ratio (CAS) between the number of cells showing alterations at different phases of the cycle for the number of cells in division. The relative indices could be calculated comparing the mitotic index (MI; the ratio between the number of cells in division by the number total of cells), the alteration index for each treatment, and the values obtained for the negative control. This type of genotoxicity test can also be used to evaluate the monomer of the polymer, as well as, the products of degradation of the polymers and its composites as described in Table 5.1.

Comet assays

The comet test is used to indicate the capacity of the material to cause DNA lesions. However, this test is considered a pre-test of the damage capacity of the material once it is not possible to identify any repair process, since during the test there is no cell division (the phase in which most of the repair of the genetic material occurs). Moreover, this test is considered fast, simple, and less expensive when compared, for example, with the *Allium cepa* test. The comet assays can be applied *in vivo* as well as *in vitro*. The test requires the application of negative and positive controls. The cells exposed at the material should be immobilized in agarose gel; its genetic material is exposed after the lyse process. The material is analyzed by electrophoresis and may resemble a comet with a tail. This phenomena is explained by the presence of fragments of DNA with different sizes; when the result of the test is positive, small fragments migrate faster than large fragments.

5.4 Biocompatible coatings

In modern medicine, artificial biocompatible coating are used in a wide range of applications. SMPs have gained increased attention over the last several years as a proposed biomaterial to prevent biofilm growth on medical devices, such as catheters, for minimally invasive surgical devices as stents and drug delivery system.

Table 5.1 Results of published works that used the *Allium cepa* test to evaluate the toxic effects of polymers, monomers, and their composites

Substance/material	Main results of *Allium cepa* test	References
Commercial detergents	One of the ecologically labeled detergents presented a reduction at the MI	Pedrazzani et al. (2012)
Mineral water packed in polyethylene terephthalate (PET) and glass bottles	The water studied does not present any type of mutagenic capacity, even that which underwent storage at 40 °C. However, the polymers were not tested and the samples were not submitted to previous aging tests before the *Allium cepa* test	Ceretti et al. (2010)
PLA and organoclays nanocomposites	The products of degradation of PLA and organoclays (Cloisite 20A and 40A) presented genotoxicity effects confirmed by the *Allium cepa* test. The genotoxicity of the PLA is not well studied in the literature. Moreover, these results suggested that the ecotoxicity of the PLA and its products of degradation should be better investigated	Souza et al. (2013)

5.4.1 Stents

A number of investigators have worked diligently over the past several years to explore the feasibility of a completely bioabsorbable stent (vanderGiessen et al., 1996). The impetus for this approach was the perception that the long-term implantation of metallic stents might result in a chronic inflammatory stimulus (Yakacki et al., 2007; Fischman et al., 1994). The excellent long-term biocompatibility of stainless steel stents, combined with the substantive difficulties in developing a polymeric stent with competitive structural characteristics, have led previously enthusiastic polymer stent proponents to focus on developing biocompatible polymeric coatings for metal stents. Such a hybrid medical device (metal backbone with polymer coating) would provide the mechanical advantages of stenting and a platform for local drug delivery to increase stent hemocompatibility.

The feasibility and biocompatibility of polymer stents have been deemed uncertain, especially after an early study showed an inflammation response to biodegradable SMP coatings on stents, such as polyglycolic acid/polylactic acid, polycaprolactone, polyhydroxybutarate valerate, polyorthoester, and polyethylenoxide/polybutylene terephthalate as well as nonbiodegradable polymers, such as PU, silicone, and PET. The authors found that all the implanted polymer coatings were associated with a significant inflammatory and exaggerated neointimal proliferative response. In addition, their data suggest that at least some of the polymer coatings may have provoked an enhanced thrombotic response (vanderGiessen et al., 1996; Fischell, 1996). Although the biocompatibility of polymer stents in animal studies has been controversial, some reports suggest that high-molecular-weight poly-L-lactic acid (PLLA) is biocompatible in porcine coronary models (Lincoff et al., 1997; Yamawaki et al., 1998). The Igaki-Tamai PLLA polymer stent was the first to be implanted in human coronary arteries, in 1999 (Tamai et al., 2000). The majority of biocompatibility studies of SMP coatings of stents are limited to *in vitro* studies and subcutaneous implant assays (Cho et al., 2008). The intravascular environment is indeed unforgiving and does not readily tolerate foreign bodies. In addition to the usual tissue biocompatability issues, the exposure to flowing blood with the potential for activation of platelets, the extrinsic clotting cascade, or both, provide a challenge to identify a compound that could be used in a hybrid stent design without aggravating the thrombotic risks (Fischell, 1996). The obvious advantages of SMP on stents are the increase of drug-loading and biodegradation capabilities (Yakacki et al., 2007).

5.4.2 Catheters

Intravascular catheters, urinary catheters, and ventilator tubes allow clinicians to deliver drugs and nutritional fluids into the body, to expel fluids out of the body, and to monitor the status of critically ill patients. It is well known that microorganisms can colonize these medical devices, which can often put patients at risk for local and systemic infectious complications, including local site infection, catheter-related bloodstream infection (BSI), and endocarditis (Bouza et al., 2002; O'Grady et al., 2002). Improving the performance and the effectiveness of catheters is mainly based on the reduction of infections due to biofilm formation on their surfaces. Chemical modifications of polymers have improved either the anti-adhesive properties or biocompatibility of existing biomaterials. Early studies showed that the introduction of phosphonate groups in PUs, by the use of glycerophosphorylcholine as a polymer chain extender, produced a strong effect on cell adhesion. Results indicated that hydrophilic surfaces were less colonized by bacteria than hydrophobic surfaces due to the increased ability of the phosphonate PU to absorb water (Baumgartner et al., 1997; Gottenbos et al., 2000; Park et al., 2002). Poly(ethylene glycol) derivatives (Roosjen et al., 2004; Kingshott et al., 2003; Tegoulia and Cooper, 2002) or zwitterionic polymers (Hirota et al., 2005; Patel et al., 2005; Cheng et al., 2007) have been extensively used as nonfouling materials to reduce bacterial attachment and biofilm formation on catheters. However, the susceptibility of PEG to oxidation damage has limited its long-term application in complex media (Roosjen et al., 2004; Ostuni et al., 2001). Cheng and his collaborators showed that zwitterionic materials, such as poly(sulfobetaine methacrylate) (pSBMA), dramatically reduced bacterial attachment and biofilm formation (Cheng et al., 2007) and were highly resistant to nonspecific protein adsorption, even from undiluted blood plasma and serum (Ladd et al., 2008).

5.4.3 Drug delivery

Active pharmaceutical ingredients are almost never administered alone but rather in dosage forms that generally include other substances called excipients. The latter are added to formulations in order to improve the bioavailability and acceptance of the drug on the part of patients. It is currently upheld that excipients influence the speed and extent of drug absorption; therefore, the pharmaceutical form of these substances affects drug bioavailability. In this regard, recent years have seen intense research on the modification of drug release and absorption. Due to a variety of drugs and their physicochemical properties, an appropriate drug carrier must be chosen. The growing interest in the bioresorbable polymers contributed to the development of a number of commercially available controlled drug delivery systems. The main function of polymeric carriers is to transport drugs to the site of action. Moreover, polymeric carriers avoid the interaction of the drug with macromolecules such as proteins, which could sequester the active ingredient preventing its arrival at the action place. The majority of polymer DDSs are in the form of microparticles such as Risperdal Consta, Nutropin Depot, or Lupron Depot, consisting of poly(L-lactide-*co*-glycolide); the most studied forms of polymer DDSs are nano- and microspheres, nano- and microcapsules. In general, their low molecular weight enables them to cross various body compartments and access numerous cell types and subcellular organelles (Musial-Kulik et al., 2014). Many different polymers have been developed to control the release of drugs. High-molecular weight, cross-linked polymers of acrylic acids constitute the carbomer matrices that are commonly used in release tablet formulations (Khan and Zhu, 1999; Zurita et al., 2006). Hard composite systems based on Al_2O_3, polylactide, and poly(methyl methacrylate) have been designed for use in orthopedic surgery and dental applications (Vallet-Regi et al., 1998). pH-sensitive systems for site-specific delivery have also been developed by using lipophilic polymers obtained from the substitution of poly[(methacrylic acid)-*co*-(methyl methacrylate)] with fatty acids (Luppi et al., 2003). Rencently, terpolymer with SMP made of L-lactide, glycolide, and oligo-trimethylene carbonate served as a drug carrier (Musial-Kulik et al., 2014).

5.5 Conclusion

SMPs published to date have sufficient thermo-mechanical and shape-memory properties to succeed as medical devices. Many industrial and academic groups are pursuing medical applications of these SMPs. The first FDA approval of a medical SMP device was granted in 2008 for an orthopedic anchor (Medshape Solutions, Inc.; www.medshapesolutions.com). The primary hurdles for the early applications of SMPs in medicine will be limited to chemistry challenges and business. The synthesis method and composition of SMPs must be carefully designed for the appropriate biological reactions. Even in the short term, however, poor biocompatibility could have long-term negative consequences on the adoption of SMP as a biomedical material. Ultimately, SMP devices will need to pass many rigorous testing protocols to be approved by the regulatory agencies, such as the FDA, before being allowed on the market.

References

Ahmed, S.A., Gogal Jr., R.M., Walsh, J.E., 1994. A new rapid and simple non-radioactive assay to monitor and determine the proliferation of lymphocytes: an alternative to [3H]thymidine incorporation assay. J. Immunol. Methods 170, 211–224.

Andre, N.D., Barbosa, D.S., Munhoz, E., Estevao, D., Cecchini, R., Watanabe, M.A., 2004. Measurement of cytotoxic activity in experimental cancer. J. Clin. Lab. Anal. 18, 27–30.

Baer, G., Wilson, T., Maitland, D., Matthews, D., 2006. Shape memory polymer neurovascular stents. J. Invest. Med. 54, S162.

Bakker, D., van Blitterswijk, C.A., Hesseling, S.C., Daems, W.T., Grote, J.J., 1990. Tissue/biomaterial interface characteristics of four elastomers. A transmission electron microscopical study. J. Biomed. Mater. Res. 24, 277–293.

Baumgartner, J.N., Yang, C.Z., Cooper, S.L., 1997. Physical property analysis and bacterial adhesion on a series of phosphonated polyurethanes. Biomaterials 18, 831–837.

Belanger, M.C., Marois, Y., 2001. Hemocompatibility, biocompatibility, inflammatory and in vivo studies of primary reference materials low-density polyethylene and polydimethylsiloxane: a review. J. Biomed. Mater. Res. 58, 467–477.

Binzen, E., Lendlein, A., Kelch, S., Rickert, D., Franke, R.P., 2004. Biomaterial-microvasculature interaction on polymers after implantation in mice. Clin. Hemorheol. Microcirc. 30, 283–288.

Bouza, E., Burillo, A., Munoz, P., 2002. Catheter-related infections: diagnosis and intravascular treatment. Clin. Microbiol. Infect. 8, 265–274.

Cabanlit, M., Maitland, D., Wilson, T., Simon, S., Wun, T., Gershwin, M.E., Van de Water, J., 2007. Polyurethane shape-memory polymers demonstrate functional biocompatibility in vitro. Macromol. Biosci. 7, 48–55. http://dx.doi.org/10.1002/mabi.200600177.

Cabrera, G.L., Rodriguez, D.M.G., 1999. Genotoxicity of soil from farmland irrigated with wastewater using three plant bioassays. Mutat. Res. Fund. Mol. Mech. 426, 211–214. http://dx.doi.org/10.1016/S0027-5107(99)00070-6.

Ceretti, E., Zani, C., Zerbini, I., Guzzella, L., Scaglia, M., Berna, V., Donato, F., Monarca, S., Feretti, D., 2010. Water Res. 44, 1462–1470.

Chan-Chan, L.H., Solis-Correa, R., Vargas-Coronado, R.F., Cervantes-Uc, J.M., Cauich-Rodriguez, J.V., Quintana, P., Bartolo-Perez, P., 2010. Degradation studies on segmented polyurethanes prepared with HMDI, PCL and different chain extenders. Acta Biomater. 6, 2035–2044. http://dx.doi.org/10.1016/j.actbio.2009.12.010.

Cheng, G., Zhang, Z., Chen, S., Bryers, J.D., Jiang, S., 2007. Inhibition of bacterial adhesion and biofilm formation on zwitterionic surfaces. Biomaterials 28, 4192–4199. http://dx.doi.org/10.1016/j.biomaterials.2007.05.041.

Cho, H.H., Han, D.W., Matsumura, K., Tsutsumi, S., Hyon, S.H., 2008. The behavior of vascular smooth muscle cells and platelets onto epigallocatechin gallate-releasing poly (l-lactide-co-epsilon-caprolactone) as stent-coating materials. Biomaterials 29, 884–893. http://dx.doi.org/10.1016/j.biomaterials.2007.10.052.

Dattani, R., 2007. Femoral osteolysis following total hip replacement. Postgrad. Med. J. 83, 312–316. http://dx.doi.org/10.1136/pgmj.2006.053215.

De Lima, R., Fraceto, L.F., 2014. Genetic studies on the effects of nanomaterials. Nanomed. Nanotoxicol, 1, 177–199.

De Lima, R., Feitosa, L., do Espirito Santo Pereira, A., de Moura, M.R., Ahmad Aouada, F., Henrique Capparelli Mattoso, L., Fernandes Fraceto, L., 2010. Evaluation of the genotoxicity of chitosan nanoparticles for use in food packaging films. J. Food Sci. 75 (6), N89–N96. http://dx.doi.org/10.1111/j.1750-3841.2010.01682.x.

De Nardo, L., Alberti, R., Cigada, A., Yahia, L., Tanzi, M.C., Fare, S., 2009. Shape memory polymer foams for cerebral aneurysm reparation: effects of plasma sterilization on physical properties and cytocompatibility. Acta Biomater. 5, 1508–1518. http://dx.doi.org/10.1016/j.actbio.2008.11.017.

Decker, T., Lohmann-Matthes, M.L., 1988. A quick and simple method for the quantitation of lactate dehydrogenase release in measurements of cellular cytotoxicity and tumor necrosis factor (TNF) activity. J. Immunol. Methods 115, 61–69.

Deka, H., Karak, N., Kalita, R.D., Buragohain, A.K., 2010. Biocompatible hyperbranched polyurethane/multi-walled carbon nanotube composites as shape memory materials. Carbon 48 (7), 2013–2022. http://dx.doi.org/10.1016/j.carbon.2010.02.009.

El Feninat, F., Laroche, G., Fiset, M., Mantovani, D., 2002. Shape memory materials for biomedical applications. Adv. Eng. Mater. 4, 91–104.

Fare, S., Valtulina, V., Petrini, P., Alessandrini, E., Pietrocola, G., Tanzi, M.C., Speziale, P., Visai, L., 2005. In vitro interaction of human fibroblasts and platelets with a shape-memory polyurethane. J. Biomed. Mater. Res. A 73, 1–11. http://dx.doi.org/10.1002/jbm.a.30193.

Fischell, T.A., 1996. Polymer coatings for stents. Can we judge a stent by its cover? Circulation 94, 1494–1495.

Fischman, D.L., Leon, M.B., Baim, D.S., Schatz, R.A., Savage, M.P., Penn, I., Detre, K., Veltri, L., Ricci, D., Nobuyoshi, M., et al., 1994. A randomized comparison of coronary-stent placement and balloon angioplasty in the treatment of coronary artery disease. Stent Restenosis Study Investigators. N. Engl. J. Med. 331, 496–501. http://dx.doi.org/10.1056/NEJM199408253310802.

Gottenbos, B., van der Mei, H.C., Busscher, H.J., 2000. Initial adhesion and surface growth of *Staphylococcus epidermidis* and *Pseudomonas aeruginosa* on biomedical polymers. J. Biomed. Mater. Res. 50, 208–214.

Hansen, M.B., Nielsen, S.E., Berg, K., 1989. Re-examination and further development of a precise and rapid dye method for measuring cell growth/cell kill. J. Immunol. Methods 119 (2), 203–210.

Hester Jr., T.R., Ford, N.F., Gale, P.J., Hammett, J.L., Raymond, R., Turnbull, D., Frankos, V.H., Cohen, M.B., 1997. Measurement of 2,4-toluenediamine in urine and serum samples from women with Meme or Replicon breast implants. Plast. Reconstr. Surg. 100 (5), 1291–1298.

Hirota, K., Murakami, K., Nemoto, K., Miyake, Y., 2005. Coating of a surface with 2-methacryloyloxyethyl phosphorylcholine (MPC) co-polymer significantly reduces retention of human pathogenic microorganisms. FEMS Microbiol. Lett. 248 (1), 37–45. http://dx.doi.org/10.1016/j.femsle.2005.05.019.

Irie, M., 1990. Photoresponsive polymers. Adv. Polym. Sci. 94, 27–67.

Jacobs, J.J., Roebuck, K.A., Archibeck, M., Hallab, N.J., Glant, T.T., 2001. Osteolysis: basic science. Clin. Orthop. Relat. Res. 393, 71–77.

Ji, W., Yang, F., Seyednejad, H., Chen, Z., Hennink, W.E., Anderson, J.M., van den Beucken, J.J., Jansen, J.A., 2012. Biocompatibility and degradation characteristics of PLGA-based electrospun nanofibrous scaffolds with nanoapatite incorporation. Biomaterials 33 (28), 6604–6614. http://dx.doi.org/10.1016/j.biomaterials.2012.06.018.

Khan, G.M., Zhu, J.B., 1999. Studies on drug release kinetics from ibuprofen-carbomer hydrophilic matrix tablets: influence of co-excipients on release rate of the drug. J. Control. Release 57 (2), 197–203.

Kim, B.K., Lee, S.Y., Xu, M., 1996. Polyurethanes having shape memory effects. Polymer 37, 5781–5793. http://dx.doi.org/10.1016/S0032-3861(96)00442-9.

Kingshott, P., Wei, J., Bagge-Ravn, D., Gadegaard, N., Gram, L., 2003. Covalent attachment of poly(ethylene glycol) to surfaces, critical for reducing bacterial adhesion. Langmuir 19 (17), 6912–6921. http://dx.doi.org/10.1021/La034032m.

Kuzma, L., Wysokinska, H., Rozalski, M., Krajewska, U., Kisiel, W., 2012. An unusual taxodione derivative from hairy roots of Salvia austriaca. Fitoterapia 83 (4), 770–773. http://dx.doi.org/10.1016/j.fitote.2012.03.006.

Ladd, J., Zhang, Z., Chen, S., Hower, J.C., Jiang, S., 2008. Zwitterionic polymers exhibiting high resistance to nonspecific protein adsorption from human serum and plasma. Biomacromolecules 9 (5), 1357–1361. http://dx.doi.org/10.1021/Bm701301s.

Lamba, N.M.K., Woodhouse, K.A., Cooper, S.L., Lelah, M.D., 1997. Polyurethanes in Medical Application. CRC Press, Boca Raton, FL, USA.

Lelah, M.D., Lambrecht, L.K., Young, B.R., Cooper, S.L., 1983. Physicochemical characterization and in vivo blood tolerability of cast and extruded Biomer. J. Biomed. Mater. Res. 17 (1), 1–22. http://dx.doi.org/10.1002/jbm.820170102.

Lendlein, A., Langer, R., 2002. Biodegradable, elastic shape-memory polymers for potential biomedical applications. Science 296 (5573), 1673–1676. http://dx.doi.org/10.1126/science.1066102.

Lendlein, A., Behl, M., Hiebl, B., Wischke, C., 2010. Shape-memory polymers as a technology platform for biomedical applications. Expert Rev. Med. Devices 7 (3), 357–379.

Lincoff, A.M., Furst, J.G., Ellis, S.G., Tuch, R.J., Topol, E.J., 1997. Sustained local delivery of dexamethasone by a novel intravascular eluting stent to prevent restenosis in the porcine coronary injury model. J. Am. Coll. Cardiol. 29 (4), 808–816.

Luppi, B., Cerchiara, T., Bigucci, F., Orienti, I., Zecchi, V., 2003. pH-sensitive polymeric physical-mixture for possible site-specific delivery of ibuprofen. Eur. J. Pharm. Biopharm. 55 (2), 199–202.

Metcalfe, A., Desfaits, A.C., Salazkin, I., Yahia, L., Sokolowski, W.M., Raymond, J., 2003. Cold hibernated elastic memory foams for endovascular interventions. Biomaterials 24, 491–497.

Metzger, M.F., Wilson, T.S., Schumann, D., Matthews, D.L., Maitland, D.J., 2002. Mechanical properties of mechanical actuator for treating ischemic stroke. Biomed. Microdevices 4 (2), 89–96. http://dx.doi.org/10.1023/A:1014674912979.

Miao, D.S., Scutt, A., 2002. Histochemical localization of alkaline phosphatase activity in decalcified bone and cartilage. J. Histochem. Cytochem. 50 (3), 333–340.

Miret, S., De Groene, E.M., Klaffke, W., 2006. Comparison of in vitro assays of cellular toxicity in the human hepatic cell line HepG2. J. Biomol. Screen. 11 (2), 184–193. http://dx.doi.org/10.1177/1087057105283787.

Monk, P.N., Scola, A.M., Madala, P., Fairlie, D.P., 2007. Function, structure and therapeutic potential of complement C5a receptors. Br. J. Pharmacol. 152 (4), 429–448. http://dx.doi.org/10.1038/sj.bjp.0707332.

Mosmann, T., 1983. Rapid colorimetric assay for cellular growth and survival: application to proliferation and cytotoxicity assays. J. Immunol. Methods 65 (1–2), 55–63.

Musial-Kulik, M., Kasperczyk, J., Smola, A., Dobrzynski, P., 2014. Double layer paclitaxel delivery systems based on bioresorbable terpolymer with shape memory properties. Int. J. Pharmaceut. 465 (1–2), 291–298. http://dx.doi.org/10.1016/j.ijpharm.2014.01.029.

Neuss, S., Blomenkamp, I., Stainforth, R., Boltersdorf, D., Jansen, M., Butz, N., Perez-Bouza, A., Knuchel, R., 2009. The use of a shape-memory poly(epsilon-caprolactone) dimethacrylate network as a tissue engineering scaffold. Biomaterials 30 (9), 1697–1705. http://dx.doi.org/10.1016/j.biomaterials.2008.12.027.

O'Grady, N.P., Alexander, M., Dellinger, E.P., Gerberding, J.L., Heard, S.O., Maki, D.G., Masur, H., McCormick, R.D., Mermel, L.A., Pearson, M.L., Raad, I.I., Randolph, A.,

Weinstein, R.A., 2002. Guidelines for the prevention of intravascular catheter-related infections. MMWR Recomm. Rep. 9, 1–29.

Ostuni, E., Chapman, R.G., Holmlin, R.E., Takayama, S., Whitesides, G.M., 2001. A survey of structure-property relationships of surfaces that resist the adsorption of protein. Langmuir 17 (18), 5605–5620. http://dx.doi.org/10.1021/La010384m.

Park, J.H., Cho, Y.W., Kwon, I.C., Jeong, S.Y., Bae, Y.H., 2002. Assessment of PEO/PTMO multiblock copolymer/segmented polyurethane blends as coating materials for urinary catheters: in vitro bacterial adhesion and encrustation behavior. Biomaterials 23 (19), 3991–4000.

Parween, S., Nahar, P., 2013. Image-based ELISA on an activated polypropylene microtest plate—a spectrophotometer-free low cost assay technique. Biosens. Bioelectron. 48, 287–292. http://dx.doi.org/10.1016/j.bios.2013.04.020.

Patel, J.D., Iwasaki, Y., Ishihara, K., Anderson, J.M., 2005. Phospholipid polymer surfaces reduce bacteria and leukocyte adhesion under dynamic flow conditions. J. Biomed. Mater. Res. A 73A (3), 359–366. http://dx.doi.org/10.1002/Jbm.A.30302.

Pedrazzani, R., Ceretti, E., Zerbini, I., Casale, R., Gozio, E., Bertanza, G., Gelatti, U., Donato, F., Feretti, D., 2012. Biodegradability, toxicity and mutagenicity of detergents: integrated experimental evaluations. Ecotoxicol. Environ. Saf. 84, 274–281.

Rainer, W.C., Redding, E.M., Hitov, J.J., Sloan, A.W., Stewart, W.D., 1964. Irradiated, cross-linked polyethylene copolymer. USA Patent No. US 3097150 A.

Ratner, B.D., Hoffman, A.S., Schoen, F., Lemons, J.E., 2004. Biomaterials Science: An Introduction to Materials in Medicine, second ed. Elsevier Academic Press, London, UK.

Roosjen, A., van der Mei, H.C., Busscher, H.J., Norde, W., 2004. Microbial adhesion to poly (ethylene oxide) brushes: influence of polymer chain length and temperature. Langmuir 20 (25), 10949–10955. http://dx.doi.org/10.1021/la048469l.

Sepai, O., Henschler, D., Czech, S., Eckert, P., Sabbioni, G., 1995. Exposure to toluenediamines from polyurethane-covered breast implants. Toxicol. Lett. 77 (1–3), 371–378.

Sieminski, A.L., Gooch, K.J., 2000. Biomaterial-microvasculature interactions. Biomaterials 21 (22), 2233–2241. http://dx.doi.org/10.1016/S0142-9612(00)00149-6.

Singhal, P., Small, W., Cosgriff-Hernandez, E., Maitland, D.J., Wilson, T.S., 2014. Low density biodegradable shape memory polyurethane foams for embolic biomedical applications. Acta Biomater. 10 (1), 67–76. http://dx.doi.org/10.1016/j.actbio.2013.09.027.

Small, W., Wilson, T.S., Benett, W.J., Loge, J.M., Maitland, D.J., 2005. Laser-activated shape memory polymer intravascular thrombectomy device. Opt. Express 13 (20), 8204–8213. http://dx.doi.org/10.1364/Opex.13.008204.

Small, W.T., Singhal, P., Wilson, T.S., Maitland, D.J., 2010. Biomedical applications of thermally activated shape memory polymers. J. Mater. Chem. 20 (18), 3356–3366. http://dx.doi.org/10.1039/B923717H.

Souza, P.M.S., Corroqué, N.A., Morales, A.R., Marin-Morales, M.A., Mei, L.H.I., 2013. PLA and organoclays nanocomposites: degradation process and evaluation of ecotoxicity using allium cepa as test organism. J. Polym. Environ 21, 1052–1063.

Tamai, H., Igaki, K., Kyo, E., Kosuga, K., Kawashima, A., Matsui, S., Komori, H., Tsuji, T., Motohara, S., Uehata, H., 2000. Initial and 6-month results of biodegradable poly-l-lactic acid coronary stents in humans. Circulation 102 (4), 399–404.

Tegoulia, V.A., Cooper, S.L., 2002. *Staphylococcus aureus* adhesion to self-assembled monolayers: effect of surface chemistry and fibrinogen presence. Colloid Surf. B 24 (3–4), 217–228. http://dx.doi.org/Pii S0927-7765(01)00240-5.

Tobushi, H., Hara, H., Yamada, E., Hayashi, S., 1996. Properties in a thin film of shape memory polymer of polyurethane series. Smart Mater. Struct. 5, 483–491.

Vallet-Regi, M., Granado, S., Arcos, D., Gordo, M., Cabanas, M.V., Ragel, C.V., Salinas, A.J., Doadrio, A.L., San Roman, J., 1998. Preparation, characterization, and in vitro release of ibuprofen from Al2O3/PLA/PMMA composites. J. Biomed. Mater. Res. 39 (3), 423–428.

van Blitterswijk, C.A., Bakker, D., Hesseling, S.C., Koerten, H.K., 1991. Reactions of cells at implant surfaces. Biomaterials 12 (2), 187–193.

vanderGiessen, W.J., Lincoff, A.M., Schwartz, R.S., vanBeusekom, H.M.M., Serruys, P.W., Holmes, D.R., Ellis, S.G., Topol, E.J., 1996. Marked inflammatory sequelae to implantation of biodegradable and nonbiodegradable polymers in porcine coronary arteries. Circulation 94 (7), 1690–1697.

Ventura-Sobrevilla, J., Boone-Villa, V.D., Aguilar, C.N., Roman-Ramos, R., Vega-Avila, E., Campos-Sepulveda, E., Alarcon-Aguilar, F., 2011. Effect of varying dose and administration of streptozotocin on blood sugar in male CD1 mice. Proc. West. Pharmacol. Soc. 54, 5–9.

Vorotnikova, E., Rosenthal, R.A., Tries, M., Doctrow, S.R., Braunhut, S.J., 2010. Novel synthetic SOD/catalase mimetics can mitigate capillary endothelial cell apoptosis caused by ionizing radiation. Radiat. Res. 173, 748–759.

Wache, H.M., Tartakowska, D.J., Hentrich, A., Wagner, M.H., 2003. Development of a polymer stent with shape memory effect as a drug delivery system. J. Mater. Sci. Mater. Med. 14 (2), 109–112. http://dx.doi.org/10.1023/A:1022007510352.

Wei, Z.G., Sandstrom, R., Miyazaki, S., 1998. Shape-memory materials and hybrid composites for smart systems—Part I Shape-memory materials. J. Mater. Sci. 33 (15), 3743–3762. http://dx.doi.org/10.1023/A:1004692329247.

Williams, D., 2003. Revisiting the definition of biocompatibility. Med. Device Technol. 14 (8), 10–13.

Williams, D.F., 2008. On the mechanisms of biocompatibility. Biomaterials 29 (20), 2941–2953. http://dx.doi.org/10.1016/j.biomaterials.2008.04.023.

Woodruff, M.A., Hutmacher, D.W., 2010. The return of a forgotten polymer-polycaprolactone in the 21st century. Prog. Polym. Sci. 35 (10), 1217–1256. http://dx.doi.org/10.1016/j.progpolymsci.2010.04.002.

Woodward, S.C., Brewer, P.S., Moatamed, F., Schindler, A., Pitt, C.G., 1985. The intracellular degradation of poly(epsilon-caprolactone). J. Biomed. Mater. Res. 19 (4), 437–444. http://dx.doi.org/10.1002/jbm.820190408.

Yakacki, C.M., Shandas, R., Lanning, C., Rech, B., Eckstein, A., Gall, K., 2007. Unconstrained recovery characterization of shape-memory polymer networks for cardiovascular applications. Biomaterials 28 (14), 2255–2263. http://dx.doi.org/10.1016/j.biomaterials.2007.01.030.

Yakacki, C.M., Shandas, R., Safranski, D., Ortega, A.M., Sassaman, K., Gall, K., 2008. Strong, tailored, biocompatible shape-memory polymer networks. Adv. Funct. Mater. 18 (16), 2428–2435. http://dx.doi.org/10.1002/adfm.200701049.

Yamawaki, T., Shimokawa, H., Kozai, T., Miyata, K., Higo, T., Tanaka, E., Egashira, K., Shiraishi, T., Tamai, H., Igaki, K., Takeshita, A., 1998. Intramural delivery of a specific tyrosine kinase inhibitor with biodegradable stent suppresses the restenotic changes of the coronary artery in pigs in vivo. J. Am. Coll. Cardiol. 32 (3), 780–786.

Zhou, H.Y., Zhang, Y.P., Zhang, W.F., Chen, X.G., 2011. Biocompatibility and characteristics of injectable chitosan-based thermosensitive hydrogel for drug delivery. Carbohyd. Polym. 83 (4), 1643–1651. http://dx.doi.org/10.1016/j.carbpol.2010.10.022.

Zhou, X.F., Zhang, T.Z., Guo, D.W., Gu, N., 2014. A facile preparation of poly(ethylene oxide)-modified medical polyurethane to improve hemocompatibility. Colloid Surf. A 441, 34–42. http://dx.doi.org/10.1016/j.colsurfa.2013.08.070.

Zilla, P., Wolf, M., Rafiee, N., Moodley, L., Bezuidenhout, D., Black, M., Human, P., Franz, T., 2009. Utilization of shape memory in external vein-graft meshes allows extreme diameter constriction for suppressing intimal hyperplasia: a non-human primate study. J. Vasc. Surg. 49, 1532–1542. http://dx.doi.org/10.1016/j.jvs.2009.01.068.

Zurita, R., Puiggali, J., Rodriguez-Galan, A., 2006. Loading and release of ibuprofen in multi- and monofilament surgical sutures. Macromol. Biosci. 6, 767–775. http://dx.doi.org/10.1002/mabi.200600084.

Part Two

Technologies and materials for biomedical shape-memory polymers

Chemo-responsive shape-memory polymers for biomedical applications

6

H. Lu[1], *W.M. Huang*[2]
[1]Harbin Institute of Technology, Harbin, China; [2]Nanyang Technological University, Singapore

6.1 Introduction

Shape-memory materials (SMMs) are fascinating, with promising potential in a range of applications as stimulus-responsive materials (SRMs), which can change their shape in a predefined manner between/among shapes with the presence of the right stimulus (Behl and Lendlein, 2007). Among them, shape memory polymers (SMPs) have recently gained widespread attention all over the world. They are lightweight, capable of high-magnitude shape recovery, and easy to manufacture and tune for tailored properties to precisely meet the need(s) of a particular application (Lendlein and Kelch, 2002). As pointed out by Prof. Irie (1998), essentially all SMPs fall into three categories according to the nature of the stimulus they respond to; namely, thermo-responsive SMP, chemo-responsive SMP, and photo-responsive SMP (Sun et al., 2012). It should be pointed out that almost by default, thermo-responsive SMP is traditionally meant only for heating-induced shape recovery, even by means of applying many unconventional heating techniques, such as inductive heating, joule heating, light heating (within the whole light wavelength range, from ultraviolent to infrared), and ultrasonic/acoustic heating etc., which seemingly help to expand the number of SMP categories (Mather et al., 2009; Ratna and Karger-Kocsis, 2008; Lendlein and Langer, 2002; Dietsch and Tong, 2007). In order to achieve true "light-induced" shape recovery (i.e., without any heat involved), polymers should have a special chemical structure that reacts to light by means of altering the molecular structure (Lendlein et al., 2005; Jiang et al., 2006). A recently developed polymer that is able to disassemble by means of near infrared irradiation may provide a supplementary approach to traditional triggering methods (Fomina et al., 2011). So far, we can say that the photo-responsive shape-memory effect (SME) is not a commonly observed feature but limited to certain special polymers that need to be purposely designed/synthesized in order to have such a function.

As a matter of fact, shape-memory materials fall into the category of SRMs, which have one or more properties that can be significantly changed in a controllable fashion upon applying the right external stimuli, such as heat (thermo-responsive), electricity (electro-active), light (photo-responsive), and chemical (chemo-responsive), etc. (Sun

Shape Memory Polymers for Biomedical Applications. http://dx.doi.org/10.1016/B978-0-85709-698-2.00006-4

et al., 2012) There are a number of types of SRMs: some are already well known and/or have been investigated extensively, such as piezoelectric materials, magnetostrictive materials, electro-/magneto-rheostatic materials, pH-sensitive materials, chromic materials, photomechanical materials, self-healing materials, and dielectric elastomers. In Table 6.1, the classification of SRMs is presented based on their major responsive behaviors. Each individual type of SRM has a different property that can be significantly altered. This property determines the kind of application a SRM can be utilized for. Some daily/engineering applications, from aerospace engineering to biomedicine engineering, have already incorporated a range of different SRMs (Behl et al., 2010). We have seen that the number of applications of SRMs is exponentially growing due to their powerful stimulus-responsive feature.

SMMs are featured by their SME, in which the temporary shape can be virtually held forever unless the right stimulus is applied to trigger the shape recovery. In addition to motion generation (for actuation), SMMs are able to alter other properties, such as stiffness, natural frequency, damping, and other thermo-mechanical characteristics, in a pre-determined manner in response to the applied stimulus. To date, the SME has been observed in a variety of alloys, ceramics, polymers, and gels, etc. (Huang et al., 2011). Both the fundamentals and properties for engineering applications of SMMs have been investigated extensively and have consequently been in implementation in true engineering applications. Some SMMs can be easily fabricated into thin films, fibers/wires, and even foams and can thus be incorporated with other materials to become a composite and/or utilized at micro/nano scale applications.

As one of the most popular SMMs, SMPs are attracting great research interest at present, and we have seen good progress in the development of SMPs for engineering applications, including biomedical engineering (Rousseau, 2008). SMPs also have comparable SMEs to traditional shape-memory alloys (SMAs). However, they promise a greater impact in a far greater range of applications, because SMPs take the advantages of many existing polymer processing techniques, e.g., extrusion and molding, which make SMP processing much less expensive when compared with SMAs. Other major advantages of SMPs are low density, ease in producing a high-quality complicated shape, high recoverable strain, ease in tailoring thermo-mechanical properties, possibility of always being transparent, wide shape-recovery temperature range, functionally gradient properties, multiple stimulation methods, high potential for recycle and reuse at a low cost, and multiple-shape-recovery ability, etc. Furthermore, excellent chemical stability, biocompatibility, and even biodegradability (in which the degradation rate may be adjusted if required) render SMPs as the right candidate for many biomedical applications (Leng et al., 2009).

The great potential of SMPs in biomedical applications has become well recognized only in the last few years, as evidenced by a number of SMP biomedical devices, especially those based on polyurethane SMPs, which are biocompatible, nontoxic, and nonmutagenic (Small et al., 2010); furthermore, their thermo-mechanical properties can be tailored.

In this chapter, Sections 6.2 and 6.3 discuss the fundamentals and theories behind the chemo-responsive SME in SMPs. Typical biomedical applications of the chemo-responsive SMPs are presented in Section 6.4. Section 6.5 presents conclusions.

Table 6.1 Classification of SRMs

Response stimulus	Thermal	Optical	Electrical	Magnetic	Mechanical	Chemical
Thermal		Thermo-chromic, Thermo-luminescent	Thermo-electric, Super-conductor	Curie point	Shape-memory	
Optical	Photothermic		Photo conductive	Opto-magnetic	Opto-mechanical, Photoacoustic	Photo-chemical, Photo-catalyst
Electrical	Peltier	Electro-chromic, Electro-optic,		Magneto-electronics	Piezo-electric, Electro-rheological	Electro-chemical, Electrolysis
Magnetic	Magneto-thermal	Magneto-optic, Piezo-chromic	Magneto-electronics		Magnetostrictive, Magneto-rheological	Magneto-chemical
Mechanical		Rheo-chromic		Magneto-strictive		
Chemical	Endo-thermic	Litmus		Magneto-chemical	Chemo-mechanical	Catalysis

6.2 Thermodynamic mechanism

6.2.1 Polymer solution and solubility parameter

The thermal properties of a polymer solution are different from those of an ideal solution in two major aspects. The first is that the interaction among polymer macromolecules is different from that between polymer macromolecule and solvent molecule, resulting in the enthalpy of the polymer solution $\Delta H_m \neq 0$. The second is the polymer macromolecules, which are flexible and composed of repeated molecules that contribute to the entropy of the polymer solution (ΔS_m). When a polymer is dissolved within a solvent, the entropy of the polymer/solvent mixture may be expressed as (Flory, 1942),

$$\Delta S_m = -R(n_1 \ln \phi_1 + n_2 \ln \phi_2), \tag{6.1}$$

where n_1 and n_2 are the molar numbers of the solvent and polymer, respectively. Hereinafter, subscripts 1 and 2 represent solvent and polymer, respectively. From Equation (6.1), we can see that ΔS_m is due to the change in entropy in the polymer/solvent system before and after mixing with the solvent.

According to the statistics, the entropy S of a polymer has a relationship with the state constant Ω as follows (Flory, 1942),

$$S = k \ln \Omega, \tag{6.2}$$

where k is the Boltzmann's constant that equals the gas constant R over the Avogadro constant $\widetilde{N}$, i.e., $k = R/\widetilde{N}$.

As for the interaction between a solvent and a polymer, if both the temperature and air pressure are kept constant, some essential factors in the change of the Gibbs free energy must be satisfied during mixing. According to the Hildebrand equation, the change in enthalpy may be written as (Flory, 1942),

$$\Delta H_m = V\phi_1\phi_2 \left[\left(\Delta E_1/_{V_1}\right)^{1/2} + \left(\Delta E_2/_{V_2}\right)^{1/2} \right]^2, \tag{6.3}$$

where ϕ_1 and ϕ_2 represent the volume fractions of solvent and polymer, respectively. ΔE is the activation energy of chain mobility, V is the total volume of mixture, and $\Delta E/V$ is defined as the cohesive energy density. According to Equation (6.3), it is obvious that the difference in cohesive energy density results in the change in enthalpy. If δ^2, where δ is the solubility parameter, is defined as the cohesive energy density, the Hildebrand equation may be expressed as (Flory, 1942),

$$\Delta H_M = V\phi_1\phi_2[\delta_1 - \delta_2]^2. \tag{6.4}$$

If the polymer is a polar polymer, Equation (6.4) should be revised as,

$$\Delta H_M = V\phi_1\phi_2\left[(\omega_1-\omega_2)^2+(\Omega_1-\Omega_2)^2\right], \tag{6.5}$$

where ω represents the solubility parameter of the polarity part, Ω stands for the solubility parameter of the non-polarity part.

Before discussing the effect of solubility parameter on the shape recovery behavior, the relaxation theory and Eyring equation should be introduced (Lu et al., 2009). As we know, the shape-recovery behavior essentially follows the relaxation theory, and the relationship between the recovery time and activation may be estimated by Eyring equation as (Rubinstein and Colby, 2003),

$$\tau=\tau_0\exp(\Delta E/RT), \tag{6.6}$$

where τ is the relaxation time (defined as the shape recovery time here), T is temperature, and τ_0 is a constant. According to Equation (6.6), relaxation time may be shortened by either decreasing the activation energy or increasing temperature, or combining both of them. In the case of chemo-responsive SME, it is the first that plays the major role.

In order to work out the relationship between the solubility parameter and relaxation time, we assume that the temperature is maintained constant. As revealed by Equations (6.5) and (6.6), the solubility parameter is related to the activation energy which affects the relaxation time. As such, one has

$$\tau=\tau_0\exp\left(\frac{\Delta E-\Delta H}{RT}\right). \tag{6.7}$$

Combining Equations (6.5) and (6.7) together, the relationship between the recovery time and the solubility is obtained as follows,

$$\tau=A\exp\left(-\frac{V\phi_1\phi_2\left[(\omega_1-\omega_2)^2+(\Omega_1-\Omega_2)^2\right]}{RT}\right), \tag{6.8}$$

where $A=\tau_0\exp\left(\frac{\Delta E}{RT}\right)$ is a constant. Hence, the recovery time is only determined by the solubility parameter. $\left[(\omega_1-\omega_2)^2+(\Omega_1-\Omega_2)^2\right]$ is a constant, which can be determined experimentally. Consequently, a linear relationship between $\ln\tau$ and $\phi_1\phi_2$ can be obtained.

6.2.2 Plasticizing effect of solvent on a polymer

Previously, Dr. Lv et al. (2008) have experimentally investigated the chemo-responsive SME in a styrene-based SMP by means of immersing into dimethylformamide (DMF). This is a kind of extension of the water-induced SME in polyurethane SMPs (Yang et al., 2005). The plasticizing effect has been identified as the underlying mechanism behind the chemo-responsive SME (Leng et al., 2008), which can be briefly summarized as follows.

According to the solution theory of polymer physics, the glass transition temperature (T_g) of a polymer decreases upon its immersion into a particular liquid, such as an organic solvent or water. Subsequently, the polymer becomes soft and flexible without involving any temperature fluctuation. A close look reveals that when the polymer is immersed into the particular solvent, the solvent molecule first has a plasticizing effect on the polymer, followed by chemical or physical interaction, resulting in a lower transition temperature. It is well known that the plasticizing effect plays a more important role in the transition temperature than the chemical or physical interaction. Solution theory, free volume theory, and Fujita's diffusion theory can be applied to qualitatively separate the effects of free water molecules and bound water molecules on polyurethane SMPs. The maximum amount of free water is about 2.5% in polyurethane SMPs. However, experimental results have revealed that the total amount of absorbed water is about 3%. The difference may be explained by Fick's law of diffusion, i.e., there are two diffusion processes: one is liquid diffusion process, and the other is gaseous diffusion process. Thus, the role of bound water can be determined by the diffusion law.

To further identify the effect of a plasticizing interaction of water or other solvents on the actuation of an SMP, investigation of the interaction should be carried out. It is clear that the first interaction with the solvent molecules is to reduce the bonding strength among macromolecules. The second is to occupy the free volume within the polymer network and then block the interactive bonding among polymer macromolecules. These chemical and/or physical interactions between solvent molecules and polymer macromolecule reduce the cohesive energy density of polymer chains. It should be pointed out that the influence of the plasticizing effect on the T_g is more significant than that on the melting transition temperature (T_m) in polymers. To quantitatively separate the plasticizing effect on the T_g, the free volume theory may be applied (van der Sman and Meinders, 2011). There are several modes to construct the relationship among the transition temperature, volume concentrations of free volume, and solvent molecules. Based on these relationships, we can predict the shape-recovery behavior of an SMP according to the relaxation theory.

6.3 Working mechanisms

According to the traditional definition, after being severely and quasi-plastically distorted, SMPs, like other SMMs, are able to recover their original shape at the presence of the right stimulus, such as heat (thermo-responsive), light (photo-responsive), and chemical (including water, chemo-responsive) (Sun et al., 2012). This phenomenon is defined as the SME, which provides an alternative approach for many designs that are difficult to achieve using conventional materials/technologies.

In an SMP, there are always two segments (domains): one is elastic (elastic component), while the other is able to significantly alter its stiffness, depending on whether the right stimulus is presented (transition component). This dual-component system is essential to enable the SME in a polymer (Huang et al., 2010).

In general, the programming procedure to set up the temporary shape of an SMP for the chemo-responsive SME is essentially the same as that for the thermo-responsive SME. However, instead of heating to above the transition temperature to activate shape recovery, in a more general sense, the approach to trigger the chemo-responsive SME is to soften/dissolve the transition component and thus lower the transition temperature by means of softening, swelling, or dissolving.

6.3.1 Softening-induced SME

A few SMPs that respond to water have been developed (e.g., Mendez et al., 2011; Yang et al., 2004; Jung et al., 2006; Willett, 2008; Chen et al., 2009; Du and Zhang, 2010). Recently, some interactive solvents (e.g., N,N-dimethylformamide, toluene, methanol, etc.) have been utilized for the chemo-responsive SME (Kumpfer and Rowan, 2011), in which the shape recovery is driven by the diffusion of the solvent molecules into the polymer network. The absorbed solvent molecules work as plasticizer to depress the interaction force among macromolecules, thus increasing the flexibility of macromolecule chains, inductively depressing the cohesive energy, and lowering the transition temperature of the polymer network (Flory, 1942). As is well known, when a polymer is brought into contact with an interactive solvent, either a chemically plasticizing or physical swelling effect will occur between the polymer network and the imbibed solvent molecules originated from the polymer physics (Lu et al., 2012). During this process, a remarkable change in the transition temperature and other properties in the SMP is expected. The depression in the transition temperature and capability of storing energy results in the shape recovery.

Taking polyurethane SMP as an example, two pieces of polyurethane SMP wires (indicated as original) are immersed into 22 °C water and methanol, respectively, as shown in Figure 6.1. The wire (MM3520) immersed in water has a nominal T_g of 35 °C, while the one (MM5520) immersed in methanol has a nominal T_g of 55 °C, which is 20 °C higher. Although the T_g of the one immersed in water (Figure 6.1a) is lower than the other piece, it takes about 40 min to straighten; the other, immersed in room temperature methanol (Figure 6.1b), reacts much faster (its shape recovery is complete within about 30 s only) (Huang et al., 2012).

According to previous studies (Yang et al., 2006; Huang et al., 2010), upon immersion into room temperature water (about 22 °C), the T_gs of both polyurethanes can be gradually reduced by up to 30 °C due to the plasticizing effect of the absorbed (bound) water on the hydrogen bonding (evidenced by the shift of C=O stretching and N-H stretching measured by Fourier transform infrared (FTIR) spectroscopy, as revealed in Figure 6.2 [for MM3520]). Figure 6.2 also reveals a similar shift in C=O stretching and N-H stretching in polyurethane (MM5520) after being immersed in ethanol and methanol. Note that upon immersion into methanol, this type of polyurethane, which is thermo-plastic, quickly dissolves.

The influence of water absorption on T_g can be quantitatively determined (Huang et al., 2005). A typical example of MM3520 is revealed in Figure 6.3. It is obvious that with a longer immersion time in water, T_g reduces further (as evidenced by the shift in C=O stretching and N-H stretching in Figure 6.2). Upon gradually heating, the SMP

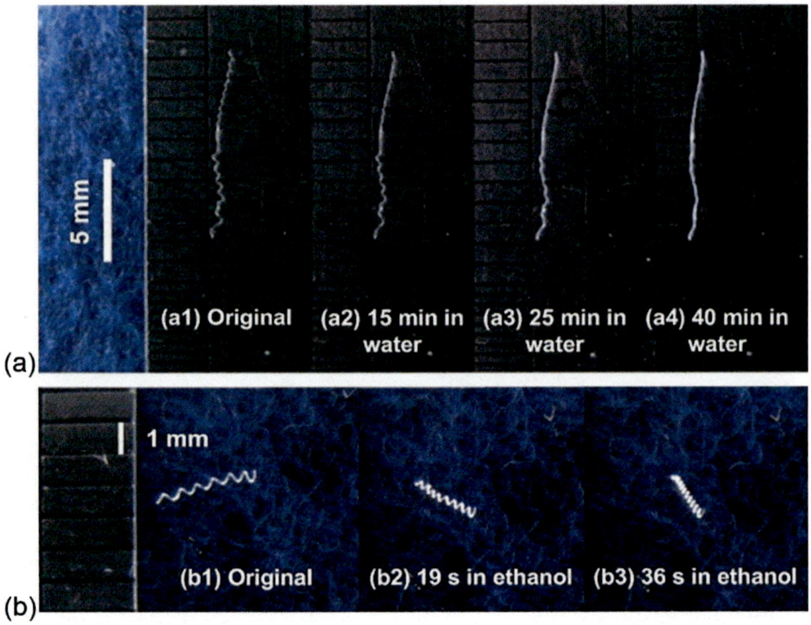

Figure 6.1 Chemo-responsive SME in polyurethane SMP; (a) in 22 °C water; (b) in 22 °C ethanol.
Reproduced from Huang et al. (2012) with permission.

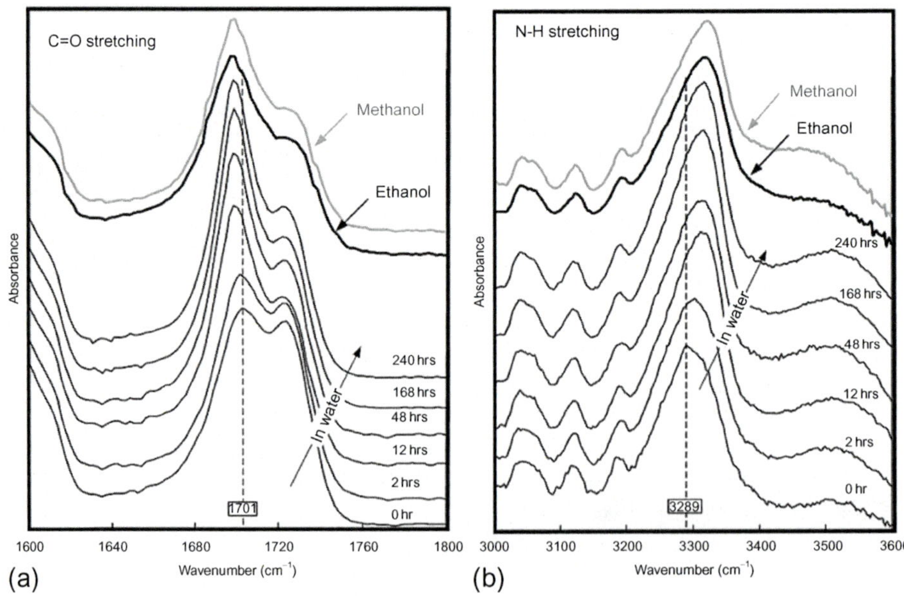

Figure 6.2 Shift in C=O stretching (a) and N-H stretching (b) upon immersing into room temperature water (MM3520) and ethanol/methanol (MM5520).
Reproduced from Huang et al. (2012) with permission.

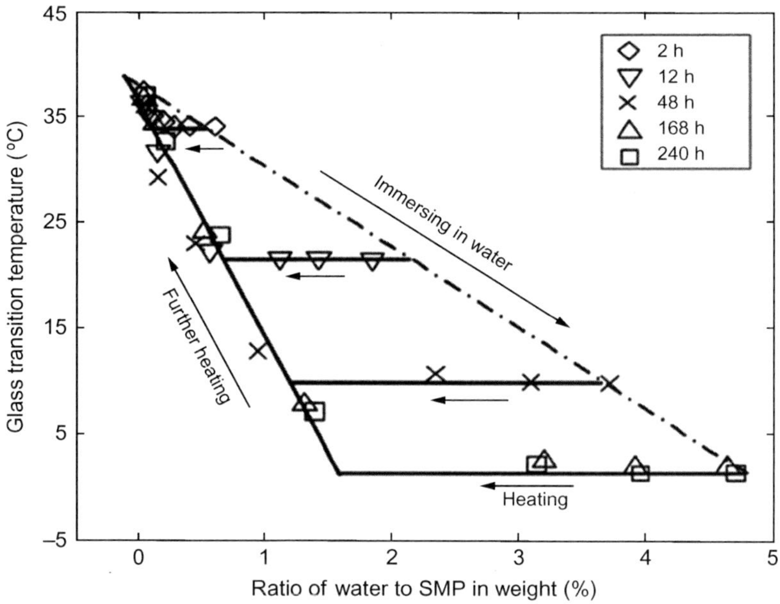

Figure 6.3 T_g vs. ratio of water to SMP in weight %.
Reproduced from Yang et al. (2006) with permission.

becomes lighter; however, there is not much change in T_g at all until it is heated above a certain temperature. From then on, with a further increase in temperature, the weight of SMP drops while T_g increases continuously. The weight ratios of the free water and bound water against immersion time are plotted in Figure 6.4. Although free water does not affect T_g, and can be removed upon heating to below 120 °C, bound water has strong influence on T_g and can only be removed upon heating to over 120 °C. The latter indicates that after heating to fully remove the absorbed water, the SMP can return to its original state/condition (as evidenced by a series of experimental results reported in Yang et al. (2006)).

The influence of water on T_g can be utilized for water-activated SME, for programmed shape recovery by means of introducing a gradient T_g into the SMP, or for reducing T_g before applying a lower heating temperature for activation (i.e., chemically tuning T_g, without altering the chemical composition).

As shown in Figure 6.5, a piece of polyurethane SMP (MM5520) is straightened first. Because its nominal T_g is 55 °C, it is relatively strong and can be easily inserted into a cluster of toad eggs at room temperature (between 20 °C and 22 °C). After 7 days, its T_g is expected to drop by as much as 30 °C, which is still above the ambient temperature, so that shape recovery is not significant. By slightly heating to 37.5 °C, remarkable shape recovery is observed. This experiment demonstrates that by selecting the right chemical, one may tailor the transition temperature of a polymer. This approach may be applied as an alternative to the chemical composition tuning, which is a rather standard practice at present, to modify the transition temperatures.

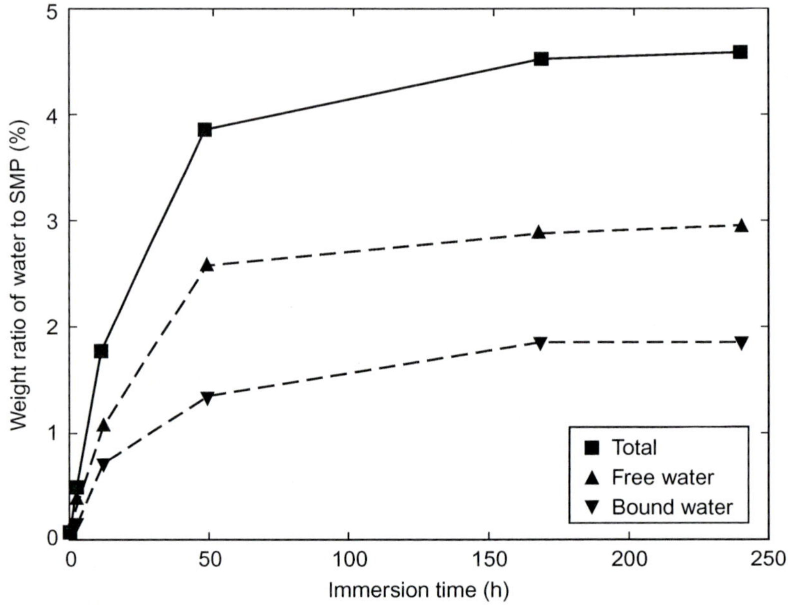

Figure 6.4 Ratio of water to SMP in weight percentage vs. immersion time.
Reproduced from Yang et al. (2006) with permission.

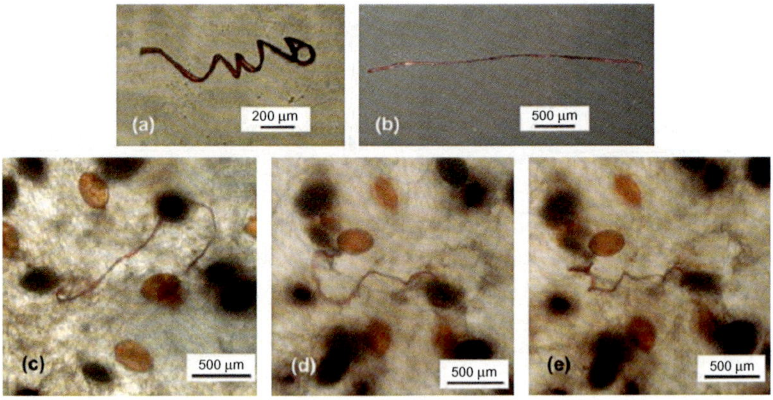

Figure 6.5 (a) Original shape; (b) after straightening; (c) after inserting into a cluster of toad eggs; (d) after 7 days in room temperature water; (e) after heating to 37.5 °C.
Reproduced from Huang et al. (2012) with permission.

Recently, a covalently cross-linked metallo-supramolecular polymer has been demonstrated to achieve methanol-induced SME (Chaunier and Lourdin, 2009). This result is consistent with the plasticizing effect of methanol on the metal-ligand hard phase of polymer. In addition, this polymer is able to respond to other chemicals, such as acetone and triethylamine. Moisture-responsive SME is also observed in hydrogel (without apparent swelling), potato starch (Chaunier and Lourdin, 2009), and translucent keratin (such as human nail or silk), and so on.

6.3.2 Swelling-induced SME

Utilizing the thermo-responsive SME, various types of polystyrene (PS) have been used in a range of applications, from traditional packaging to surface patterning and micro-machining of microchannels (Hidber et al., 1996; Liu et al., 2007, 2008, 2010; Zhao et al., 1998, 2011a; Grimes et al., 2008). Previously, the chemo-responsive SME in PS has been achieved by means of immersion into dimethylformamide (DMF) through chemical conjunct interaction (Lv et al., 2008). When a polymer is brought into contact with a solvent, the polymer network may imbibe solvent molecules progressively; it then swells, resulting in aggregation of solvent molecules, known as gel (Miyazaki et al., 2009; Leng and Du, 2010). A gel is able to undergo a large deformation due to long-range migration of the solvent molecules, resulting in a significant change in volume, until reaching an equilibrium state (for a given environment). Simultaneously, a significant change in the transition temperature of the polymer is expected. The change in the transition temperature affects the relative motion in the transition segment, which is the primary mechanism for the SME in SMPs.

Toluene has been used to trigger shape recovery in a piece of PS by means of physical swelling effect. As shown in Figure 6.6(a), a piece of straight SMP strip (original shape) is bent into an "N"-like shape at 85 °C (T_g+20 °C) and then cooled back to 45 °C (T_g – 20 °C). Only some slight shape recovery is observed after it is kept in the air for more than 6 hours. After immersion in toluene at 45 °C for 40 min, the sample starts to return to its original shape. After another 90 min, the sample becomes straight again. Swelling is revealed in Figure 6.6(b), which is apparent, but not very significant (Lu et al., 2012).

Dynamic mechanical analysis (DMA) and FTIR tests have been conducted to characterize the thermo-mechanical properties and chemical structures of the SMP after its immersion for a period of time. DMA results reveal a lower T_g after immersion. A decrease from 55.77 °C to 35.82 °C is observed after 60 min of immersion. Meanwhile, the modulus gradually depresses. The result of FTIR spectroscopy reveals no significant chemical interaction between the polymer and solvent, because the characteristic peaks of O-H and C=O bonds virtually do not shift (Lu et al., 2009). We may conclude that there is not much remarkable chemical and polar interaction between the polymer and solvent molecules. Note that the solvent molecules contain no polar group that can interact with the characteristic polar group in the SMP molecules. It is clear that shape recovery in this styrene-based SMP upon immersion into the toluene solvent is the result of the effect of physical swelling effect (Lu et al., 2010a).

Apart from experimental verification, the rubber elastic theory of Young's modulus has been used to theoretically investigate the effect of physical swelling on the actuation of SMP. According to the rubber elastic theory, the force per unit area and the concentration of chain segment in the polymer network are reduced when

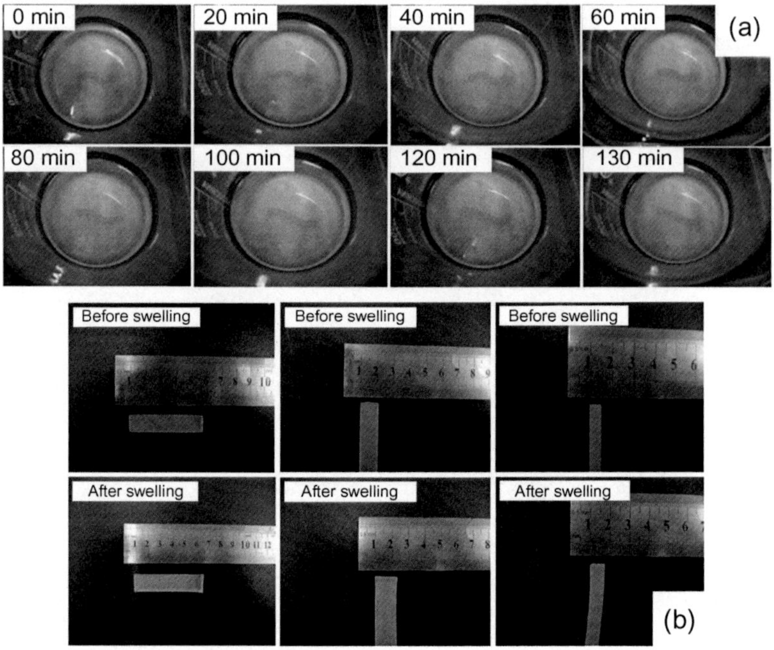

Figure 6.6 (a) Shape recovery in a styrene-based SMP (induced by swelling); (b) change in dimensions before and after swelling.
Reproduced from Lu et al. (2012) with permission.

the polymer network swells in an interactive solvent. These changes result in the reduction in elastic modulus. On the other hand, the volume of polymer increases. The elastic modulus of the polymer network decreases gradually with an increase in the expansion (i.e., stretch) in a bulky piece of SMP. In the case of a cubic-shaped SMP, the effect of stretch on the decrease in Young's modulus is revealed in Figure 6.7 (Lu et al., 2010a).

On the other hand, free-energy function is applicable to study swelling-induced deformation and shape recovery in SMPs. When a piece of polymer (which is a non-ionic solvent-swollen polymer) is subject to a solvent and then stressed, the free energy in the polymer/solvent system (W) is a function of the stretching free energy (W_s), mixing free energy (W_m), and polarizing free energy (W_c), as shown by (Lu et al., 2010b):

$$W = W_s + W_m + W_c. \tag{6.9}$$

As a result of the physical swelling effect due to the interaction between the polymer and solvent, the polarizing potential may be assumed to be zero. Subsequently, Equation (6.9) may be reduced to:

$$W = W_s + W_m. \tag{6.10}$$

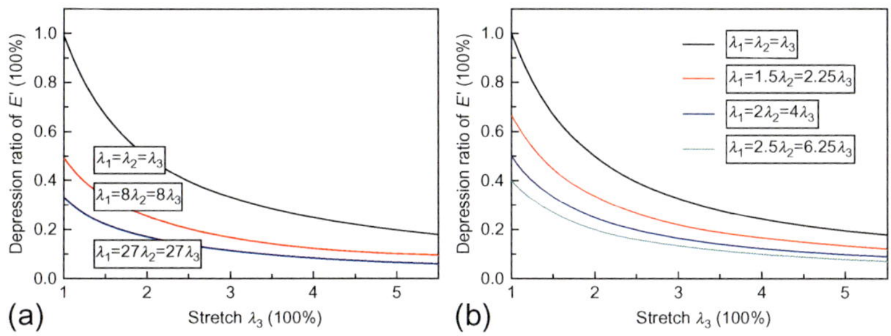

Figure 6.7 (a) Inhomogeneous deformation in two stretches $\lambda_2 = \lambda_3$ in a cubic SMP and (b) inhomogeneous deformation in a cubic SMP with stretches $\lambda_1 = \lambda_2 = \lambda_3$ induced by physical swelling effect in solvent.
Reproduced from Lu et al. (2010a) with permission.

The stretching free energy and mixing free energy of polymers may be taken as (Flory, 1953),

$$W = \frac{1}{2}NkT\left(\lambda_1{}^2 + \lambda_2{}^2 + \lambda_3{}^2 - 3 - 2\log\lambda_1\lambda_2\lambda_3\right) - \frac{kT}{v}\left[vC\log\left(1 + \frac{1}{vC}\right) + \frac{\chi}{(1+vC)}\right], \tag{6.11}$$

where N is the number of chains in the polymer divided by the volume of the polymer block in the referenced state. k is the Boltzmann's constant. T is the temperature in the unit of energy. λ_1, λ_2, and λ_3 are the generalized coordinates of a cubic block in three directions. v is the volume of solvent. C is the number of solvent molecules in the polymeric network. χ is the Flory-Huggins interaction parameter.

λ, which is denoted to be free-swelling stretch, is related to the chemical potential μ. The differential potential change of polymer is equal to the negative value of solvent. Assume that there are two states: (a) and (b). In state (a), the molar numbers of polymer and solvent are x_p^a and x_s^a, respectively, in the system (where $x_p^a + x_s^a = 1$). In state (b), the molar numbers of polymer and solvent are x_p^b and x_s^b, respectively, in the system (where $x_p^b + x_s^b = 1$). From state (a) to (b), the change in the mole of solvent is $x_s^b - x_s^a = dC$, while the change in the mole of polymer is $x_p^b - x_p^a = \left(1 - x_s^b\right) - \left(1 - x_s^a\right) = -\left(x_s^b - x_s^a\right) = -dC$.

Considering a cubic piece of solvent-swollen polymer subjected to stretching in three directions in the same amount, i.e., $\lambda_1 = \lambda_2 = \lambda_3 = \lambda$, $1 + vC$ may be calculated by substituting λ into Equation (6.11), namely $1 + vC = \lambda^3$.

Hence,

$$W = \frac{3}{2}NkT\left(\lambda^2 - 1 - 2\log\lambda\right) - \frac{kT}{v}\left[\left(\lambda^3 - 1\right)\log\left(\frac{\lambda^3}{\lambda^3 - 1}\right) + \frac{\chi}{\lambda^3}\right]. \tag{6.12}$$

Here, the change in chemical potential of polymer μ_2 may be expressed as

$$\mu_p = \frac{\partial W}{\partial(-C)} = -\left(\frac{\partial W_s}{\partial C} + \frac{\partial W_m}{\partial C}\right) \tag{6.13}$$

and

$$\begin{aligned}\mu_p &= \frac{\partial W}{\partial(-C)} = -\left(\frac{\partial W_s}{\partial C} + \frac{\partial W_m}{\partial C}\right)\\ &= -NkTv\left(\frac{1}{\lambda} - \frac{1}{\lambda^3}\right) - kT\left[\log\frac{\lambda^3 - 1}{\lambda^3} + \frac{1}{\lambda^3} + \frac{\chi}{\lambda^6}\right].\end{aligned} \tag{6.14}$$

Equation (6.14) may be rewritten as

$$\frac{\mu_p}{kT} = -Nv\left(\frac{1}{\lambda} - \frac{1}{\lambda^3}\right) - \left[\log\frac{\lambda^3 - 1}{\lambda^3} + \frac{1}{\lambda^3} + \frac{\chi}{\lambda^6}\right]. \tag{6.15}$$

We may normalize the chemical potential by kT. The value of v for a representative volume per solvent molecule is 10^{-28} m^3 (Lu et al., 2012). In the Flory-Rehner free-energy function, two dimensionless material parameters, Nv and χ, are included. Nv ranges from 10^{-4} to 10^{-1} (Lu et al., 2012). Here, we assume $Nv = 10^{-3}$. χ is a measure of enthalpy change in the mixture and ranges from 0 to 1.2. In an application, which prefers a solvent-swollen polymer with a large swelling ratio, a mixture with proper values of Nv and χ are used. The chemical potential as a function of swelling stretch with some typical χ values is shown in Figure 6.8.

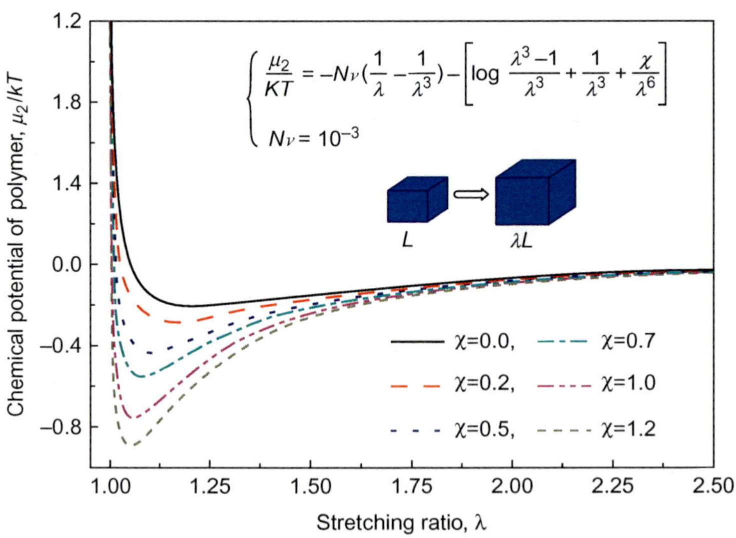

Figure 6.8 Chemical potential of a solvent-swollen polymer as a function of λ with some representative χ values.
Reproduced from Lu et al. (2012) with permission.

In the next step, a uniaxial stress is applied to examine swelling-induced shape recovery in response to the right solvent. Based on Equation (6.12), the constitutive relationship between stress and strain in a polymer/solvent system can be obtained,

$$\frac{vS_1}{kT}=\frac{v}{kT}\cdot\left(\frac{\partial W}{\lambda_1}\right)=Nv\left[\lambda_1\left(1+\frac{2}{\lambda_2^2}\right)-\frac{3}{\lambda_1}\right]+\left[\frac{3\lambda_1^2}{\lambda_2^2}\log\left(1-\frac{B^2}{\lambda_1^3}\right)+\frac{3}{\lambda_1}+\frac{3\chi B^2}{\lambda_1^4}\right]. \tag{6.16}$$

Equation (6.16) is the equilibrium condition in a solvent-swollen polymer subjected to longitudinal stretching. The left-hand side of Equation (6.16) corresponds to λ_1, λ_2, and parameter χ. The characteristic of vS_1/kT in terms of χ and stretch ratio λ_1/λ_2 are revealed in Figure 6.9. Figures 6.9(a) and (b) reveal the relationship between vS_1/kT and λ_1/λ_2. For a given parameter, e.g., $\chi=0$ or $\chi=0.5$, vS_1/kT gradually decreases with the increase in stretching, λ_1. On the other hand, while stretching ratio λ_1/λ_2 increases from 2 to 3, vS_1/kT decreases rather slowly. This numerical study reveals that with the increase in λ_1/λ_2, the peak value of vS_1/kT is reduced at the same stretch value of λ_1.

Figures 6.9(c) and (d) reveal the effects of χ on vS_1/kT at two fixed (λ_1/λ_2) of 2.0 and 3.0; vS_1/kT gradually increases when λ ($\lambda=\lambda_2$) increases. On the other hand,

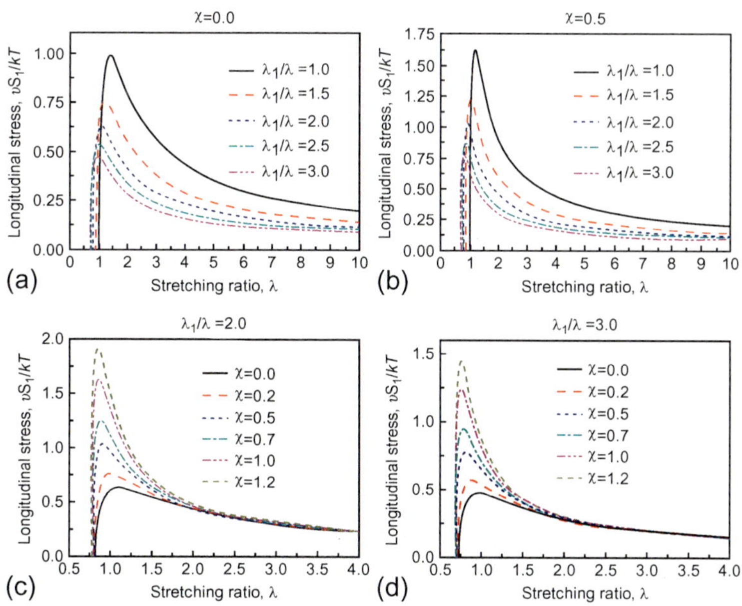

Figure 6.9 Parametrical study of swelling in a piece of SMP immersed into a solvent. (a) Relationship of vS_1/kT versus λ_1/λ_2 at $\chi=0$; (b) relationship of vS_1/kT versus λ_1/λ_2, at $\chi=0.5$; (c) relationship of vS_1/kT versus χ at $\lambda_1/\lambda_2=2.0$; (d) relationship of vS_1/kT versus χ at $\lambda_1/\lambda_2=3.0$.
Reproduced from Lu et al. (2012) with permission.

vS_1/kT also increases with the increase in χ, because a higher stress is required to achieve the amount of stretch if χ is increased.

Based on the experimental investigation and theoretical analysis above, we may conclude that the physical swelling effect between the imbibed solvent molecules and SMP molecules results in the volume expansion in polymer and subsequently lowers the transition temperature of the polymer, triggering shape recovery. Fundamentally, according to the relaxation theory, the chemo-responsive SME in SMPs is a result of the decrease in the cohesive energy density in polymers. It should be reasonable to say that the physical swelling effect is applicable to all SMPs for the chemo-responsive SME.

Polymer gel is another good example to demonstrate the swelling-induced SME. Gels are defined as a substantially diluted cross-linked system, without any flow in the steady-state (http://en.wikipedia.org/wiki/Gel). They behave like a solid due to a three-dimensional cross-linked network within the liquid. It is the crosslinks within the fluid that give a gel its structure (hardness) and contribute to its stiffness.

Polymer gels are able to dramatically change their volume in response to the change in an externally applied particular stimulus, such as chemical, temperature, electrical/magnetic field, and light, etc. (Hu et al., 1995; Osada and Gong, 1998; Ju et al., 2001; Roy et al., 2010; Wang et al., 2011; Xing et al., 2011; Li et al., 2011). As demonstrated in Figure 6.10, a silicone strip with hydrogel embedded in the middle part of one side is able to bend significantly upon its immersion into room temperature water and return to its original straight shape upon drying. On the other hand, Figure 6.11 reveals the feasibility to achieve wetting for shrinkage in a straw with a piece of spherical-shaped hydrogel embedded inside (Sun and Huang, 2009), in which the swelling of the hydrogel causes the length of the straw (with cuts) to decrease.

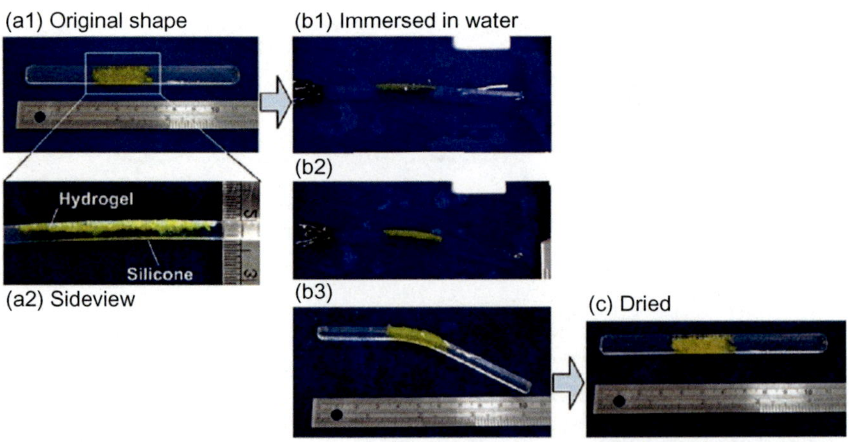

Figure 6.10 Shape change in a silicone strip with embedded hydrogel in a part of it. (a) Original straight shape; (b) bending upon immersing in room temperature water; (c) shape recovery after drying.
Reproduced from Huang et al. (2010) with permission.

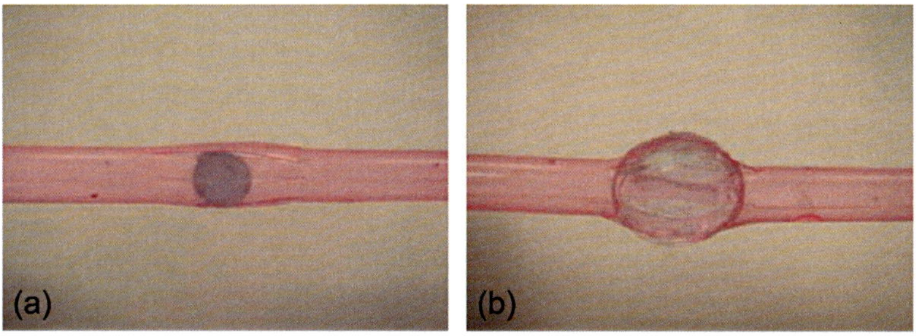

Figure 6.11 Swelling of a piece of spherical-shaped hydrogel inside a straw (with some local cuts). (a) Partially halfway wetted; (b) fully wetted.
Reproduced from Sun and Huang (2009) with permission.

6.3.3 Dissolving-induced SME

A polyurethane block copolymer synthesized from polyhedral oligomeric silsesquioxane molecules and poly(ethylene glycol) (PEG) is able to achieve over 70% shape recovery upon immersing into 30 °C water, due to dissolution of PEG in water (Xu and Song, 2010). Such water-responsive SME is originated from dissolving the transition component in an SMP, so that the elastic component can freely release the elastic energy stored during programming.

It is well known that sodium acetate trihydrate is highly dissolvable in water and has a melting temperature at about 60 °C. As shown in Figure 6.12, a ring made of silicone and sodium acetate trihydrate is programmed at above 60 °C into a star shape (Fan et al., 2011). After being immersed into room temperature water, the ring gradually recovers its original circular shape. The actual recovery speed can be controlled

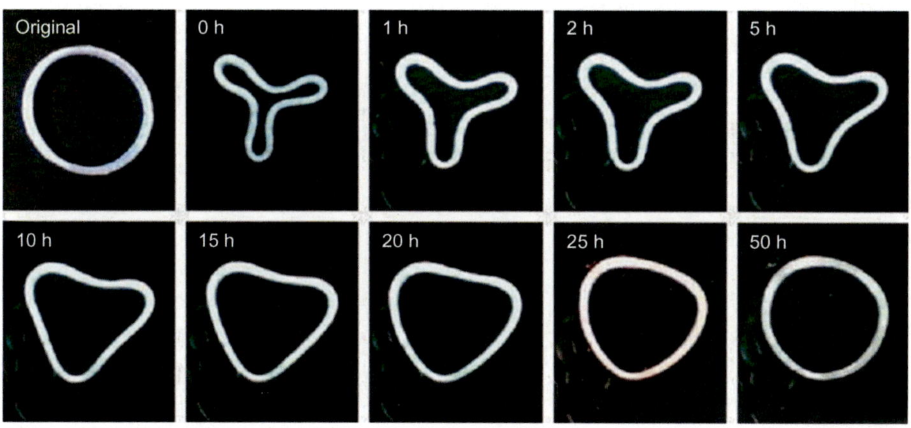

Figure 6.12 Shape recovery in a silicone ring filled with 50 vol% of sodium acetate trihydrate upon immersing in room temperature water.
Reproduced from Fan et al. (2011) with permission.

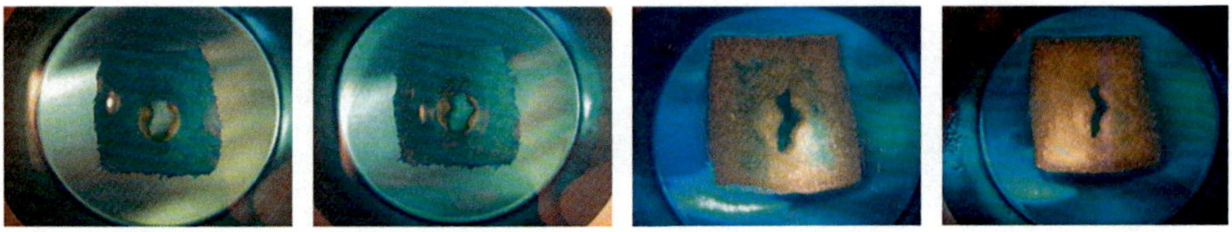

Figure 6.13 Shape recovery (hole closure) of sponge/cupric sulphate pentahydrate hybrid upon immersing in room temperature water.
Reproduced from Fan et al. (2011) with permission.

by varying the volume fraction of sodium acetate trihydrate. Different from that in Figure 6.12, the transition component in Figure 6.13 is cupric sulphate pentahydrate, which, in the programming stage, grows (by means of ctystalization) inside a piece of pre-distorted elastic sponge. Upon immersion into room temperature, cupric sulphate pentahydrate quickly dissolves and, thus, the hole is largely closed within 6 min.

Dissolving-induced SME may be considered as a kind of extension of the swelling-induced SME, in which the volume expansion of the transition component is infinite.

6.4 Biomedical applications

Chemo-responsive SME, in particular water-induced SME, provides a powerful feature for novel device design and may be utilized to supplement, if not to replace, the well-known thermo-responsive SME in a range of biomedical applications; in particular, in minimally invasive surgery, which has become widely accepted at present. Although the chemo-responsive SME is a relatively new concept, the examples presented in this section demonstrate the feasibility of utilizing this effect in a number of biomedical applications, especially minimally invasive surgery.

6.4.1 Retractable stent

Conventional stents are normally designed to be delivered to the required location through, for instance, a catheter and then released there to keep the working shape forever or gradually degraded later on. However, retractable stents are actually in high demand in many surgical applications; for instance, in patients recovering from complications of bladder and prostate cancer operations (Gibbs et al., 1994; Farrell and Sack, 2008; Agrawal and Habr, 2009). The retraction function is also a great advantage: if severe infection or other situations occur within 1 to 2 weeks after installation, the stent can shrink and be brought into a catheter for quick and easy removal in a minimally invasive fashion.

Utilizing the plasticizing effect upon its immersion into water, which reduces the T_g of polyurethane as discussed above, we can achieve a retractable stent (Huang et al., 2007). As shown in Figure 6.14, a polyurethane stent is pre-expanded

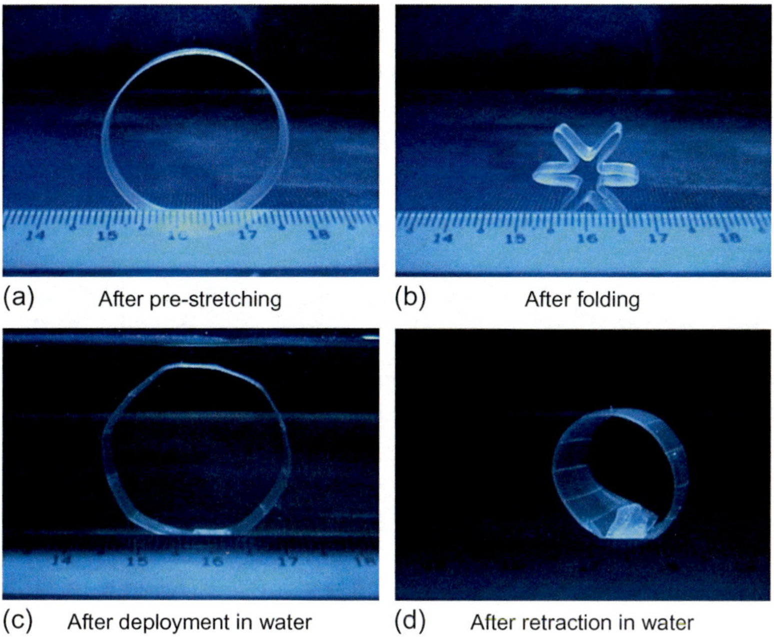

Figure 6.14 Retraction of polyurethane SMP stent in water.
Reproduced from Huang et al. (2007) with permission.

and then deformed into a star shape so it can be packed into a catheter and then delivered to the required location. After being mechanically expanded into a circular shape, as in many conventional stents, it will stay there for a certain period of time, which can be controlled. Due to the gradual absorption of water, the stent later shrinks and can be brought back into the catheter again for removal. Such a concept is mostly applicable to temporary non-cardiovascular stents.

On the other hand, one may design shape-memory hybrids in which an embedded drug functions as the transition component. The shape of the device changes accordingly after the drug is released. Figure 6.15 demonstrates this concept, in which the originally star-shaped shape memory hybrid is made of silicone (as the elastic component) and sodium acetate trihydrate (as the transition component) (Fan et al., 2011). It is heated above the melting temperature of sodium acetate trihydrate (about 70 °C) to expand it to a larger size. Upon its immersion into room temperature water, sodium acetate trihydrate gradually dissolves into water and the shape-memory hybrid gradually returns to its original shape.

In practice, an SMP foam can be designed with an embedded drug, so that the device can be deformed at high temperatures and then let the drug solidify to fix the temporary shape, as revealed in Figure 6.13.

Ethylene vinyl acetate (EVA) is a copolymer made of ethylenen and vinyl acetate. It is commonly used as an implant material to carry and gradually release a drug. EVA itself has excellent SME, in which ethylenen and vinyl acetate serve as the elastic and

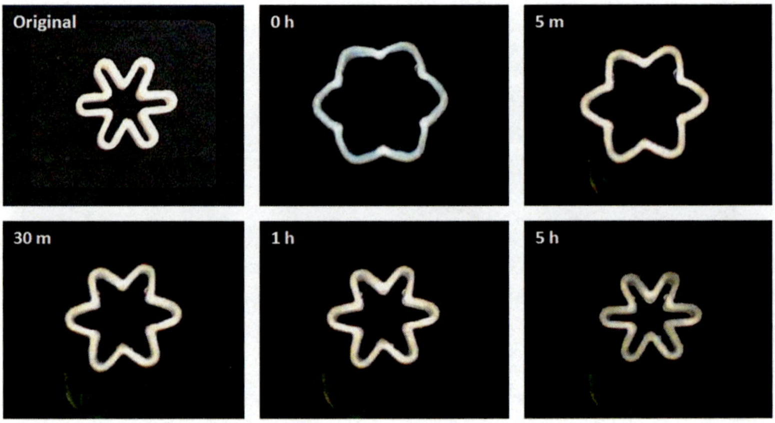

Figure 6.15 Retractable shape memory hybrid stent upon immersing in room temperature water.
Reproduced from (Huang et al., 2012) with permission.

transition segments, respectively. However, the transition temperature of EVA is normally well above our body temperature. Using EVA as the elastic component and the drug as the transition component, a nice combination of a controlled drug release and shape recovery becomes achievable.

6.4.2 Self-tightening suture

In minimally invasive surgery, tissue suturing becomes a difficult task and requires special training and a great deal of practice. Even with improved suturing devices, suturing by hand during minimally invasive surgery is still time-consuming, and the quality of sutures varies depending on the experience and skill of the surgeon (Cuschieri and Szabo, 1995).

An SMP suture that self-sutures upon heating (as demonstrated in Figure 6.16) provides an easy solution (Lendlein and Langer, 2002). Instead of using heat to tighten based on the thermally induced SME, Figure 6.17 reveals that upon immersion into room temperature water (about 22 °C), a polyurethane SMP (MM3520) knot is tightened gradually. Similarly, without heating, a knot can be self-unraveled (Figure 6.18), and a suture can be automatically tightened (Figure 6.19) upon immersion into room temperature water, all because of the water-responsive SME.

As mentioned above, the influence of moisture on the T_g in polyurethane SMPs can be applied not only for actuation, i.e., shape recovery, but also for tuning T_g. In Figure 6.20, there are two pieces of polyurethane SMP wires (MM3520) with the same diameter of 0.4 mm. The left piece of SMP wire has been pre-immersed into water so that it has a lower T_g, while the right one has been kept dry (as such, its T_g remains the same). After pre-stretching and making a loosely tightened knot, both wires are immersed into room temperature water. As we can see, the knot in the left piece of wire tightens at a much higher speed than that in the right wire (Huang et al., 2011).

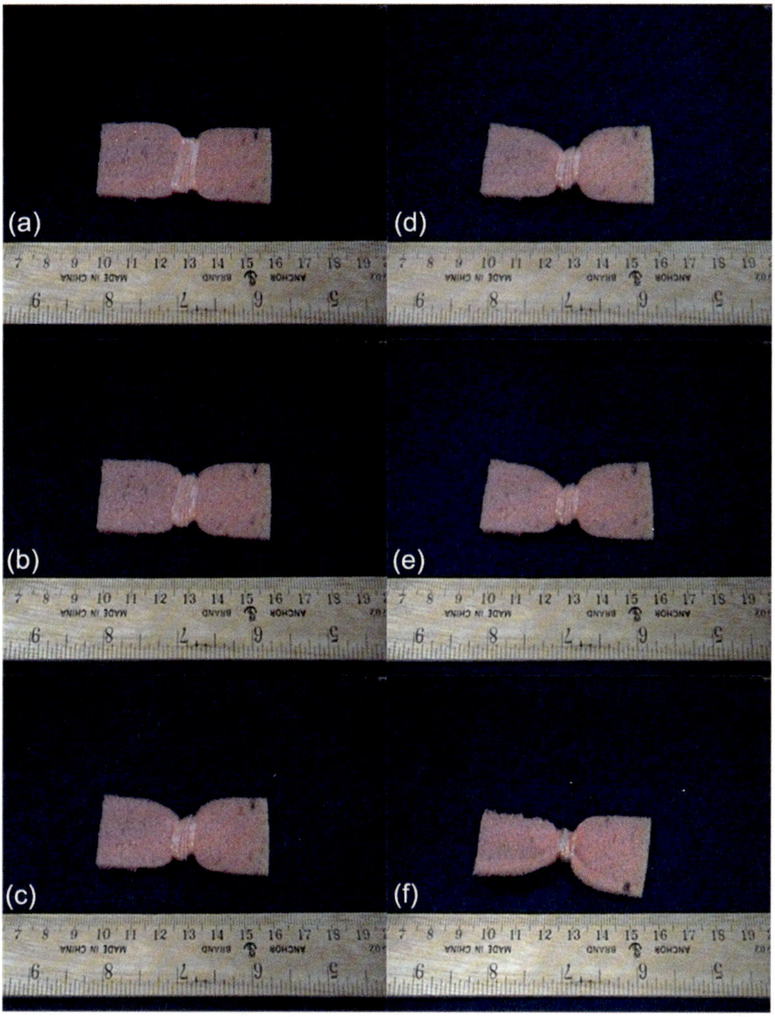

Figure 6.16 (a–f) Tightening of an SMP wire wrapped around a sponge upon gradual heating. Adapted with permission from Huang et al. (2007). Copyright 2007 SPIE.

Fillers may be used to enhance the performance of SMPs not only for strengthening them, but also for adjusting the shape recovery speed (Huang et al., 2011). Attapulgite is a kind of biocompatible clay with a great capacity for water absorption. As revealed in Figure 6.21, treated attapulgite clay (i.e., heated close to 1000 °C) does not have much effect on the recovery speed in the water-induced SME, while the original clay does. This is because after heat treatment, the clay largely loses its ability to absorb moisture/water. In addition, with more clay loaded into the SMP, water penetrates more easily into the SMP through the embedded clay, which functions as micro channels and thus speeds up the shape recovery.

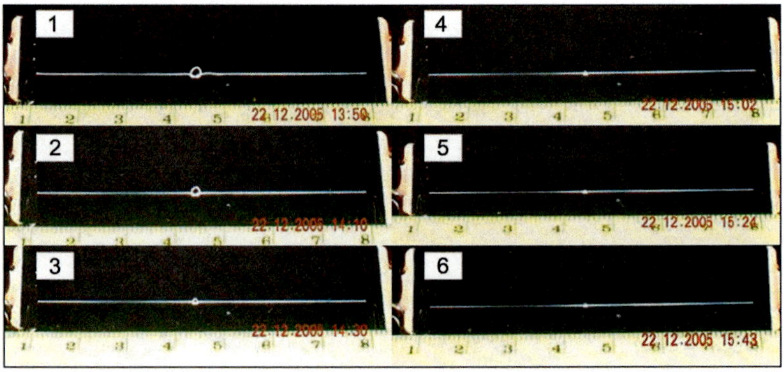

Figure 6.17 Self-tightening of an SMP knot upon immersing in room temperature water. Adapted with permission from Huang et al. (2007). Copyright 2007 SPIE.

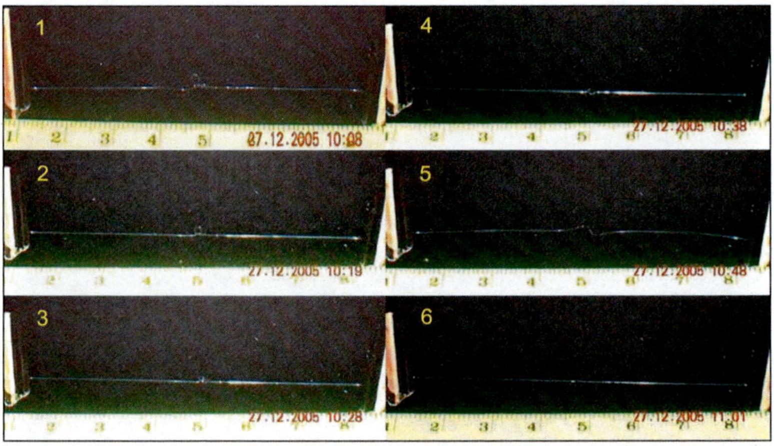

Figure 6.18 Self-unraveling of an SMP wire upon immersing in room temperature water. Adapted with permission from Huang et al. (2007). Copyright 2007 SPIE.

It should be pointed out that in addition to conventional SMPs, many natural materials intrinsically have the moisture/water-responsive SME as well. Hence, they may be used in biomedical engineering.

Figure 6.22 reveals the water-responsive SME in a silk thread (Huang et al., 2012). A piece of silk thread with a diameter of about 80 μm is wound around a cylinder with a diameter of 2.5 mm and then placed into 25 °C water for 30 min. After drying in the open air for 3 hours, a spiral-shaped silk spring is produced Figure 6.22(a). Subsequently, the silk spring is cut into two pieces. We place one piece into 25 °C water, which becomes straight within about 1 minute Figure 6.22(c1). The other piece is first heated to 80 °C for 30 min. After heating, the spring is only distorted slightly Figure 6.22(c2). In the next

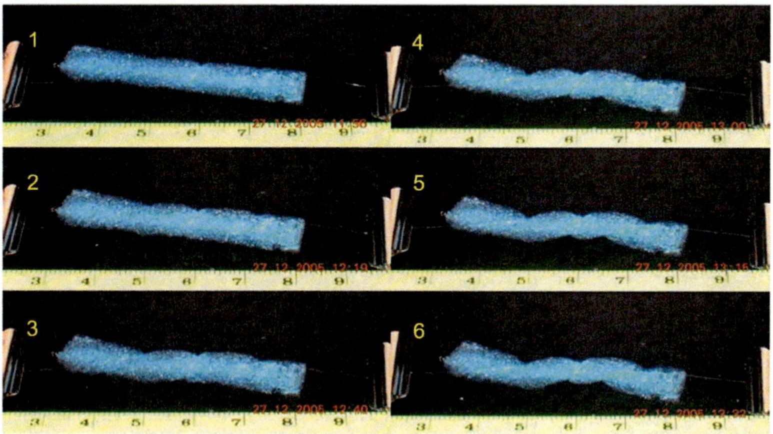

Figure 6.19 Self-tightening of an SMP wire wrapped around a sponge upon immersing in room temperature water.
Adapted with permission from Huang et al. (2007). Copyright 2007 SPIE.

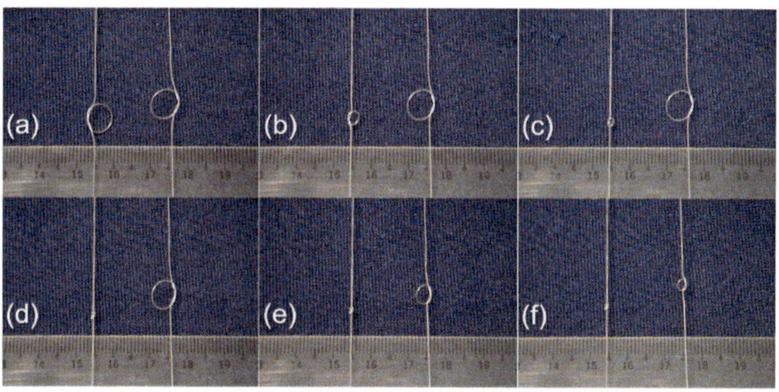

Figure 6.20 Self-tightening of two pieces of SMP wire (MM3520) (a–f) upon immersion into room temperature water. In each panel, the left piece has been pre-immersed in water to reduce its T_g.
Adapted with permission from Huang et al. (2007). Copyright 2007 SPIE.

step, it is placed into 25 °C water as was the other piece of silk spring. Figure 6.22(d2) reveals that it also straightens within about 1 minute.

6.4.3 Cellular surgery

In the 1966 film *Fantastic Voyage*, a miniaturized submarine, the *Proteus*, was injected into a scientist's body to remove a blood clot in his brain and save his life. Although there are a number of surgical techniques available today to remove a blood

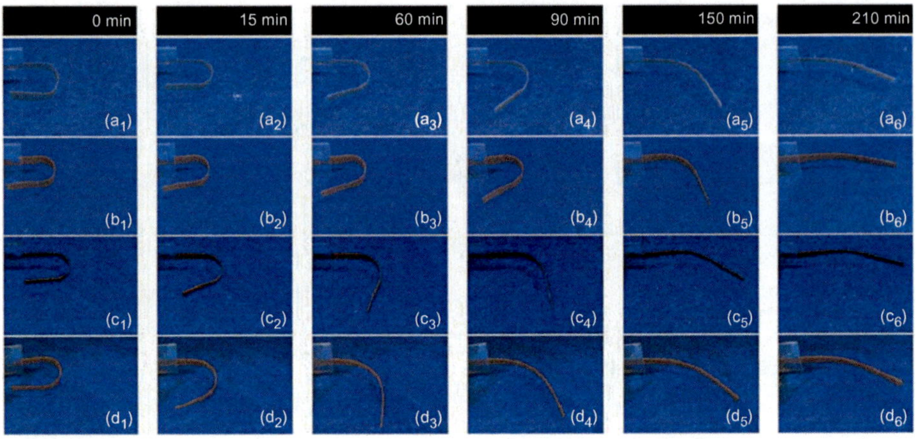

Figure 6.21 Shape recovery in polyurethane SMP/attapulgite composites upon immersing in room temperature water. (a) SMP (MM3520) without clay; (b) with 5 vol% of treated clay; (c) with 5 vol% of original clay; (d) with 10 vol% of original clay.
Reproduced from Behl and Lendlein (2007) with permission.

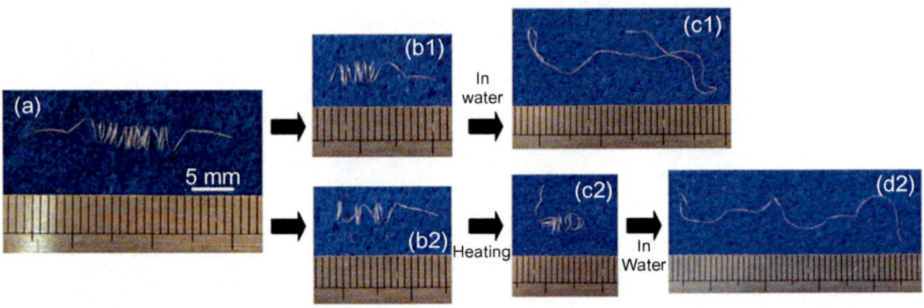

Figure 6.22 Water-responsive SME in a silk thread. See text for explanation.
Reproduced from Huang et al. (2012) with permission.

clot in a minimally invasive fashion, we are still far from being able to shrink a real ship into a size of a few micrometers. However, from an engineering point of view, we have almost all the necessary techniques to deliver a micro vehicle made of SMPs into a living cell (Sun et al., 2012).

As illustrated in Figure 6.23, a tiny vehicle is deformed into a wire shape and then inserted into a cell. If this vehicle is made of the thermo/moisture-responsive SMP, it is going to recover its original shape after absorbing enough water inside the cell. Subsequently, it can be operated within the living cell using, for instance, a laser beam from outside of the cell to control its motion (Sun et al., 2012).

The SME in micron and submicron-sized SMMs (Behl and Lendlein, 2007; Sun et al., 2012; Huang et al., 2011; Zhao and Huang, 2011; Nespoli et al., 2010) enables

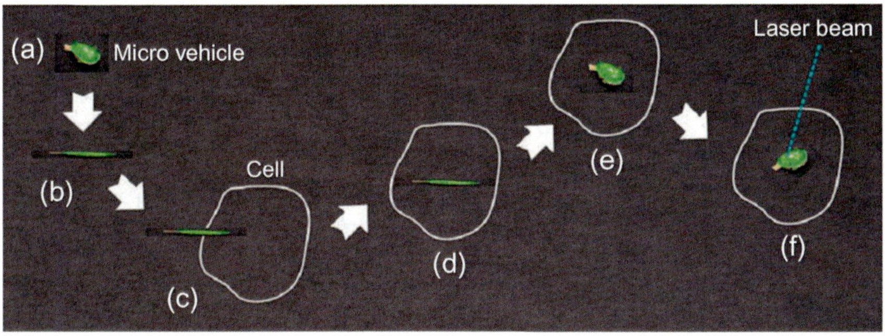

Figure 6.23 Delivery of a micro vehicle into a living cell for an inside-cell operation controlled by a laser beam (illustration). (a) The original shape of the micro vehicle; (b) the shape of the vehicle after reshaping; (c) inserting the deformed vehicle into a cell; (d) the vehicle fully inside the cell; (e) shape recovery of the vehicle; (f) the vehicle in operation powered by a laser beam from outside.
Reproduced from Sun et al. (2012) with permission.

the shrinkage of surgical devices to a much smaller size. Such miniature surgical devices are in high demand in, for instance, endovascular repair and even cellular surgery (Sun et al., 2012; Fernandes and Gracias, 2009). The concept of delivering a micro-device by injection is demonstrated in Figure 6.24 using a piece of polyurethane SMP spiral spring.

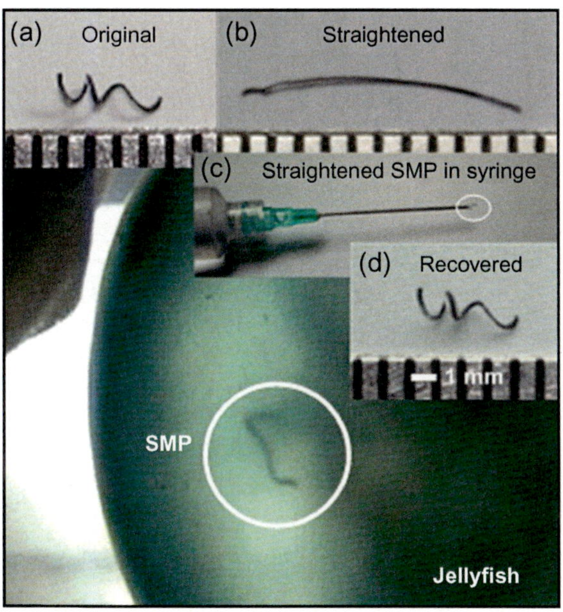

Figure 6.24 Delivery of a polyurethane SMP coil into a jellyfish by injection. (a) Original coiled shape; (b) after being straightened at high temperatures; (c) ready for injection; (d) recovered shape.
Reproduced from Behl and Lendlein (2007) with permission.

6.4.4 Surface patterning for controlled cell adhesion/growth

Cell culture substrates with a defined topography have been applied in the investigation of cell mechanobiology. In addition, well-defined surface topographies have found an application in biomedical device design to enhance implant cell adhesion and tissue in-growth (Anselme, 2000). SMPs appear as a promising material for the study of the influence of the change in surface topography on cell culture (Davis et al., 2011).

Self-assembly is a fundamental process to drive structural organization in both inanimate and living systems that is under strict genetic control; however, physical mechanisms ultimately bring about the complex structures (Jakab et al., 2004). How to control the shape of an organ in its early growth stage, in, for instance, organ printing in computer-aided jet-based 3-dimensional tissue generation (Mironov et al., 2003), has become a critical issue.

Micro/nano-sized surface wrinkles (e.g., in Figure 6.25) and micro/nano-sized protrusion/indentation arrays (e.g., in Figure 6.26) using the chemo-responsive SME provide an effective approach to further enhance the influence of surface morphology. This can result in different cell dispersion pattern and growth rates at different locations, depending on the exact surface morphology underneath (Huang et al., 2012).

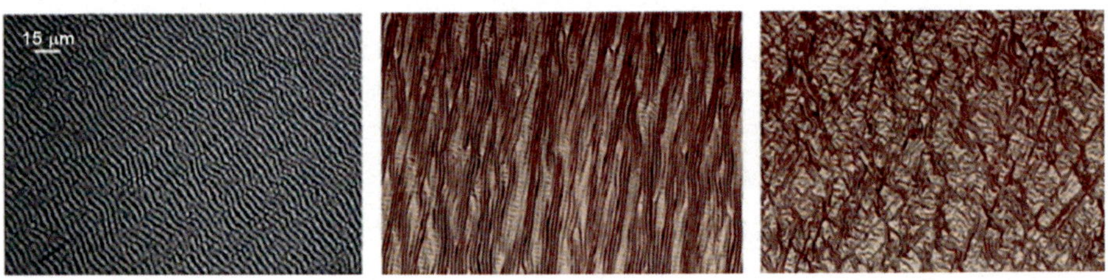

Figure 6.25 Typical types of wrinkles on polyurethane SMP.
Reproduced from Huang et al. (2012) with permission.

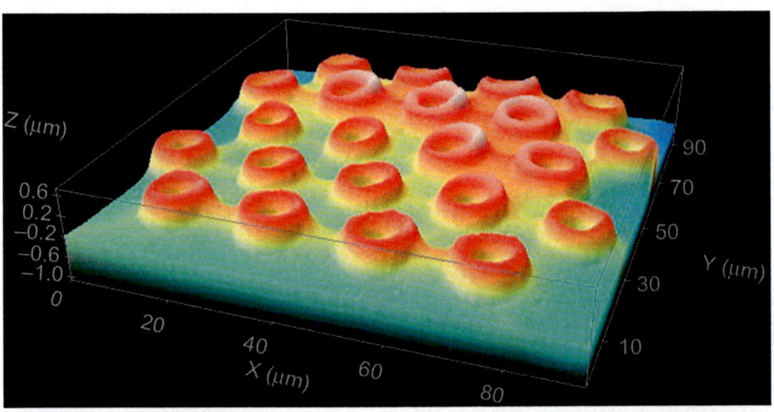

Figure 6.26 Micro surface pattern on PMMA.
Reproduced from Huang et al. (2012) with permission.

6.4.5 Micro lens array for a new generation of endoscopes

Lytro, the first generation of light field cameras, is bringing a revolution by enabling us to "Shoot first, focus later." In addition to the theory in data/image processing, a microlens array is required to taken a series of images simultaneously. Such cameras could have a significant impact on endoscopes and tablet inspection devices by providing clear images with minimal time and effort.

PMMA is one of the conventional optical polymers for the macro/micro lens. The chemo-responsive SME can be utilized to fabricate a disposable PMMA microlens array in a nonconventional way and at very low cost. The fabrication procedure of such a microlens array has only two major steps (Zhao et al., 2011b). In the first step, an array of micro-indents is produced using a spherical-shape micro indenter (Figure 6.27a). The exact pattern of the indents may vary, and the indents may be closely packed. In the second step, the PMMA is immersed in ethanol. A few hours later, an array of crown-shaped protrusions is produced (Figure 6.27b).

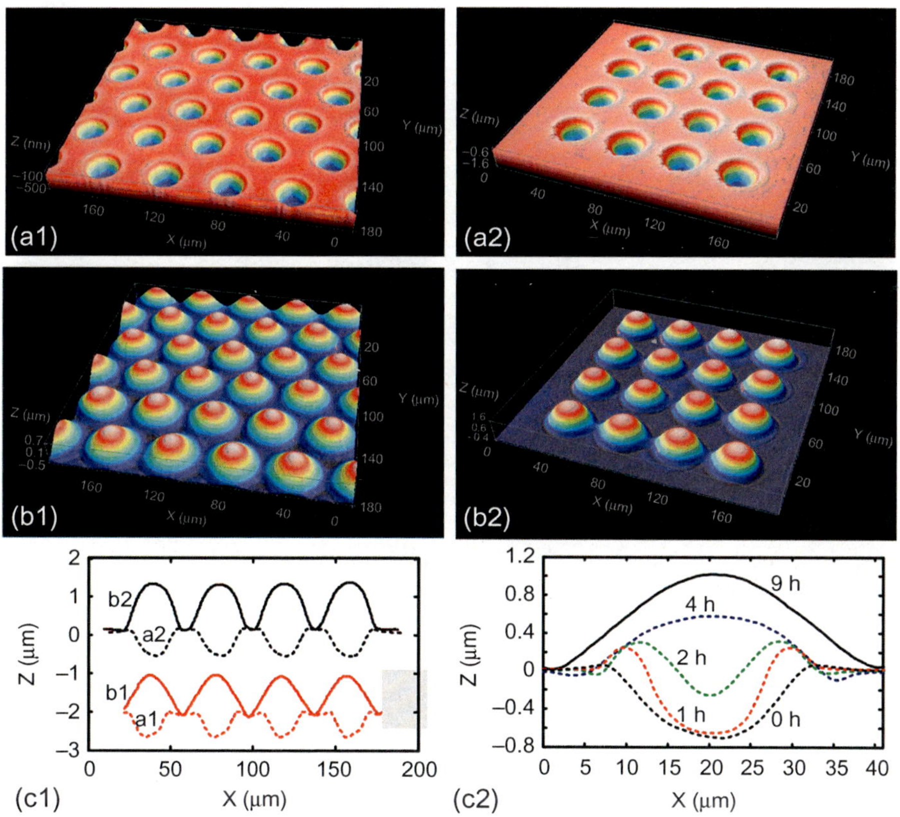

Figure 6.27 2-D microlens array and surface profile. (a) After indentation; (b) after immersion in ethanol; (c1) comparison of cross-sections; (c2) comparison of cross-sections upon immersion in ethanol for different time periods (hours).
Reproduced from Zhao et al. (2011b) with permission.

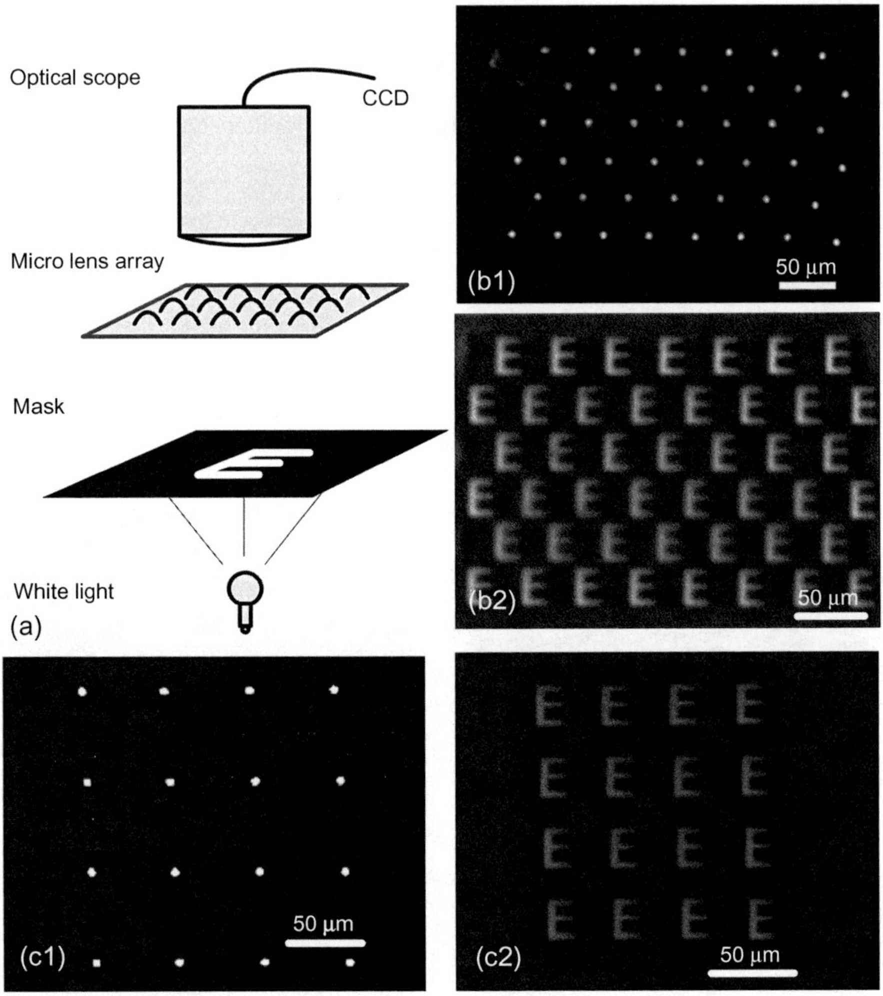

Figure 6.28 Projection experiment and results. (a) Illustration of the experimental setup; (b and c) the focus spot and projected images through two different MLAs. Reproduced from Zhao et al. (2011b) with permission.

Figure 6.28 reveals typical optical experimental results of a PMMA microlens array. The images are less than 50 μm in size. The exact dimensions of a lens can be controlled by using different-sized indenters to compress into different depths and adjusting the time of immersion. Figure 6.29 shows different-sized lenses produced atop one piece of PMMA.

A 3-D compound lens, i.e., insect eye (lens atop lens), has the advantage of large-view angle. This is a feature highly in demand in endoscopes (in particular hard endoscopes, in which tip-turning is restricted) and tablet inspection devices. Combining the thermo-responsive and chemo-responsive SMEs in PMMAs (Zhao et al., 2011c), 3-D PMMA microlens arrays have been produced (Figure 6.30).

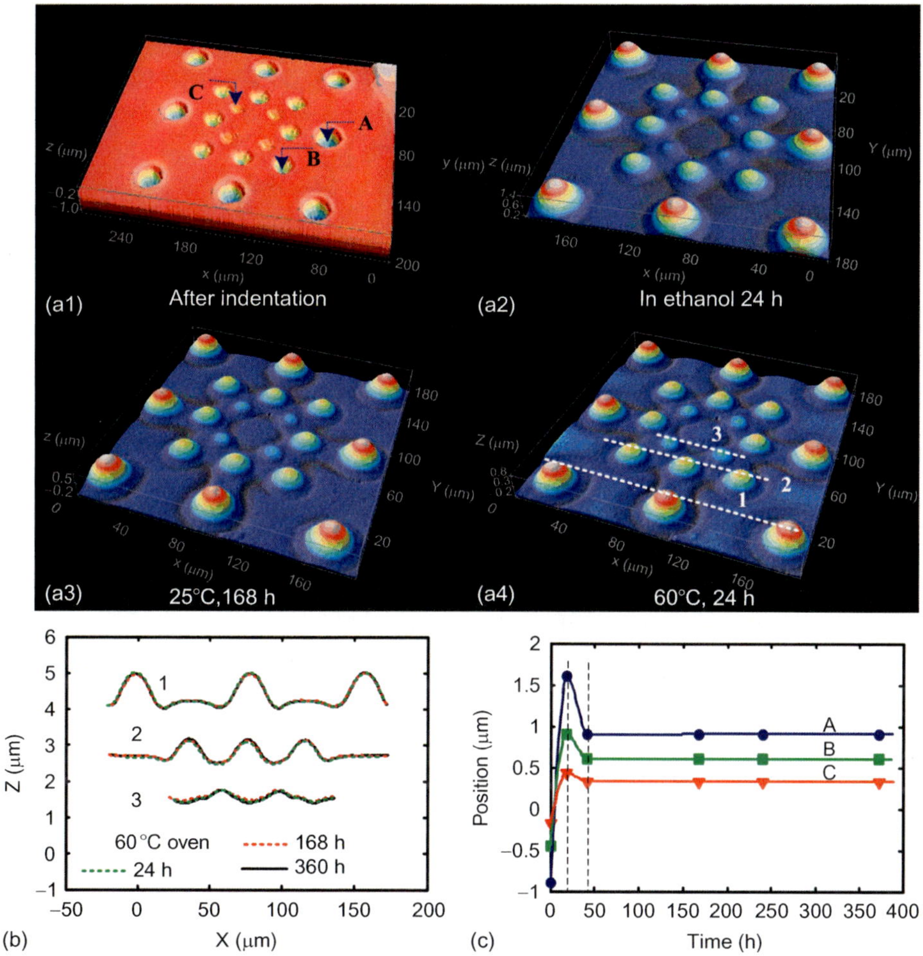

Figure 6.29 Different-sized/shaped 2-D microlens array. (a1) Surface profile of an indent array, in which three different-sized indents were made by a 20 μm spherical under three different maximum loads; (a2) surface profile of MLA after immersion in ethanol for 24 hours; (a3 and a4) two typical MLA surface profiles after being kept inside an oven for thermal stability test; (b) comparison of surface profile of MLA after immersion in ethanol for 24 hours; (c) evolution of the center points of three different-sized indents/protrusions (depth/height) against time in the whole process (i.e., after indentation, immersed in ethanol and placed in 60°C oven). Reproduced from Zhao et al. (2011b) with permission.

6.5 Conclusion

In this chapter, we introduce the basic mechanisms and theories behind the chemo-responsive SME in polymers. A number of examples are presented to reveal the potential of utilizing the softening-, swelling-, and dissolving-induced SMEs, either individually or jointly, in biomedical engineering. As we can see, together with other types of SMEs, chemo-responsive SMEs can reshape the design of biomedical devices in many ways.

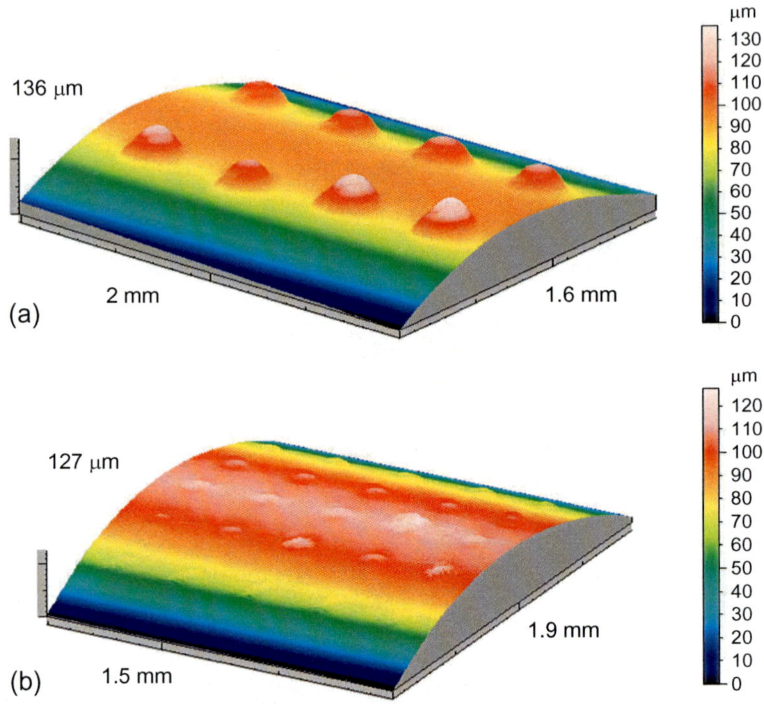

Figure 6.30 (a–b) 3D profile of two PMMA microlens array produced. Reproduced from Zhao et al. (2011b) with permission.

Acknowledgments

We would like to thank Y. Zhao, C. Tang, Z. Ding, and Dr C.C. Wang for conducting some of the experiments reported here.

References

Agrawal, D., Habr, F.G., 2009. Removable self-expandable plastic stent to treat postphotodynamic therapy esophageal stricture. Gastrointest. Endosc. 69, 27–30. http://dx.doi.org/10.1016/j.gie.2008.08.037.

Anselme, K., 2000. Osteoblast adhesion on biomaterials. Biomaterials 21, 667–681. http://dx.doi.org/10.1016/S0142-9612(99)00242-2.

Behl, M., Lendlein, A., 2007. Shape-memory polymers. Mater. Today 10, 20–28. http://dx.doi.org/10.1016/S1369-7021(07)70047-0.

Behl, M., Zotzmann, J., Lendlein, A., 2010. Shape-memory polymers and shape-changing polymers. Adv. Polym. Sci. 226, 1–40. http://dx.doi.org/10.1007/12_2009_26.

Chaunier, L., Lourdin, D., 2009. The shape memory of starch. Starch-Starke 61, 116–118. http://dx.doi.org/10.1002/star.200800074.

Chen, S.J., Hu, J.L., Yuen, C.W.M., Chan, L.K., 2009. Novel moisture-sensitive shape memory polyurethanes containing pyridine moieties. Polymer 50, 4424–4428. http://dx.doi.org/10.1016/j.polymer.2009.07.031.

Cuschieri, A., Szabo, Z., 1995. Tissue approximation in endoscopic surgery. Oxford: Isis Medical Media ISBN-13, 978–1899066032.

Davis, K.A., Burke, K.A., Mather, P.T., Henderson, J.H., 2011. Dynamic cell behavior on shape memory polymer substrates. Biomaterials 32, 2285–2293. http://dx.doi.org/10.1016/j.biomaterials.2010.12.006.

Dietsch, B., Tong, T., 2007. A review—features and benefits of shape memory polymers (SMPs). J. Adv. Mater. 39, 3–12.

Du, H.Y., Zhang, J.H., 2010. Solvent induced shape recovery of shape memory polymer based on chemically cross-linked poly(vinyl alcohol). Soft Matter 6, 3370–3376. http://dx.doi.org/10.1039/B922220K.

Fan, K., Huang, W.M., Wang, C.C., Ding, Z., Zhao, Y., Purnawali, H., Liew, K.C., Zheng, L.X., 2011. Water-responsive shape memory hybrid: Design concept and demonstration. eXPRESS Polym. Lett. 5, 409–416. http://dx.doi.org/10.3144/expresspolymlett.2011.40.

Farrell, J.J., Sack, J., 2008. Removable colonic stenting: time to expand the indications? Gastrointest. Endosc. 68, 721–723. http://dx.doi.org/10.1016/j.gie.2008.04.044.

Fernandes, R., Gracias, D.H., 2009. Toward a miniaturized mechanical surgeon. Mater. Today 12, 14–20. http://dx.doi.org/10.1016/S1369-7021(09)70272-X.

Flory, P.J., 1942. Thermodynamics of high polymer solutions. J. Chem. Phys. 10, 51–61. http://dx.doi.org/10.1063/1.1723621.

Flory, P.J., 1953. Principles of Polymer Chemistry. Ithaca, New York, ISBN: 9780801401343.

Fomina, N., McFearin, C.L., Sermsakdi, M., Morachis, J.M., Almutairi, A., 2011. Low power, biologically benign NIR light triggers polymer disassembly. Macromolecules 44, 8590–8597. http://dx.doi.org/10.1021/ma201850q.

Gibbs, J.S., Sigwart, U., Buller, N.P., 1994. Temporary stent as a bail-out device during percutaneous transluminal coronary angioplasty—preliminary clinical-experience. Brit. Heart J. 71, 372–377. http://dx.doi.org/10.1016/PMC483691.

Grimes, A., Breslauer, D.N., Long, M., Pegan, J., Lee, L.P., Khine, M., 2008. Shrinky-dink microfluidics: rapid generation of deep and rounded patterns. Lab Chip 8, 170–172. http://dx.doi.org/10.1039/B711622E.

Hidber, P.C., Nealey, P.F., Helbig, W., Whitesides, G.M., 1996. New strategy for controlling the size and shape of metallic features formed by electroless deposition of copper: Microcontact printing of catalysts on oriented polymers, followed by thermal shrinkage. Langmuir 12, 5209–5215. http://dx.doi.org/10.1021/la960238u.

Hu, Z., Zhang, X., Li, Y., 1995. Synthesis and application of modulated polymer gels. Science 269, 525–527. http://dx.doi.org/10.1126/science.269.5223.525.

Huang, W.M., Yang, B., An, L., Li, C., Chan, Y.S., 2005. Water-driven programmable polyurethane shape memory polymer: Demonstration and mechanism. Appl. Phys. Lett. 86, 114105. http://dx.doi.org/10.1063/1.1880448.

Huang, W.M., Yang, B., Liu, N., Phee, S.J., 2007. Water-responsive programmable shape memory polymer devices. Int. Conf. Smart Mater. Nanotechnol. Eng. 6423, 64231–64237. http://dx.doi.org/10.1117/12.779663.

Huang, W.M., Yang, B., Zhao, Y., Ding, Z., 2010. Thermo-moisture responsive polyurethane shape-memory polymer and composites: a review. J. Mater. Chem. 20, 3367–3381. http://dx.doi.org/10.1039/B922943D.

Huang, W.M., Yang, B., Fu, Y.Q., 2011. Polyurethane Shape Memory Polymers. CRC Press, Boca Raton, ISBN: 978-1439838006.

Huang, W.M., Zhao, Y., Wang, C.C., Ding, Z., Purnawali, H., Tang, C., Zhang, J.L. (2012). Thermo/chemo-responsive shape memory effect in polymers: working mechanisms, fundamentals and optimization. Submitted for publication. J. Polym. Res. 19, 9952. http://dx.doi.org/10.1007/s10965-012-9952-z.

Irie, M., 1998. In: Otsuka, K., Wayman, C.M. (Eds.), Shape Memory Polymers. Cambridge University Press, Cambridge, ISBN: 0521663849.

Jakab, K., Neagu, A., Mironov, V., Markwald, R.R., Forgacs, G., 2004. Engineering biological structures of prescribed shape using self-assembling multicellular systems. Proc. Natl. Acad. Sci. U. S. A. 101, 2864–2869. http://dx.doi.org/10.1073/pnas.0400164101.

Jiang, H.Y., Kelch, S., Lendlein, A., 2006. Polymers move in response to light. Adv. Mater. 18, 1471–1475. http://dx.doi.org/10.1002/adma.200502266.

Ju, H.K., Kim, S.Y., Lee, Y.M., 2001. pH/temperature-responsive behaviors of semi-IPN and comb-type graft hydrogels composited of alginate and poly(N-isopropylacrylamide). Polymer 42, 6851–6857. http://dx.doi.org/10.1016/S0032-3861(01)00143-4.

Jung, Y.C., So, H.H., Cho, J.W., 2006. Water-responsive shape memory polyurethane block copolymer modified with polyhedral oligomeric silsesquioxane. J. Macromol. Sci. B 45, 453–461. http://dx.doi.org/10.1080/00222340600767513.

Kumpfer, J.R., Rowan, S.J., 2011. Thermo-, photo-, and chemo-responsive shape-memory properties from photo-cross-linked metallo-supramolecular polymers. J. Am. Chem. Soc. 133, 12866–12874. http://dx.doi.org/10.1021/ja205332w.

Lendlein, A., Kelch, S., 2002. Shape-memory polymers. Angew. Chem. Int. 41, 2034–2057. http://dx.doi.org/10.1002/1521-3773(20020617).

Lendlein, A., Langer, R., 2002. Biodegradable, elastic shape-memory polymers for potential biomedical applications. Science 296, 1673–1676. http://dx.doi.org/10.1126/science.1066102.

Lendlein, A., Jiang, H.Y., Junger, O., Langer, R., 2005. Light-induced shape-memory polymers. Nature (London) 434, 879–882. http://dx.doi.org/10.1038/nature03496.

Leng, J., Du, S., 2010. Shape-Memory Polymers and Multifunctional Composites. CRC Press/ Taylor & Francis, Boca Raton, ISBN: 1420090194.

Leng, J.S., Lu, H.B., Liu, Y.J., Du, S.Y., 2008. Comment on "Water-driven programable polyurethane shape memory polymer: Demonstration and mechanism" [Appl. Phys. Lett. 86, 114105 (2005)]. Appl. Phys. Lett. 92, 206105. http://dx.doi.org/10.1063/1.2936288.

Leng, J.S., Lu, H.B., Liu, Y.J., Huang, W.M., Du, S.Y., 2009. Shape-memory polymers—a class of novel smart materials. MRS Bull. 34, 848–855. http://dx.doi.org/10.1557/mrs2009.235.

Li, Y., Maciel, D., Tomas, H., Rodrigues, J., Ma, H., Shi, X., 2011. pH sensitive Laponite/alginate hybrid hydrogels: swelling behavior and release mechanism. Soft Matter 7, 6231–6238. http://dx.doi.org/10.1039/C1SM05345K.

Liu, N., Huang, W.M., Phee, S.J., Fan, H., Chew, K.L., 2007. A generic approach for producing various protrusive shapes on different size using shape-memory polymer. Smart Mater. Struct. 16, N47–N50. http://dx.doi.org/10.1088/0964-1726/16/6/N01.

Liu, N., Xie, Q., Huang, W.M., Phee, S.J., Guo, N.Q., 2008. Formation of micro protrusion arrays atop shape memory polymer. J. Micromech. Microeng. 18, 027001. http://dx.doi.org/10.1088/0960-1317/18/2/027001.

Liu, X.C., Chakraborty, A., Luo, C., 2010. Fabrication of micropatterns on the sidewalls of a thermal shape memory polystyrene block. J. Micromech. Microeng. 20, 095025. http://dx.doi.org/10.1088/0960-1317/20/9/095025.

Lu, H.B., Liu, Y.J., Leng, J.S., Du, S.Y., 2009. Qualitative separation of the effect of solubility parameter on the recovery behavior of shape-memory polymer. Smart Mater. Struct. 18, 085003. http://dx.doi.org/10.1088/0964-1726/18/8/085003.

Lu, H.B., Liu, Y.J., Leng, J.S., Du, S.Y., 2010a. Qualitative separation of the physical swelling effect on the recovery behavior of shape memory polymer. Eur. Polym. J. 46, 1908–1914. http://dx.doi.org/10.1016/j.eurpolymj.2010.06.013.

Lu, H.B., Liu, Y.J., Leng, J.S., Du, S.Y., 2010b. Comment on "Water-driven programable polyurethane shape memory polymer: Demonstration and mechanism" [Appl. Phys. Lett. 86, 114105 (2005)]. Appl. Phys. Lett. 97, 056101. http://dx.doi.org/10.1063/1.3421393.

Lu, H.B., Liu, Y.J., Leng, J.S., Du, S.Y., 2012. A simulation method to analyze chemo-mechanical behavior of swelling-induced shape-memory polymer in response to solvent. J. Appl. Polym. Sci. 123, 1137–1146. http://dx.doi.org/10.1002/app.34597.

Lv, H.B., Leng, J.S., Liu, Y.J., Du, S.Y., 2008. Shape-memory polymer in response to solution. Adv. Eng. Mater. 10, 592–595. http://dx.doi.org/10.1002/adem.200800002.

Mather, P.T., Luo, X.F., Rousseau, I.A., 2009. Shape memory polymer research. Annu. Rev. Mater. Res. 39, 445–471. http://dx.doi.org/10.1146/annurev-matsci-082908-145419.

Mendez, J., Annamalai, P.K., Eichhorn, S.J., Rusli, R., Rowan, S.J., Foster, E.J., et al., 2011. Bioinspired mechanically adaptive polymer nanocomposites with water-activated shape-memory effect. Macromolecules 44, 6827–6835. http://dx.doi.org/10.1021/ma201502k.

Mironov, V., Boland, T., Trusk, T., Forgacs, G., Markwald, R.R., 2003. Organ printing: computer-aided jet-based 3D tissue engineering. Trends Biotechnol. 21, 157–161. http://dx.doi.org/10.1016/S0167-7799(03)00033-7.

Miyazaki, S., Fu, Y.Q., Huang, W.M., 2009. Thin Film Shape Memory Alloys: Fundamentals and Device Applications. Cambridge University Press, New York, ISBN: 0521885760.

Nespoli, A., Besseghini, S., Pittaccio, S., Villa, E., Viscuso, S., 2010. The high potential of shape memory alloys in developing miniature mechanical devices: A review on shape memory alloy mini-actuators. Sensor Actuat. A-Phys. 158, 149–160. http://dx.doi.org/10.1016/j.sna.2009.12.020.

Osada, Y., Gong, J.P., 1998. Soft and wet materials: polymer gels. Adv. Mater. 10, 827–837.

Ratna, D., Karger-Kocsis, J., 2008. Recent advances in shape memory polymers and composites: a review. J. Mater. Sci. 43, 254–269. http://dx.doi.org/10.1007/s10853-007-2176-7.

Rousseau, I.A., 2008. Challenges of shape memory polymers: a review of the progress toward overcoming SMP's limitations. Polym. Eng. Sci. 48, 2075–2089. http://dx.doi.org/10.1002/pen.21213.

Roy, D., Cambre, J.N., Sumerlin, B.S., 2010. Future perspectives and recent advances in stimuli-responsive materials. Prog. Polym. Sci. 35, 278–301. http://dx.doi.org/10.1016/j.progpolymsci.2009.10.008.

Rubinstein, M., Colby, R.H., 2003. Polymer Physics. Oxford University Press, Oxford, ISBN: 019852059X.

Small, W., Singhal, P., Wilsona, T.S., Maitland, D.J., 2010. Biomedical applications of thermally activated shape memory polymers. J. Mater. Chem. 20, 3356–3366. http://dx.doi.org/10.1039/B923717H.

Sun, L., Huang, W.M., 2009. Wet to shrink: an approach to realize negative expansion upon wetting. Adv. Compos. Mater. 18, 95–103. http://dx.doi.org/10.1163/156855109X428763.

Sun, L., Huang, W.M., Ding, Z., Zhao, Y., Wang, C.C., Purnawali, H., Tang, C., 2012. Stimulus-responsive shape memory materials: A review. Mater. Design 33, 577–640. http://dx.doi.org/10.1016/j.matdes.2011.04.065.

van der Sman, R.G.M., Meinders, M.B.J., 2011. Prediction of the state diagram of starch water mixtures using the Flory–Huggins free volume theory. Soft Matter 7, 429–442. http://dx.doi.org/10.1039/C0SM00280A.

Wang, W.B., Xu, J.X., Wang, A.Q., 2011. A pH-, salt- and solvent-responsive carboxymethylcellulose-g-poly(sodium acrylate)/medical stone superabsorbent composite with enhanced swelling and responsive properties. eXPRESS Polym. Lett. 5, 385–400. http://dx.doi.org/10.3144/expresspolymlett.2011.38.

Willett, J.L., 2008. Humidity-responsive starch-poly(methyl acrylate) films. Macromol. Chem. Phys. 209, 764–772. http://dx.doi.org/10.1002/macp.200700495.

Xing, S., Guan, Y., Zhang, Y., 2011. Kinetics of glucose-induced swelling of P(NIPAM-AAPBA) microgels. Macromolecules 44, 4479–4486. http://dx.doi.org/10.1021/ma200586w.

Xu, J.W., Song, J., 2010. High performance shape memory polymer networks based on rigid nanoparticle cores. Proc. Natl. Acad. Sci. U. S. A. 107, 7652–7657. http://dx.doi.org/10.1073/pnas.0912481107.

Yang, B., Huang, W.M., Li, C., Lee, C.M., Li, L., 2004. On the effects of moisture in a polyurethane shape memory polymer. Smart Mater. Struct. 13, 191–195. http://dx.doi.org/10.1088/0964-1726/13/1/022.

Yang, B., Huang, W.M., Li, C., Li, L., Chor, J.H., 2005. Qualitative separation of the effects of carbon nano-powder and moisture on the glass transition temperature of polyurethane shape memory polymer. Scripta Mater. 53, 105–107. http://dx.doi.org/10.1016/j.scriptamat.2005.03.009.

Yang, B., Huang, W.M., Li, C., Li, L., 2006. Effects of moisture on the thermomechanical properties of a polyurethane shape memory polymer. Polymer 47, 1348–1356. http://dx.doi.org/10.1016/j.polymer.2005.12.051.

Zhao, Y., Huang, W.M., 2011. Micron sized polyurethane shape-memory polymer beads. Adv. Mater. Res. 239–242, 2675–2678. http://dx.doi.org/10.4028/www.scientific.net/AMR.239-242.2675.

Zhao, X.M., Xia, Y.N., Schueller, O.J.A., Qin, D., Whitesides, G.M., 1998. Fabrication of microstructures using shrinkable polystyrene films. Sensor Actuat. A-Phys. 65, 209–217. http://dx.doi.org/10.1016/S0924-4247(97)01692-0.

Zhao, Y., Huang, W.M., Fu, Y.Q., 2011a. Formation of micro/nano-scale wrinkling patterns atop shape memory polymers. J. Micromech. Microeng. 21, 067007. http://dx.doi.org/10.1088/0960-1317/21/6/067007.

Zhao, Y., Wang, C.C., Huang, W.M., Purnawali, H., An, L., 2011b. Formation of micro protrusive lens arrays atop poly(methyl methacrylate). Opt. Express 19, 26000–26005. http://dx.doi.org/10.1364/OE.19.026000.

Zhao, Y., Wang, C.C., Huang, W.M., Purnawali, H., 2011c. Buckling of poly(methyl methacrylate) in stimulus-responsive shape recovery. Appl. Phys. Lett. 99, 131911. http://dx.doi.org/10.1063/1.3645005.

Shape-memory polyurethane cellular solids for minimally invasive surgical procedures

7

M.C. Tanzi[1], *L. De Nardo*[2], *S. Bertoldi*[2], *S. Farè*[2]
[1]INSTM, Politecnico di Milano, Italy; [2]Materials and Chemical Engineering 'G. Natta', Milano, Italy

7.1 Introduction

Minimally invasive surgery represents a beneficial alternative to traditional surgical procedures for the implantation of medical devices, allowing for such procedures to be carried out through natural body cavities or small artificial incisions. In the past years, mini-invasive procedures have introduced novel therapeutic opportunities, with a significant improvement in quality of life and a decrease in health costs. Such improvements create new opportunities, but also new challenges, particularly for the materials.

Stimuli-responsive (SR) materials have a high potential in minimally invasive implant surgery, permitting the design of devices that can appropriately modify their macroscopic properties when receiving a stimulus by the human body. Among the SR materials, shape-memory polymers (SMPs) have the ability to "remember" a permanent shape, which can significantly differ from a functional temporary shape. The transition from the temporary to the permanent shape can be activated by an external stimulus, such as a temperature increase above the switching transition temperature (T_{trans}) of the polymer (Lendlein et al., 2010).

The thermally induced shape-memory effect has been described both for metal alloys and polymer systems. Shape-memory alloys (SMAs), primarily nickel-titanium alloys, have already been introduced in clinical practice (Yahia, 2000), whereas a number of shape-memory polymeric systems are described in literature (Lendlein and Langer, 2002; Metcalfe et al., 2003). Compared to SMAs, SMPs show the ability to recover larger deformations (up to 800%). In addition, SMPs offer other interesting properties, such as a good biocompatibility (Kim et al., 1996; Farè et al., 2005), low cost, and easy processability (Huang et al., 2011). Due to these advantageous properties, the development of SMPs is actively promoted and their use is being proposed in different areas for the design of innovative devices (Huang et al., 2011).

SMPs could be beneficially used in the fabrication of various medical devices, and in particular for minimally invasive applications. As an example, SMP stents can be preprogrammed to activate at body temperature, facilitating the delivery of larger devices through smaller transport vehicles, resulting in natural deployment with no

Shape Memory Polymers for Biomedical Applications. http://dx.doi.org/10.1016/B978-0-85709-698-2.00007-6

need for auxiliary devices and devoid of the adverse strain-hardening effects found in metal stent expansion (Yakacki et al., 2007).

Specifically tailored SMP foams are useful tools for the design of novel scaffolding biomedical devices. For instance, they would be profitable in the repair of bone defects, where a filler made of an SMP, and possibly carrying bioactive molecules, could be miniaturized and appropriately shaped so they can be introduced through a small diameter catheter in a compact (i.e., non-invasive) temporary shape and delivered in the site that needs to be repaired. When reaching the body temperature in situ, the filler would be able to expand, thus recovering a larger predetermined permanent shape, effectively filling the bone defect and releasing appropriate signals for bone cells recruitment.

Among the polymer systems with shape-memory properties that can be designed for this purpose, polyurethane copolymers are materials in which the transition temperature can be modified by specific tailoring of molecular parameters. Furthermore, physical and mechanical properties of shape-memory polyurethanes (SMPUs) can be customized by small changes in their chemical composition and structure, making it possible to combine the shape-memory properties with those required for a specific application (Li et al., 1997; Lin and Chen, 1998).

Pioneering work on shape-memory polyurethane foams has been performed by Hayashi and Sokolowski (Sokolowski et al., 1999, 2007; Tobushi et al., 2001), and their application in medical devices by the latter with L. H. Yahia (Metcalfe et al., 2003; Sokolowski et al., 2007; Tey et al., 2001). Such a preliminary work was based on cold hibernated elastic memory (CHEM), a polyurethane-based porous structure (Metcalfe et al., 2003; Sokolowski et al., 2007; Tobushi et al., 2001, 2004; Tey et al., 2001; Sokolowski, 2004). More recently, Lee et al. (Lee et al., 2007) proposed polyurethane flexible foams in which shape fixability and pore size can be tuned with no major effects on shape recoverability.

In this chapter, we describe some methods to prepare cellular solids made of SMPUs to be used in a minimally invasive approach for tissue repair in regenerative medicine.

Porosity is often obtained during the polyurethane synthesis by gas foaming. However, the shape-memory effect relies on the molecular architecture and results from a combination of polymer morphology and specific processing, being understood as a polymer functionalization (Behl and Lendlein, 2007).

Our work was aimed at obtaining porous structures with tunable thermo-mechanical properties via three different methods, based on conventional polymer processing: (i) co-extrusion with chemical blowing agents; (ii) co-extrusion with sodium chloride (NaCl), followed by salt particulate leaching; and (iii) solvent casting/particulate leaching (SC/PL).

The SMPUs selected were CaloMER™ and MM-4520 shape-memory polyurethanes. CaloMER™ is represented by a thermoplastic polyurethane copolymer system firstly developed by The Polymer Technology Group (PTG, Berkeley, CA, U.S.) with the idea that shape memory is triggered by a glass transition temperature ($T_{trans} = T_g$) that can be adjusted in the range of the body temperature. Heating above T_g activates shape-memory effects and produces a dramatic change in the elastic modulus

(White and Ward, 2002). MM-4520 is an aromatic polyetherurethane with shape-memory properties developed at the Nagoya R&D Center, Mitsubishi H.I. Ltd., Japan.

The obtained porous structures were compared to CHEM, a class of shape-memory polyurethane foams developed by Jet Propulsion Laboratory in cooperation with Mitsubishi H.I. Ltd. (Metcalfe et al., 2003).

Microscopy and micro-computed tomography (micro-CT) observations were performed to evaluate the morphological features of SMPU cellular solids. Thermo-mechanical and shape-memory recovery tests were carried out to correlate the properties of the obtained cellular solids with their morphological features. The effect of two recently introduced methods for sterilization (cold plasma and ozone) were analyzed, and preliminary tests on cytocompatibility of the selected cellular solids were performed with murine fibroblasts of the L929 cell line.

7.2 Methods for obtaining cellular solids

7.2.1 Porous materials by co-extrusion with foaming agents

Co-extrusion with chemical blowing agents, a conventional polymer processing, was applied for the design of CaloMER™ SMPU foams, as described in De Nardo et al., 2011.

Briefly, CaloMER™ 48 (C48) pellets, with a declared $T_{trans} = T_g = 48$ °C, were kindly provided by The Polymer Technology Group (PTG, Berkeley, CA, U.S.). The material was preconditioned for 48 h at 80 °C and porous samples were extruded into strips by a four-zone horizontal micro-extruder (GiMac Srl, Castronno, VA, Italy) with a coaxial screw. Different extrusion parameters were set up to obtain the optimal working conditions as described in De Nardo et al., 2011.

Two different foaming agents were used to obtain porous SMPU structures: Plastronfoam BSH and W16, provided by Ferroplast Srl (Vimodrone, MI, Italy). BSH is an endothermic multi-component blowing agent system, based on sodium bicarbonate and citric acid derivatives. W16 is composed of thermoplastic polymer shell microspheres encapsulating a liquid with a low boiling point. The foaming agents were mixed to C48 pellets before the extrusion process and the micro-extrusion process was optimized for weight fractions of 30% (w/w) for BSH and 4% and 12% (w/w) for W16.

7.2.2 Porous materials by co-extrusion/particulate leaching

This method consisted of co-extruding the SMPU with salt particles (usually sodium chloride), that after extrusion can be leached out by dissolution in an appropriate solvent (usually water), leaving pores inside the polymer matrix. The amount of salt and the size of the particles will determine the pore percentage and morphology.

CaloMER™ 48 pellets were mixed with NaCl salt crystals (200–400 μm size) previously desiccated and sifted with a metal sieve. The extrusion process was optimized for three weight fractions: 20%, 50%, and 70% w/w (C48 S20, C48 S50, and C48 S70, respectively). The blends were extruded into strips using the same four-heat-zone micro-extruder described above. Rectangular samples (2 mm width), for thermo-mechanical and shape recovery characterizations, and disks ($\phi = 5$ mm), for morphological observations, were cut out by manual die.

To remove NaCl, the extruded samples were immersed in distilled water in an ultrasonic bath for 48 h. The leaching procedure was optimized for a complete leaching out of the salt particles.

7.2.3 Porous material by solvent casting/particulate leaching (SC/PL)

In this method, microspheres are fabricated with a dispersion method and bonded together through a heat treatment to form a three-dimensional assembly in a mold. The selected polymer is dissolved in a suitable solvent and cast onto the microsphere assembly. The porous polymer scaffold is then formed by dissolving the microspheres in an appropriate solvent that does not dissolve the polymer itself.

Porous structures were produced by SC/PL using MM-4520 raw material (Mitsubishi H.I. Ltd), by a solvent casting/particulate leaching technique, using gelatin microspheres, according to a previously developed protocol (Draghi et al., 2005). Briefly, gelatin was dissolved in distilled water at a very high concentration, and the solution was added to a beaker containing soybean oil, heated up to 60 °C under stirring. After few minutes, the emulsion was cooled down to 15 °C in an ice bath, and gelatin microspheres were formed and then dehydrated by adding cold acetone. The microspheres were then removed from the soybean oil, washed several times with acetone, and dried. The microspheres were sieved to obtain two different size ranges: $\phi < 150$ μm (to be used for foams with smaller pores, MM-4520 SP), and 150 μm $< \phi <$ 400 μm (to be used for foams with larger pores, MM-4520 LP). The microspheres were then leveled in a glass mold to a 3 mm thickness. To attain their reciprocal adhesion, the mold was placed in an oven for 96 h at 50 °C and 95% relative humidity.

MM-4520 was dissolved in chloroform (3% w/v solution) and cast into a mold containing the previously compacted gelatin microspheres. After vacuum drying, 5 mm diameter cylindrical samples were punched out from the sheets before dissolving the porogen by washing the foams several times with deionized water. All samples were dried in air and kept in a desiccator until characterization.

7.2.4 Cold hibernated elastic memory foams

Two cold hibernated elastic memory foams (CHEM 3520, $T_g = 35$ °C, and CHEM 5520, $T_g = 55$ °C), were kindly provided by W. Sokolowski from Jet Propulsion Laboratory (Pasadena, CA, U.S.) and synthesized by Nagoya R&D Center, Mitsubishi H.I. (Nagoya, JP). CHEM are poly(ether urethane) foams produced by a gas-foaming process by adding to the polyurethane prepolymer a blowing agent together with the chain extender (Hayashi, 1991). Slices 3 mm thick were cut from the CHEM foams, and then 5 and 10 mm diameter samples were punched out for further characterization.

7.3 Morphological characterization

7.3.1 *Scanning electron microscopy (SEM)*

The porous morphology of the different samples was evaluated by scanning electron microscopy (SEM). Samples ($\phi = 5$ mm) were gold sputter coated (Edwards S150B) and observed at SEM (StereoScan 360, Cambridge) at 10 kV.

7.3.2 *Micro-computed tomography (micro-CT)*

The porous structures were analyzed with a 1172 micro-CT imaging system (Skyscan, Aartselaar, Belgium) desktop X-ray CT scanner, as previously described in De Nardo et al., 2011. The morphological characterization was performed using the software CTAn and CTvol (Skyscan, Aartselaar, Belgium) to evaluate scaffold porosity, average pore size, and pore interconnection.

7.3.3 *Results of morphological characterization*

7.3.3.1 SEM observations, co-extrusion with blowing agents

Co-extrusion with W16 blowing agent resulted in CaloMER™ samples with pores of 200–600 μm, poorly oriented along the extrusion axis (Figure 7.1a). The morphology of C48 samples extruded with BSH resulted in an anisotropic distribution of pore dimensions (50–600 μm), with a strong orientation along the longitudinal extrusion axis (Figure 7.1b).

7.3.3.2 SEM observations, co-extrusion/particulate leaching

By salt co-extrusion, it was possible to obtain a complete salt leaching with good pore interconnection only with a 70% w/w NaCl concentration. No preferential orientation of the pores was observed for these samples, the pore dimensions being in the range of 50–500 μm, with a homogeneous distribution within the polymer matrix. An example is shown in Figure 7.1c.

7.3.3.3 SEM observations, solvent casting/particulate leaching

By solvent casting/particulate leaching, the different size of gelatin microspheres ($\phi < 150$ μm and $\phi = 150$–400 μm) allowed us to obtain MM-4520 scaffolds with corresponding different pore dimensions, as shown in Figure 7.2. Both scaffolds showed a regular pore morphology, with pores of controlled dimensions and spherical shape.

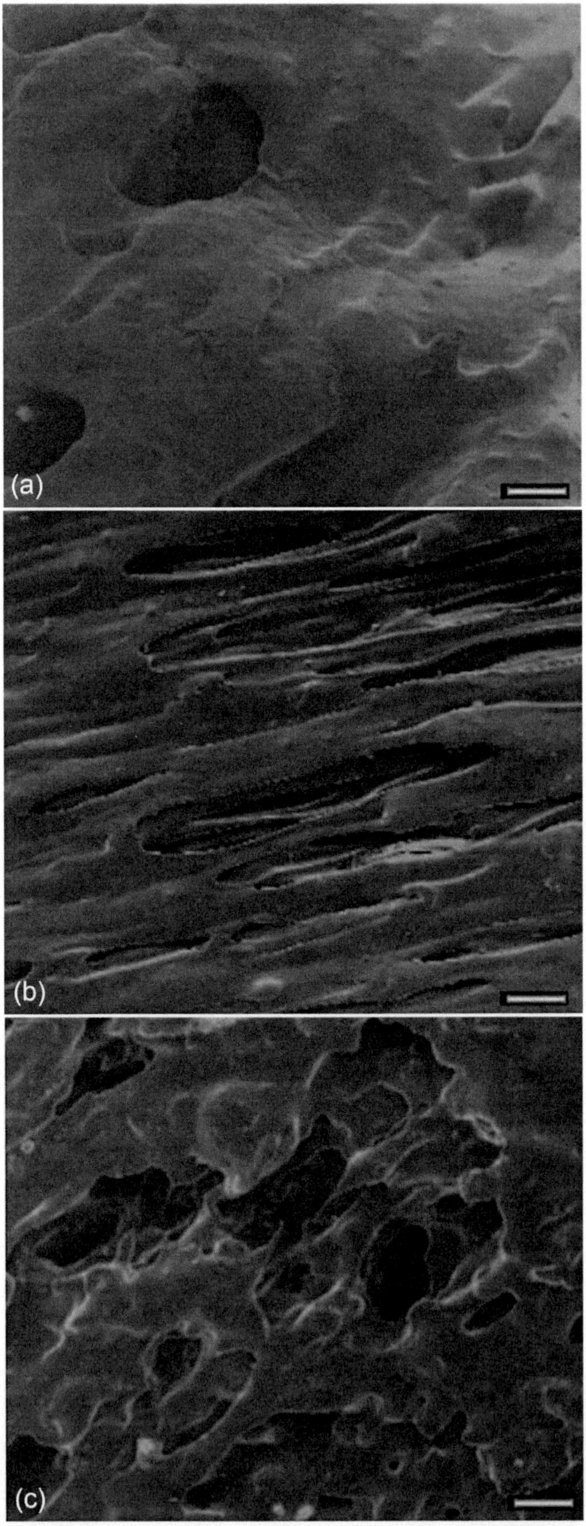

Figure 7.1 SEM micrographs of foams obtained by Calo·MER™ 48 co-extrusion with blowing agents (a: W16, b: BSH), and with 70% w/w salt co-extrusion (c) [b and c: © IOP Publishing. Reproduced with permission. All rights reserved]. Scale bar 200 μm.

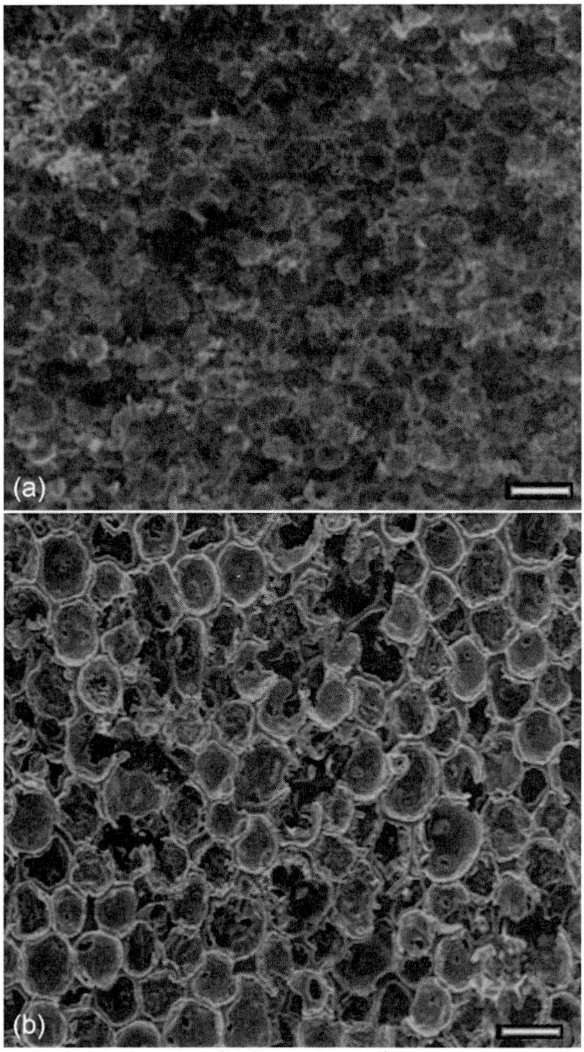

Figure 7.2 SEM micrographs of MM-4520 porous structures obtained via solvent casting/particulate leaching of gelatin microspheres $\phi < 150$ μm (a: smaller pores, MM-4520-SP) and $\phi = 150–400$ μm (b: larger pores, MM-4520-LP) [b: © IOP Publishing. Reproduced with permission. All rights reserved]. Scale bar 200 μm.

7.3.3.4 SEM observations, CHEM foams

CHEM foams exhibited a regular pore morphology, a large pore dimension distribution and thin pore walls. For both CHEM-3520 (Figure 7.3a) and CHEM-5520 (Figure 7.3b) the pores were found to be in the range of 200–600 μm.

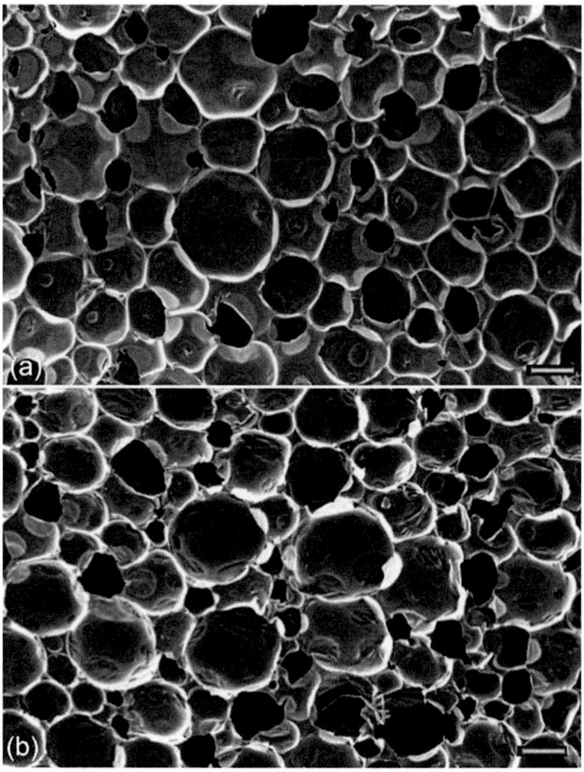

Figure 7.3 SEM micrographs of CHEM-3520 (a) and CHEM-5520 (b) foams. Scale bar 200 μm.

7.3.3.5 Micro-CT characterization

Data of percentage open porosity and pore size obtained by micro-CT for all the examined porous samples are presented in Figure 7.4.

7.3.4 Discussion

In our study, the results obtained by micro-CT characterization fit well with the morphological observations at SEM.

C48-based porous materials obtained by co-extrusion with blowing agents showed a low porosity, slightly higher for C48 BSH samples, either by micro-CT (Figure 7.4a) or SEM (Figure 7.1a and b). The porous structure of the foams was obtained by co-extrusion of C48 with blowing agents and their subsequent thermal decomposition during the transformation process.

With this procedure, it was generally difficult to control the pore size and the interconnectivity between the pores, as previously shown by Gomes et al., 2002.

In addition, a thin layer of solid material was observed to surround the porous inner structure of the material (Gomes et al., 2002).

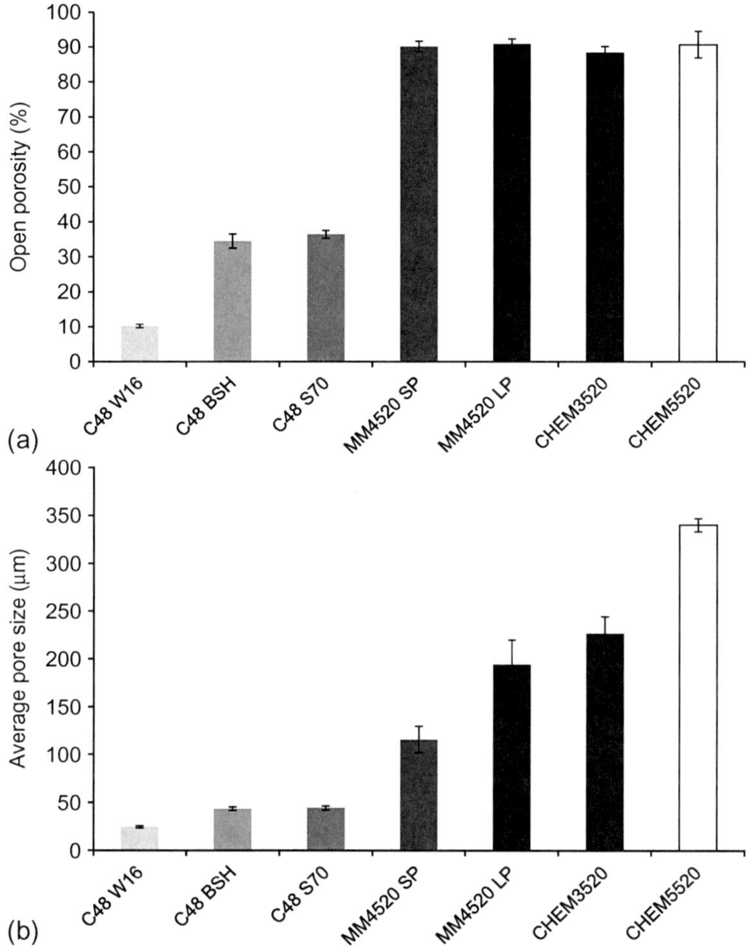

Figure 7.4 Open porosity and average pore size data obtained by micro-CT analyses.

A better control of the pore interconnection was achieved by co-extrusion/salt leaching. The resulting porosity was more evenly distributed, with an increase of pore interconnection with the increase of the salt/polymer ratio (De Nardo et al., 2011). Salt co-extrusion is a very simple processing method, even though particle leaching often results in a poor pore interconnection and irregular pore shape, as these critical variables are generally not controlled (Ma, 2004; De Nardo et al., 2010).

In both cases (chemical blowing agents or salt co-extrusion), specimens with small pores ($\phi < 50$ μm) were produced. This result can probably be related to the extrusion process, which does not allow for the growth of pores produced by the selected porogen agents.

For MM-4520 SP and MM-4520 LP, a correspondence between SEM observation and micro-CT results was detected as well. SEM micrographs (Figure 7.2) show the effect of the starting microsphere dimension on final pore dimensions. This result was also confirmed by the evaluation of pore size distribution performed by micro-CT, which detected a peak in the range of the size of gelatin microspheres, showing a homogenous pore distribution in comparison with the other porous structures. Moreover, the proposed method for microsphere leaching enabled an easy control of both porosity and pore interconnection (Figure 7.4). Such cellular solids with spherical pores are reasonably expected to improve fluid exchange and nutrient supply to cells due to their low flow resistance (Draghi et al., 2005).

Finally, the homogeneous pore distribution and the regular pore morphology of CHEM foams, qualitatively observed at SEM (Figure 7.3), was confirmed by the quantitative analysis of the average pore size distribution by micro-CT (Figure 7.4).

7.4 Physico-mechanical characterization

The use of thermally activated SMPs in the fabrication of biomedical devices can be based on two different approaches in terms of shape-memory activating forces: either the use of body temperature or an external heating source. The choice of one of these approaches affects both the device design and the material selection. The characterization of SMPs in terms of transition temperatures, mechanical properties, and shape-memory ability provides the basic information for exploiting their application.

In our work, the thermo-mechanical properties of the obtained porous structures were characterized by both dynamic mechanical analysis (DMA) and shape-memory recovery tests. DMA provides baseline state transition information for SMP materials (Gall et al., 2002), particularly in determining the temperature that activates the shape-memory recovery (T_{trans}). DMA provides some insights on the effects of porosity on the mechanical properties as well.

The shape-memory effect can be quantified by thermo-mechanical investigations. The tests are generally performed with a mechanical tester equipped with a thermo-chamber, and different test protocols can be used to evaluate the shape-memory ability.

A correct selection of the characterization procedure is a crucial point when designing such materials and structures. In our work, we performed the tests in different stress states (tension versus compression), similarly to DMA analyses.

7.4.1 Thermo-dynamic mechanical analyses

Dynamic mechanical analysis (DMA 290, TA Instrument) was performed in tensile mode for extruded CaloMER™ 48 samples. The samples were analyzed in the temperature range of 5–195 °C, as described in De Nardo et al., 2011, with a heating rate (H_R) of 1 °C min^{-1}, 1 Hz, and 15 μm strain application.

The DMA analyses were performed in compression mode for MM-4520 SP, MM-4520 LP, and CHEM foams in the temperature range of 0–180 °C (or until melting temperature), with a heating rate of 1 °C min^{-1}, 1 Hz, and 50 μm strain application, as described in De Nardo et al., 2009. The tests were duplicated, according to the standard practice ASTM 1640-99. Storage modulus (E'), loss modulus (E''), and Tan δ (Tan $\delta = E''/E'$) parameters were recorded, and T_g values were defined as the peak of Tan δ curve.

7.4.2 Shape-memory recovery tests

Shape-memory recovery tests were performed with the DMA analyzer, in tensile mode for CaloMER™ 48, in compression mode for MM-4520 SP, MM-4520 LP, and CHEM foams. In tensile mode, each specimen was heated to a temperature $T_H = 90$ °C above the transition temperature ($T_m > T_H > T_g = T_{trans}$) and stretched to $\varepsilon_m = 100\%$. While maintaining the strain constant (ε_m), the specimen was cooled down to $T_L = 15$ °C ($T_L < T_g$) to fix the temporary shape. At $T = T_L$, the stress was released and the specimen was initially allowed to recover to ε_u and then heated at a constant rate ($H_r = 1$ °C min^{-1}).

In compression mode, the samples were heated up to $T_H = T_g + 30$ °C, then compressed to $\varepsilon_m = 50\%$. While maintaining constant the strain (ε_m), the samples were cooled down to $T_L = T_g - 30$ °C to fix the temporary shape. At $T = T_L$ the stress was released; the samples were allowed to recover to ε_u and subsequently heated at a constant rate ($H_r = 1$ °C min^{-1}).

The shape-memory recovery tests were performed in triplicate.

The value of the recovered deformation as a function of temperature and the final deformation (ε_p) were recorded. The shape-memory properties of the material were quantified by determining the strain-recovery rate (R_r), the strain-fixity rate (R_f) and the recovery behavior as a function of temperature [R(T)], according to the following equations (Lendlein and Kelch, 2002):

$$R_r = \frac{\varepsilon_m - \varepsilon_p}{\varepsilon_m}, \tag{7.1}$$

$$R_f = \frac{\varepsilon_u}{\varepsilon_m}, \tag{7.2}$$

$$R(T) = \frac{\varepsilon(T) - \varepsilon_p}{\varepsilon_m}. \tag{7.3}$$

In (7.2), ε_u represents the deformation after the release of the stress, and it is a consequence of the fact that the resulting temporary shape always differs from the shape achieved by deformation (Lendlein and Kelch, 2002).

7.4.3 Results of the physico-mechanical characterization

Table 7.1 reports the most significant parameters obtained by the performed DMA and shape-memory recovery tests.

7.4.3.1 Co-extrusion with blowing agents

Dense C48 showed a thermal transition at about 190 °C and a substantial "overshoot" of Tan δ due to melting. This transition represents the stability limit of the reversible phase: at a higher temperature, it is possible to obtain a different permanent shape via conventional thermoplastic polymer processing technologies.

Table 7.1 Thermo-mechanical properties of SMPU porous structures obtained via DMA and shape-memory recovery (SMR) tests

Processing technique	Material	Type	DMA		SMR test
			T_g (°C)	T_m (°C)	R_r (%)
Co-extrusion/blowing agent	C48	Dense	82	187	56
		W16	61[a], 80[b]	187	53
		BSH	89	187	65
Co-extrusion/particulate leaching	C48	S70	89	188	76
Solvent casting/ particulate leaching	MM-4520	SP	51	—	74
		SL	48	—	95
Gas foaming	CHEM	3520	32	130	100
		5520	45	158	95

[a]First deconvoluted peak in Tan δ.
[b]Second peak in Tan δ.

C48 thermal properties were slightly affected in the case of co-extrusion with BSH blowing agent. In contrast, W16 blowing agent appeared to affect the T_{trans} of the material as two different peaks, partially overlapped, were detectable (Table 7.1). In both BSH and W16 foams, the melting transition temperature did not show significant differences compared to the control material.

The shape-memory behavior (Table 7.1) appeared to be improved by the presence of porosity: in particular, the final recovery R_r of the BSH-foam resulted in 65 versus 56% of the dense material.

7.4.3.2 Co-extrusion/particulate leaching

In the case of C48 S70 samples, in which the NaCl particles were completely leached out, the shape-memory behavior appeared to be improved by the presence of the pores. In particular, the final recovery R_r resulted to be 76%, versus 56% of the dense material (Table 7.1).

7.4.3.3 Solvent casting/particulate leaching (SC/PL)

The mechanical properties of the porous structures with small (MM-4520 SP, $\phi < 150$ μm) and large (MM-4520 LP, $\phi = 150$–400 μm) pores resulted to be two orders of magnitude lower than the extruded foams (E' values range from 1 GPa for C48 to 1 MPa for MM-4520, at T = 25 °C) due to the different hardness of the two investigated polymers. The transition temperatures were similar for the two porous structures, at about 50 °C. The scaffolds with larger porosity (LP) were characterized by a value of $R_r = 95\%$ as compared to 74% for the SP samples (Table 7.1).

7.4.3.4 CHEM foams

The mechanical properties of these foams lie between the extruded (C48-based) and SC/PL samples (MM-4520 based). A difference between the two CHEM foams was evident: both CHEM 3520 and CHEM 5520 showed the typical behavior of a semi-crystalline polymer, with glass transition values (calculated from peaks of Tan δ), respectively = 32 and 45 °C. Both cellular solids showed an optimal recovery ability, which resulted in $R_r = 100\%$ for CHEM 3520 and $R_r = 95\%$ for CHEM 5520.

7.4.4 Discussion and conclusions

C48, MM-4520, and CHEM are polyurethane-based SMPs: the differences in the obtained values of glass transition and melting temperatures can be correlated to both chemical composition and a different ratio between hard and soft segment domains. From Table 7.1, it is evident that the proposed materials and cellular solids span a wide range of transition temperatures, and that the 3D structures obtained via different processing methods resulted in a broad spectrum of size, dimension, distribution, and interconnection of pores, preserving their shape-memory properties.

In analyzing the effects of porosity on the thermal properties (T_g, T_m), variation in density seems to have a negligible effect (Table 7.1). However, in analyzing the effects of porosity on the mechanical properties, the thermo-mechanical behavior seems to strongly depend on the foam density, resulting in a lowering of the storage modulus.

As a general observation, the shape-memory recovery behavior seems to be affected by the porosity. Even though two different procedures of shape-recovery tests have been taken into account (tensile versus compression mode), depending on the specimen geometry, a clear trend in increased shape-recovery ability on increasing the foam porosity is evident (Table 7.1). However, a better understanding of the effects of porosity and pore interconnection on the recovery behavior will be reached by specifically designing the sample morphology and focusing on a particular base material.

7.5 Biocompatibility studies

7.5.1 Effect of the sterilization procedures

Sterilization is mandatory for biomedical devices, and a validation before their clinical use is necessary. In the selection of a sterilization technique among the currently used methods, it is important that the applied method does not adversely modify chemical and mechanical properties nor functionality and biocompatibility.

Traditional techniques hold limitations in terms of polymer stability (e.g., γ radiation and heat), treatment time, and patient/operator safety (e.g., ethylene oxide). To overcome these limitations, efforts have been made in developing new sterilization technologies. Plasma and ozone sterilizations, for instance, are currently employed in medical centers to decontaminate surgical equipment and devices.

The effects of plasma sterilization on chemico-physical and thermo-mechanical properties of polymers were studied by different authors (Moisan et al., 2001; Lerouge et al., 2002). On shape-memory polymers, plasma sterilization was found to determine surface oxidation with no evident effects on the thermo-mechanical behavior, but resulted in a reproducible cytotoxic response (Yakacki et al., 2008).

In our work, we studied the effects of plasma and ozone sterilization on chemico-physical, thermo-mechanical, and shape-memory recovery properties of two cold hibernated elastic memory (CHEM) shape-memory polyurethane foams.

7.5.1.1 Sterilization procedures

Cylindrical specimens ($\phi = 15$ mm) were punched from CHEM 3520 and CHEM 5520 foam slices (h = 10 mm) by a mechanical die. The obtained cylindrical specimens underwent either plasma (PL) or ozone (OZ) sterilization, according to indications of the manufacturer sterilization system. Plasma sterilization was performed in a Sterrad® system (100S, Johnson & Johnson), at the Istituto Nazionale per lo Studio e la Cura dei Tumori (MI, Italy), ozone sterilization was performed with a TSO3 system (125 L, TSO3 Inc. Québec, QC, Canada) at the Institut de Cardiologie de Montréal (Montreal, QC, Canada), as described by De Nardo et al. (De Nardo et al., 2010).

7.5.1.2 SEM analyses

Morphological characterization was carried out with a scanning electron microscopy (SEM EVO50EP, Zeiss) coupled with an energy dispersion X-ray spectroscopy for surface microanalyses (EDS, Oxford INCA 200). SEM images of plasma-sterilized foams showed a general increase of interconnections between the pores (Figure 7.5b and e) compared to the untreated CHEM (Figure 7.5a and d). Pore wall fractures were observed in plasma-treated foams whereas ozone sterilization resulted in a greater pore interconnection in both CHEM foams (Figure. 7.5c and f) in comparison to both control and plasma-sterilized samples. In addition, at higher magnification, submicrometric cracks were detected on the C3520-ozone sterilized samples. C5520-ozone sterilized samples (Figure 7.5f) showed more irregular profiles of interconnected pores, even if no cracks were observed on pore walls.

7.5.1.3 IR spectroscopy analyses

IR spectroscopy was performed with Nicolet FTIR 6700 spectrometer (Thermo Electron Co.) in ATR mode, using an ATR single bounce accessory and ZnSe crystal. ATR-FT IR spectra showed similar features for both CHEM foams, indicating the characteristic IR adsorption bands of poly(ether urethane)s, with no differences in chemical composition between the two materials.

After plasma and ozone sterilization, the presence of new bands was not detected. To investigate possible changes in phase separation at the surface of CHEM samples after sterilization, peak height analysis was performed (De Nardo et al., 2010). After plasma treatment, the peak height ratios related to both hard and soft segments showed a slight and uniform increase ($<5\%$). Because the ratio between non-hydrogen-bonded and free urethane carbonyls was unchanged versus control CHEM foams,

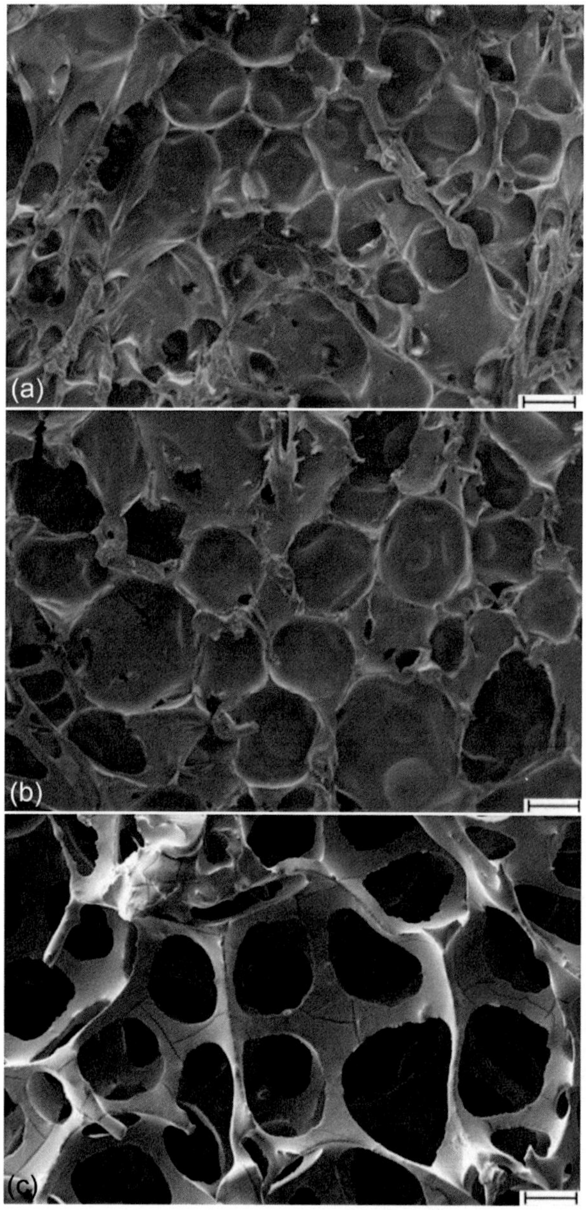

Figure 7.5 SEM micrographs of CHEM PU foams before and after plasma and ozone sterilization: (a) C3520, not sterilized, (b) C3520-PL, plasma sterilized, (c) C3520-OZ, ozone sterilized,

(Continued)

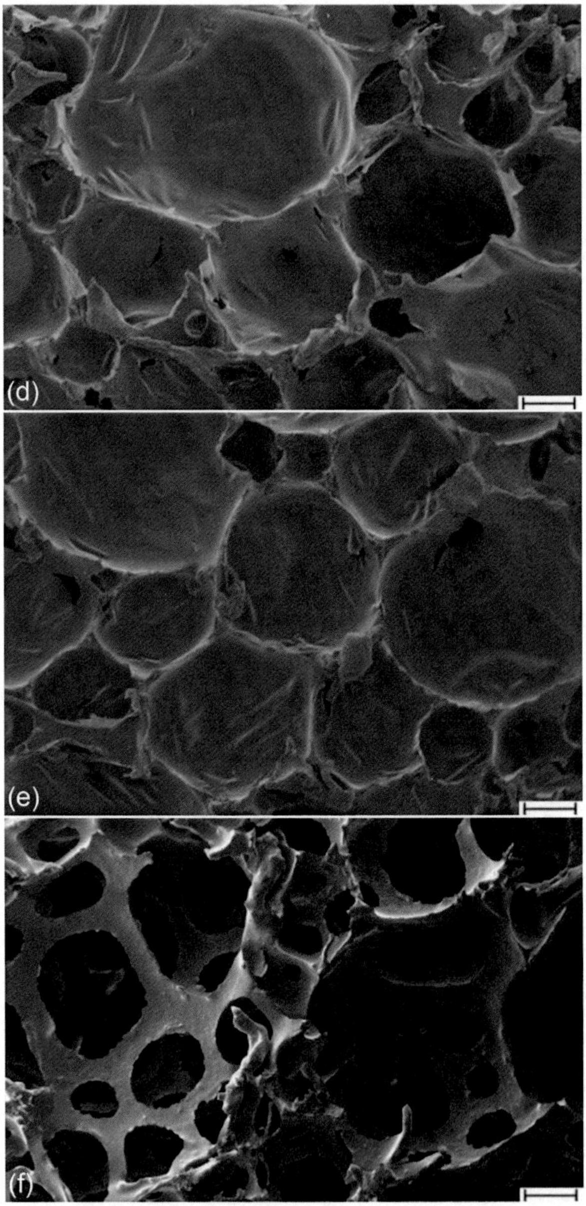

Figure 7.5 Continued. (d) C5520, not sterilized, (e) C5520-PL, plasma sterilized, (f) C5520-OZ, ozone sterilized. Scale bar = 100 μm.

it was assumed that the surface degradation was homogeneous. Conversely, ozone sterilization caused a noticeable change in all the considered peak ratios, related to both hard and soft segments, indicating a more extended phase separation on these samples, with rearrangement of hydrogen bonds.

7.5.1.4 HPLC analyses

To evaluate the possible release of low molecular weight substances from the material after the sterilization treatments, CHEM foam samples were incubated at 37 °C in phosphate-buffered saline (PBS, pH 7.4). HPLC analyses of the extracts at 2, 7, and 10 days for untreated and plasma-sterilized CHEM samples evidenced only the characteristic peak of the PBS salts; instead, chromatograms of ozone sterilized foams showed at each time point a new peak, representing a possible release of low-molecular-weight by-products.

7.5.1.5 Dynamic mechanical analysis (DMA)

DMA tests were performed in compression mode in the temperature range of 0–220 °C, with an amplitude of 50 μm at 1 Hz (DMA 2980 analyzer, TA Instrument). Shape-memory recovery tests were also performed in compression mode, as described in Section 7.4.2. The obtained results indicated that plasma sterilization had minor effects on dynamic mechanical properties as well as on transition temperatures, whereas ozone sterilization evidenced significant changes on thermo-mechanical properties (Table 7.2). Two main effects were observed after ozone sterilization: a downshift of T_g and the decrease of the rubbery plateau temperature range. The decrease in $T_{trans} = T_g$ was evident from the analysis of Tan δ, which showed a peak at 23 °C. Moreover, a downshift of melting temperature (T_m, Table 7.2) after ozone sterilization at 96 °C is evident (versus 130 °C detected for not sterilized C3520).

As expected, T_g value of C5520 foam is higher than C3520, even if CHEM 5520 foam displayed a difference between the T_g and the nominal value declared by the producer (45 versus 55 °C, respectively, Table 7.2). Effects of plasma sterilization on C5520 are negligible ($T_{trans} = T_g = 49$ °C), whereas a significant effect of ozone sterilization was detectable ($T_{trans} = T_g = 40$ °C), once again with a decrease of the T_{trans} value.

Table 7.2 Thermo-mechanical properties of CHEM foams before and after sterilization as evaluated by dynamic mechanical analysis (DMA) and shape-memory recovery (SMR) tests

		DMA		SMR test
Material	**Type**	T_g (°C)	T_m (°C)	R_r (%)
CHEM 3520	Control	32	130	100
	PL	32	117	100
	OZ	23	109	98
CHEM 5520	Control	45	158	90
	PL	49	137	89
	OZ	40	135	83

PL, plasma sterilization; OZ, ozone sterilization; SMR, shape memory recovery.

7.5.1.6 Shape-memory recovery tests

Results of shape-memory recovery tests on specimens before and after plasma and ozone sterilization are reported in Table 7.2. As for DMA analysis results, no evident differences between control and plasma sterilized samples were noticed. Conversely, C3520-ozone sterilized samples showed a different behavior: shape recovery began at 12 °C, reaching a $R_r = 98\%$ at 73 °C. For higher temperatures, the recovery decreased, resulting in a R_r lower than 94% at 100 °C.

CHEM 5520 presented a slower recovery, which occurred at higher temperatures. In fact, the shape-memory recovery began near 30 °C, and at 100 °C reached a value of about 90% (Table 7.2). In this case, the behavior of the recovery curve for ozone sterilized foams was similar to both control and plasma sterilized specimens. However, in this case, the final R_r was slightly lower (83% versus 89%, respectively for C5520-OZ and C5520-PL).

7.5.2 Evaluation of the *in vitro* interaction with cells

The *in vitro* cytotoxicity and cytocompatibility of CHEM foams were also preliminarily evaluated before and after sterilization, using murine fibroblasts of the L929 cell line (De Nardo et al., 2010). Only plasma-sterilized samples were selected due to the marked yellowing of the ozone-sterilized samples, coupled with the detection of a signal attributable to the release of low-molecular-weight substances in HPLC analyses of the PBS extracts.

7.5.2.1 Cytotoxicity tests

Briefly, *in vitro* cytotoxicity was assessed with the extracts obtained by immersing the CHEM foam samples in Dulbecco's Modified Eagle's Medium (DMEM), according to the standard practice ASTM F619. After 2 and 7 days of incubation, the extracts were added to the L929 cell culture (cell density $= 1 \times 10^5$ cells ml^{-1}), and the culture was prolonged for 48 h.

Cell viability was evaluated by MTT colorimetric biochemical assay (Sigma Tox-1 kit, Saint Louis, U.S.), that measures the activity of living cells via mitochondrial dehydrogenases. The absorbance measured at 570 nm was expressed as relative ratio over control cells cultured on tissue culture plastic (TCP).

The results of the MTT assay (Table 7.3) indicated, after 48 h, a not significant difference ($p > 0.05$) between control and plasma-sterilized CHEM samples, showing at both time points of incubation in DMEM very similar absorbance values. For this reason, *in vitro* cytocompatibility tests were performed only on plasma-sterilized samples (C3520-PL and C5520-PL).

7.5.2.2 Cytocompatibility tests

In vitro cytocompatibility was evaluated by seeding a L929 cell suspension (7.5 x 10^5 cell ml^{-1}, 100 μl/well) onto each CHEM foam sample ($n = 3$), and performing the culture in an incubator (5% CO_2, 37 °C) up to 7 days. Cell viability was assessed with the Alamar Blue® colorimetric assay (BUF012B, AbD Serotec,

Table 7.3 MTT absorbance values for L929 cells cultured in the presence of 2 and 7 days DMEM-extracts of untreated (control) and plasma sterilized (PL) CHEM foams

Material		2 days	7 days
CHEM 3520	Control	62.75 ± 3.44	86.93 ± 6.25
	PL	66.11 ± 3.39	93.52 ± 2.87
CHEM 5520	Control	55.67 ± 8.21	99.07 ± 4.80
	PL	56.77 ± 5.74	93.02 ± 6.04

Values are expressed as percentage versus control (culture medium, DMEM, only).

Oxon, UK) and cell morphology at SEM (SEM EVO50EP, Zeiss) at each time point (3 h, 1, 3 and 7 days after seeding). For SEM analyses, the samples were fixed with a glutaraldehyde solution in 0.1 M sodium cacodylate buffer (pH 7.2), dehydrated through a series of ethanol solutions (20–100% v/v ethanol in distilled water) and then air dried. The samples were gold-sputtered and observed at SEM at an accelerating voltage of 7.5 kV.

As shown in Figure 7.6, Alamar Blue assay demonstrated that 1 day after seeding, both CHEM foams and TCP (control) showed a similar cells viability; after 3 days, a general increase in cells activity was noticed ($p > 0.05$). After 7 days, the viability of cells cultured on C5520-plasma treated samples showed values almost four times higher than TCP ($p < 0.05$); compared to the values observed at 3 days, cell viability increased significantly ($p < 0.05$) also in the case of C3520-plasma treated.

The results of Alamar Blue assay were confirmed by SEM analyses. For C3520-PL samples, the few cells observed after 1 day (Figure 7.7a) began to spread and colonize the foam after 3 days (Figure 7.7b), and a homogeneous distribution of the cells, with a good spreading onto the pore walls, could be detected after 7 days (Figure 7.7c).

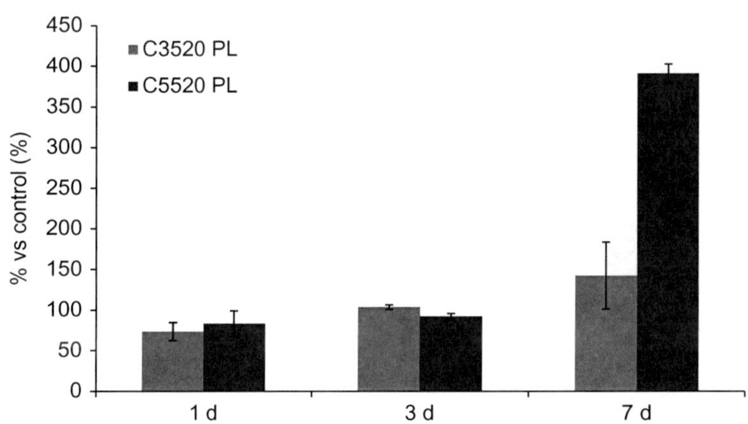

Figure 7.6 Alamar Blue values for L929 cells seeded onto plasma sterilized (PL) CHEM foams and cultured for 1, 3, and 7 days. Values are expressed as percentage versus control (TCP).

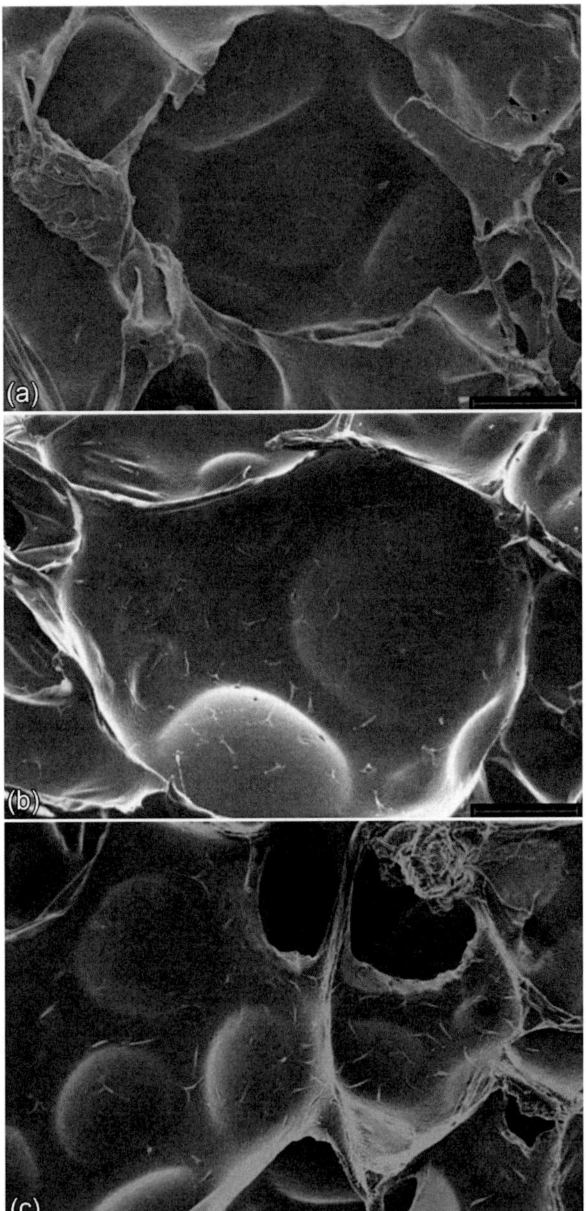

Figure 7.7 SEM micrographs of L929 cells seeded on plasma-sterilized CHEM foams and cultured for up to 7 days. (a) C3520-PL, 24 h, (b) C3520-PL, 3 days, (c) C3520-PL, 7 days,

(Continued)

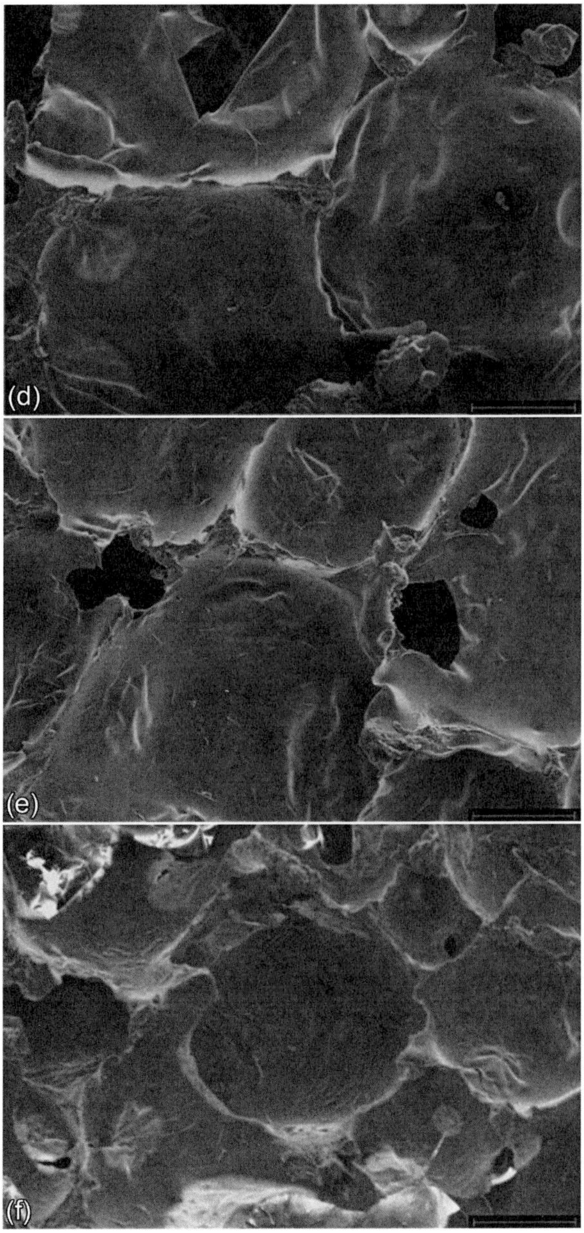

Figure 7.7 Continued. (d) C5520-PL, 24 h, (e) C5520-PL, 3 days, (f) C5520-PL, 7 days. Scale bar = 200 μm.

The behavior of L929 cells cultured on C5520-PL samples was similar to that observed on C3520-PL (Figure 7.7d, e and f), with a higher number of spherical cells at 3 days and completely colonized pore walls at 7 days.

7.5.3 Conclusions

In conclusion, in our studies, plasma and ozone sterilization were shown to affect the morphological and chemico-physical properties of both shape-memory CHEM foams, even though these properties were more severely affected by ozone sterilization (De Nardo et al., 2010).

Ozone sterilization induced both chemical and morphological changes that affected the shape-memory recovery behavior of CHEM samples; surface oxidation was indicated by ATR-IR analyses and visually confirmed by a strong yellowing of ozone-sterilized CHEM foams. Considering also the release of possible cytotoxic substances, as indicated by HPLC analysis of the extracts from ozone-sterilized samples, these samples were not tested for cytocompatibility.

However, ozone sterilization appears promising for a practical hospital use, and a specific sterilization procedure for polyurethanes and cellular solids should be intentionally developed.

For plasma sterilization, the observed increase of pore interconnection can be explained by the exposition of the porous samples to variable pressures during the sterilization cycle. However, the plasma treatment did not seem to affect both thermo-mechanical and shape-memory recovery properties. Cell proliferation tests showed that the selected CHEM 3520 and CHEM 5520 SMPUs were non-cytotoxic and highly cytocompatible after plasma sterilization.

As for the other SMPU cellular solids obtained by co-extrusion and gas foaming described here, the processing parameters should be optimized to obtain porosity values adequate for promoting cell colonization and therefore for cytocompatibility evaluation.

MM-4520 SMPU porous structures obtained by solvent casting/NaCl leaching, instead, showed a good and very interconnected porosity. MM-4520-SP and MM-4520-LP were preliminarily tested for *in vitro* cytocompatibility, demonstrating an ability to support *in vitro* cell adhesion and proliferation without cytotoxic effect (De Nardo et al., 2012). However, at this point they have not undergone ozone or plasma sterilization.

Additional studies aimed at a correct selection of advanced biomaterials, such as shape-memory polyurethanes, and at designing novel devices for minimally invasive surgery applications, should be performed, as requested by the growing clinical demand.

Acknowledgments

The authors acknowledge the sources of the text that they have used for preparing this work, namely: IOP Publishing Ltd, UK; Elsevier Ltd, UK; Trans Tech Publications Ltd, Switzerland; Springer Science + Business Media LLC (Springer).

References

Behl, M., Lendlein, A., 2007. Shape-memory polymers. Mater. Today 10, 20–28.

De Nardo, L., Alberti, R., Cigada, A., Yahia, L.H., Tanzi, M.C., Farè, S., 2009. Shape memory polymer foams for cerebral aneurysms preparation: effects of plasma sterilization on physical properties and cytocompatibility. Acta Biomater. 5, 1508–1518.

De Nardo, L., Moscatelli, M., Silvi, F., Tanzi, M.C., Farè, S., 2010. Chemico-physical modifications induced by plasma and ozone sterilizations on shape memory polyurethane foams. J. Mater. Sci. Mater. Med. 21, 2067–2078.

De Nardo, L., Bertoldi, S., Tanzi, M.C., Haugen, H.J., Farè, S., 2011. Shape memory polymer cellular solid design for medical applications. Smart Mater. Struct. 20, 035004.

De Nardo, L., Bertoldi, S., Cigada, A., Tanzi, M.C., Haugen, H.J., Farè, S., 2012. Preparation and characterization of shape memory polymer scaffolds via solvent casting/particulate leaching. J. Appl. Biomater. Funct. Mater. 10, 119–126.

Draghi, L., Resta, S., Pirozzolo, M.G., Tanzi, M.C., 2005. Microspheres leaching for scaffold porosity control. J. Mater. Sci. Mater. Med. 16, 1093–1097.

Farè, S., Valtulina, V., Petrini, P., Alessandrini, E., Pietrocola, G., Tanzi, M.C., Speziale, P., Visai, L., 2005. In vitro interaction of human fibroblasts and platelets with a shape-memory polyurethane. J. Biomed. Mater. Res. A 73, 1–11.

Gall, K., Dunn, M.L., Liu, Y., Finch, D., Lake, M., Munshi, N.A., 2002. Shape memory polymer nanocomposites. Acta Mater. 50, 5115–5126.

Gomes, M.E., Godinho, J.S., Tchalamov, D., Cunha, A.M., Reis, R.L., 2002. Alternative tissue engineering scaffolds based on starch: processing methodologies, morphology, degradation and mechanical properties. Mater. Sci. Eng. C 20, 19–26.

Hayashi, S., 1991. Shape memory polymer foam, US Patent Specification 5,049,591. 1991-Sep-17.

Huang, W.H., Yang, B., Fu, Y.Q., 2011. Polyurethane Shape Memory Polymers. CRC, Boca Raton.

Kim, B.K., Lee, S.Y., Xu, M., 1996. Polyurethane having shape memory effects. Polymers 37, 5781–5793.

Lee, S.H., Jang, M.K., Kim, S.H., Kim, B.K., 2007. Shape memory effects of molded flexible polyurethane foam. Smart Mater. Struct. 16, 2486–2491.

Lendlein, A., Kelch, S., 2002. Shape-memory polymers. Angew Chem. Int. Edn. 41, 2034–2057.

Lendlein, A., Langer, R., 2002. Biodegradable, elastic shape-memory polymers for potential biomedical applications. Science 296, 1673–1676.

Lendlein, A., Behl, M., Hiebl, B., Wischke, C., 2010. Shape-memory polymers as a technology platform for biomedical applications. Expert Rev. Med. Devices 7, 357–379.

Lerouge, S., Tabrizian, M., Wertheimer, M.R., Marchand, R., Yahia, L.H., 2002. Safety of plasma-based sterilization: surface modifications of polymeric medical devices induced by Sterrad and Plazlyte processes. Bio-Med. Mater. Eng. 12, 3–13.

Li, F., Zhang, X., Hou, J., Xu, M., Luo, X., Ma, D., Kim, B.K., 1997. Studies on thermally stimulated shape memory effect of segmented polyurethanes. J. Appl. Polym. Sci. 64, 1511–1516.

Lin, J.R., Chen, L.W., 1998. Study on shape-memory behavior of polyether based polyurethanes. I. Influence of the hard-segment content. J. Appl. Polym. Sci. 69, 1563–1574.

Ma, P.X., 2004. Scaffolds for tissue fabrication. Mater. Today 7, 30–40.

Metcalfe, A., Desfaits, A.C., Salazkin, Y., Yahia, L.H., Sokolowski, W.M., Raymond, J., 2003. Cold hibernated elastic memory foams for endovascular interventions. Biomaterials 24, 491–497.

Moisan, M., Barbeau, J., Moreau, S., Pelletier, J., Tabrizian, M., Yahia, L.H., 2001. Low-temperature sterilization using gas plasmas: a review of the experiments and an analysis of the inactivation mechanisms. Int. J. Pharm. 226, 1–21.

Sokolowski, W.M., 2004. Cold hibernated elastic memory self-deployable and rigidizable structure and method therefore, US Patent Specification 6,702,976. 2004-Mar-09.

Sokolowski, W.M., Chmielewski, A.B., Hayashi, S., Yamada, T., 1999. Cold hibernated elastic memory (CHEM) self-deployable structures. Proc. SPIE—Int. Soc. Opt. Eng. 3669, 179–185.

Sokolowski, W., Metcalfe, A., Hayashi, S., Yahia, L.H., Raymond, J., 2007. Medical applications of shape memory polymers. Biomed. Mater. 2, S23–S27.

Tey, S.J., Huang, W.M., Sokolowski, W.M., 2001. Influence of long-term storage in cold hibernation on strain recovery and recovery stress of polyurethane shape memory polymer foam. Smart Mater. Struct. 10, 321–325.

Tobushi, H., Okumura, K., Endo, M., Hayashi, S., 2001. Thermomechanical properties of polyurethane-shape memory polymer foam. J. Intell. Mater. Syst. Struct. 12, 283–287.

Tobushi, H., Matsui, R., Hayashi, S., Shimada, D., 2004. The influence of shape-holding conditions on shape recovery of polyurethane-shape memory polymer foams. Smart Mater. Struct. 13, 881.

White, K.A., Ward, R.S., 2002. Softenable, shape-memory thermoplastic for biomedical applications. Trans. 28th Ann. Meet. Soc. Biomater. 25, 671.

Yahia, L., 2000. Shape Memory Implants. Springer, Berlin.

Yakacki, C.M., Shandas, R., Lanning, C., Rech, B., Eckstein, A., Gall, K., 2007. Unconstrained recovery characterization of shape-memory polymer networks for cardiovascular applications. Biomaterials 28, 2255–2263.

Yakacki, C.M., Lyons, M.B., Rech, B., Gall, K., Shandas, R., 2008. Cytotoxicity and thermo mechanical behavior of biomedical shape memory polymer networks post-sterilization. Biomed. Mater. 3, 15010.

Thiol-ene/acrylate systems for biomedical shape-memory polymers

8

T. Javanbakht[1], *W. Sokolowski*[2]
[1]Biomedical Engineering Institute, Ecole Polytechnique, Montreal, QC, Canada; [2]California Institute of Technology, Pasadena, CA, USA

8.1 Introduction

Thiol-ene/acrylate photopolymers are one of the most commonly used shape-memory polymer (SMP) systems that have significant thermo-mechanical properties due to their polymerization mechanism. Their homogeneous networks, toughness, and flexibility in comparison to the acrylic systems make them appropriate candidates for diverse applications, such as in biomedical and electronic research (Nair et al., 2010; Kasprzak et al., 2009). On the other hand, the acrylates are desirable for their relatively low cost, ready availability, ease of monomer synthesis and polymer manufacture and processing, rapid polymerization kinetics, optical clarity, toughness, and potential biocompatibility (Sawhney et al., 1993; West and Hubbell, 1995).

The thiol-ene reaction was first suggested by Posner in 1905 (Posner, 1905). In the last two decades, the advantages of thiol-ene reaction mechanism over acrylate polymerization have been discovered. For example, the shrinkage stress of thiol-ene SMPs is low (Lu et al., 2005). Other advantages are that they have no oxygen inhibition (Jacobine, 1993; O'Brien et al., 2006; Lu et al., 2005) but high optical clarity. The thiol-ene reaction has a unique characteristic: various chemical groups (e.g., phenolic rings, ethylene glycol groups, ester groups) can be incorporated into the main chain backbones (Kasprzak et al., 2009). Kharasch and his colleagues were the first researchers to propose the thiol-ene polymerization reaction (Kharasch et al., 1938). Several studies have previously been carried out on the reaction kinetics of thiol-ene/acrylate systems. A thiol-ene system composed of stoichiometrically mixed triallyl-1,3,5-triazine-2,4,6-trione (TATATO) and pentaerythritol tetra(3-mercaptopropionate) (PETMP) was compared with a dimethacrylate (Lu et al., 2005), revealing that the polymerization of stoichiometrically mixed PETMP/TATATO occurred at a much higher rate and significantly higher functional group conversion than the dimethacrylate system. In another study, Cramer and Bowman (2001) showed that for thiol-ene polymerizations, the conversion of ene functional groups was greater than that of thiol functional groups. The studies on the thermo-mechanical properties of these polymers have been focused on the effect of acrylate structure on the properties of various ternary

Shape Memory Polymers for Biomedical Applications. http://dx.doi.org/10.1016/B978-0-85709-698-2.00008-8

copolymers as well as those of monomer structure on these systems formed via mixed-mode polymerization (Jacobine et al., 1992; Hoyle et al., 2004; Kasprzak et al., 2009).

The glass transition temperature (T_g) and rubbery modulus (E_r) of acrylates can be tailored independently to suit a particular application. Hence, these polymers are also used as SMPs (Gall et al., 2005; Ortega et al., 2008). Several studies on the memory effect of thiol-ene polymers showed the possibility of tailoring these systems to fit bone defects and maintain the tailored shape (Nair et al., 2010).

Thiol-ene polymers have great potential for biomedical applications, such as in drug delivery and tissue engineering (Xiao et al., 2011; Zhang et al., 2012; Shih and Lin, 2013). They can be used as catheters and vascular stents for accurate manipulation by a physician. Their application as orthopedic braces and splints has also been investigated. The deformation capacity of these materials has made them good candidates for dental application (Sokolowski et al., 2007).

The effects of temperature on a step-growth photopolymerization with small amounts of chain growth reactions has been studied (Johnson et al., 2008). The authors reported that the ene chain growth conversion was separated from the step-growth polymerization, which allowed for analysis of chain growth within a predominately step-growth polymerization. They added this gradient to previous techniques in order to make the effects of composition, temperature, and exposure time on photopolymerization kinetics assessable. This technique provides new possibilities to explore multiple factors in a short period of time as well as fundamental and practical information.

In this chapter, Sections 8.2 and 8.3 discuss the properties of thiol-ene/acrylate photopolymers and techniques for activating the memory effect. Medical applications for these systems are presented in Section 8.4. Section 8.5 presents conclusions and outlines.

8.2 Properties of thiol-ene/acrylate photopolymers

The thermo-physical properties of ternary thiol-ene/acrylate systems are influenced by the chemical structure of their acrylate monomer. A research team has studied these properties as well as the tensile properties of these polymers (Senyurt et al., 2007). They carried out the analysis of the mechanical relaxation spectra and the nondestructive impact energy absorption in order to establish a relationship between the chemical structure of the monomers and the mechanical properties of the final cross-linked networks. The control of the material properties was achieved by adjusting the composition of the ternary systems. They showed that all samples break in a brittle manner without yielding, and elongations are low (10–15%) due to the thermoset nature of the matrices.

8.2.1 Thermo-mechanical properties

Thiol-ene/acrylate systems behave as lightly cross-linked elastomers at the very verge of the thermoset-thermoplastic limit. At low concentrations, they are not solid enough for handling. Therefore, matching cross-linker concentrations are necessary for these materials. The "copolymer effect" and "cross-linking effect" are two concurrent effects that contribute to the resulting T_g values of networks formed by various compositions of chemically different monomers (Fox and Loshaek, 1955; Kannurpatti et al., 1998). The cross-linking effect can increase T_g and E_r as the cross-linker concentration is increased. These increases can also influence the cross-link density (Kasprzak et al., 2009). The value of T_g of a network can be raised or lowered by the copolymer, depending on the chemical rigidity of the monomers being added and subtracted. According to the ideal rubber theory (Treloar, 1958), the rubbery modulus is inversely proportional to the average molecular weight between cross-links, or directly proportional to the cross-link density. Non-ideal (meth)acrylate networks also have this mechanical property (Ortega et al., 2008). In addition, the incorporation of a monomer via the thiol-ene reaction raises the T_g of the polymer by the copolymer effect. In this case, the added monomer simply acts as a linear chain extender, and the homopolymerization route raises T_g and E_r due to both the copolymer and the cross-linking effects. If the vinyl groups exist in the structure of the copolymer, the value of E_r will decrease (Kasprzak et al., 2009).

8.2.2 Strengths/limitations

SMPs have some strengths and limitations that are important to consider. A research on these materials revealed that higher concentrations of cross-linker reduce strain at failure but increase stress at failure (Ortega et al., 2008). This behavior is due to their cross-link density. The macromolecular motion of the network is restricted by higher concentrations of cross-linker, which increases the network's load-carrying capacity. Moreover, increased cross-link density generally means increased network heterogeneity. The increased probability of a stress concentration arising corresponds to a densely cross-linked area, which causes a premature failure.

The monomer chemistry plays an important role in the network toughness of SMPs and their stress–strain behavior. The toughness of the polymers having rings in their structure is much higher than those lacking rings because of the ringed members within their monomer (Safranski and Gall, 2008).

Strain and stress at failure are strongly related to the network structure and the density of cross-linking (Ortega et al., 2008). Although the difference in the polymerization reactions are important, the overall mechanical effect of cross-linking a polymer results in similar system behaviors at T_g. More cross-linking (lower T/E_r) results in a higher stress at failure due to the increased load-carrying capacity of the cross-link points, and less cross-linking (higher T/E_r) gives little strength but significant deformability.

Thiol-ene coupling has the advantage of high yields and simplified purification requirements. Killops et al. (2008) synthesized high purity dendrimers using an accelerated procedure without the need for chromatographic purification or protecting groups. Using a combination of thiol-ene chemistry and traditional Grignard-based growth steps for carbosilanes, Rissing and Son (2009) synthesized carbosilane-thioether dendrimers. They also demonstrated that thiol-ene coupling is an ideal reaction despite the high synthetic demands of dendritic systems.

Thiol-ene coupling is a highly efficient reaction and can be used for polymer functionalization. In addition, the orthogonality of the process has permitted the chemists to use a range of starting materials from commodity polymers, such as polybutadiene homopolymers, copolymers and block copolymers, tomethacrylate- and styrenic-based systems, and poly(ethylene glycol) (PEG). For example, Gress et al. (2007) carried out the polymer functionalization by thiol-ene addition, taking advantage of a poly(oxazoline) derivative with alkene side groups prepared by cationic ring opening polymerization (ROP). This kind of reaction is based on the ability to attach a wide array of thiols onto the polymer backbone. David and Kornfield (2008) also developed a synthetic protocol in order to prepare a variety of functionalized polybutadienes. In another study, Campos et al. (2008) synthesized the styrenic, methacrylic, and caprolactone monomers, each bearing alkene-functionalities that could be combined with functional initiators and postpolymerization modifications by moving away from backbone functionalization. This reaction increased the range and architectural position of orthogonal groups, which can be built into macromolecular systems.

The ability to functionalize nanoscale objects is another important advantage of thiol-ene reactions (Polizzotti et al., 2008; Johnson et al., 2008). The authors have reported that the orthogonality between CuAAC and thiol-ene coupling allowed for the introduction of unreacted alkenes throughout the resulting hydrogel. The functionalization of alkenes was carried out by photochemical thiol-ene reaction, enabling photopatterning of the material using a variety of thiols. In another study, a multilayer coating was constructed on the surface of a silica nanoparticle (Connal et al., 2009). This layer-by-layer approach was used by alternating deposition of poly(vinyl pyrrolidone) and poly(methacrylic acid), the latter containing either alkene or thiol functional groups. The authors attached alkene-terminated PEG chains to cross-linked multilayer structures, thereby changing the surface chemistry and creating protein-resistant particles. They took advantage of the high tolerance of the reaction that allowed excess unreacted thiol or alkene units to be involved in secondary thiol-ene reactions.

8.3 Techniques for activating the memory effect

The memory effect of thiol-ene/acrylate SMPs needs to be activated by the external stimulus. The researchers (Nair et al., 2010; Bowman et al., 2011) had conducted comprehensive studies, testing, and evaluating the photopolymerized thiol-ene SMP systems for potential medical applications. The thiol-ene systems examined were designed to respond to temperature changes as the stimulus for their shape change.

Five different thiol-ene polymer systems were evaluated in comparison with a conventional acrylic polymer shape-memory system as a control (Nair et al., 2010). The polymer systems chosen for the study were significantly different in their network structures, although all exhibited glass transition temperatures in the range of 30–40 °C, making them suitable for thermally induced biomedical shape-memory applications. To obtain thiol-ene polymer systems with T_gs near physiological temperature, a tri-thiol (trimethylolpropane tris(3-mercaptopropionate)) and a tri-ene, TATATO resin was formulated. The authors demonstrated that thiol-ene-based SMP systems can be tailored to exhibit a wide range of polymer mechanical properties suitable for biomedical applications. Upon thermal stimulation, the thiol-ene polymer systems exhibited a more rapid and distinct shape-memory response as well as improved shape retention as compared to the control system.

The original shape of the medical devices made of thiol-ene polymers can be deformed or crushed into a temporary shape having a reduced profile to facilitate insertion into a vessel, lumen, or other aperture or cavity (Bowman et al., 2011). After insertion, the device can self-expand to assume a deployed configuration. The medical device may assume its deployed configuration due to changes in temperature, hydration, changes in other physiological conditions, or combinations of these parameters.

In general, the non-biodegradable polymer does not include aromatic and ester groups that are readily hydrolyzed at physiological pH and temperature (Bowman et al., 2011).

In thiol-ene systems, one or more of the monomers can be biodegradable and degrade by hydrolysis, exposure to water, or enzymes under physiological conditions. The system can be configured to degrade or dissolve with time. The onset of degradation may be configured to occur upon the delivery of some external stimulus, such as heat and/or light. Alternatively, the system may be configured such that the degradation begins at some preset time after deployment.

8.4 Medical applications of thiol-ene/acrylate photopolymers

Recently, some medical applications have been considered and investigated for thiol-ene/acrylate SMPs. These polymers were found to be biocompatible; the glass transition temperature (T_g) can be tailored for shape restoration/self-deployment of clinical devices when attached or inserted in the human body (Nair et al., 2010). In addition, the thiol-ene systems offer a unique combination of properties that are advantageous for SMP systems, including rapid polymerization, low volume shrinkage and shrinkage stress, the formation of homogeneous networks, and insensitivity to oxygen inhibition.

The thiol-ene/acrylate SMP medical devices may take a variety of forms. They can be miniaturized and deformed, inserted in the human body through small catheters, and subsequently recover a larger predetermined shape once they are in a satisfactory position (Lendlein and Kelch, 2002; Sokolowski et al., 2007). This SMP-based medical device technology provides a simple end-to-end process for storage and deployment and avoids the complexities associated with other methods for deployment of medical devices (Sokolowski et al., 2007).

The nondegradable thiol-ene systems, as a lifetime implant, could be used in a variety of different biomedical applications, such as vascular and coronary grafts, and medical prosthetics (Bowman et al., 2011).

The inherent material advantages of degradable thiol-ene systems and biomedical applications, such as drug delivery and tissue engineering, are described in the following sections.

8.4.1 Drug-delivery systems

The thiol-ene reaction has gained great research interest in the functionalization of polymers.

A recent effort has been to prepare and utilize the polymer carriers for platinum drugs. However, the side effects of small molecule platinum-based antitumor drugs narrowed their clinical use.

To reduce the toxicities of the platinum drugs, thiol-ene polymers were investigated for use as a drug-delivery carrier for protection from blood clearance and protein binding (Xiao et al., 2011). A biodegradable and amphiphilic copolymer, mPEG-b-P (LA-co-MAC/TMA), that contained pendant 1,2-bidentate carboxyl groups was synthesized by thiol-ene radical addition. It was further used to chelate with the active anticancer species (DACH-Pt) of oxaliplatin to form an mPEG-b-P(LA-co-MAC/TMA-Pt-DACH) complex. The polymer platinum complex self-assembled into micelles, showed acid-responsive drug-release kinetics beneficial to the drug release under intracellular environment. The authors showed *in vitro* evaluation that the DACH-Pt micelles displayed enhanced or comparable cytotoxicity against SKOV-3 and MCF-7 cancer cells, while they displayed reduced toxicity to HeLa cells compared with oxaliplatin. These DACH-Pt micelles are a polymeric prodrug of DACH-Pt for cancer therapy. They are more effective for SKOV-3 and other cancers. Moreover, the synthetic method of employing thiol-ene reaction to functionalize a biodegradable and amphiphilic polymer used in this study could be also utilized in other drug-delivery systems and biomedical materials.

Some research has been done on the modification of cyclodextrins (CDs) via thiol-ene reaction (Zhang et al., 2012). Cyclodextrins are cyclic oligosaccharides composed of cx-1,4-linked o-glucopyranose units and have been used in drug delivery due to their ability to form inclusion complexes with guest molecules (Uekama et al., 1998; Harada et al., 1992). The thiol-ene reaction has attracted interest due to its facile and versatile process, which fulfills the basic requirements of a click reaction.

Zhang et al. (2012) reported the modification of CD-centered star polymers via a combination of thiol-ene click and ROP. The synthesis of CD was conducted via thiol-ene addition of per-6-thio-β-cyclodextrin (CD-$(SH)_7$) with vinyl terminated polymers. The obtained thiol-ene product was employed as an initiator for ROP of ε-caprolactone. Different CD-centered macromolecular architectures and star polymers have been prepared by authors through the combination of catalytic chain transfer polymerization (CCTP), ROP, and thiol-ene click reaction. This approach introduced the thiol-ene click reaction into modification of CD for polymer synthesis and authors decided to continue the future studies on synthesis of miktoarm star polymers and polymers covalently attached to CD.

8.4.2 Tissue engineering

Radical-initiated photopolymerizations have received significant attention for *in situ* cell encapsulation and controlled delivery of biological molecules (Quick et al., 2004; Mellott et al., 2001).

Shih and Lin (2013) reported a visible-light-mediated thiol-ene hydrogelation scheme using eosin-Y as the only photoinitiator. Under visible light exposure, rapid and highly tunable step-growth gelation was achieved using PEG-norbornene and a model cross-linker dithiothreitol. In addition to investigating the gelation kinetics and properties of thiol-ene hydrogels formed by this new gelation scheme, the authors accomplished a high cytocompatibility of these hydrogels using human mesenchymal stem cells and pancreatic MIN6 β-cells (Shih and Lin, 2013).

In another research, Rydholm et al. (2005) investigated the thiol-acrylate photopolymers, and their polymerization and degradation behavior of the *in situ*-forming biomaterial. The degradable thiol-acrylate photopolymers were capable of rapidly polymerizing under physiological conditions upon exposure to UV light, with or without added photoinitiators and to depths exceeding 10 cm. The materials were formed *in situ*, and the versatility of their chemistry allowed a high degree of control over the final material properties. The variations in monomer mole fractions directly affected the final network molecular structure, the molecular weight distributions of the degradation products, and the swelling ratios and compressive moduli throughout degradation. For most tissue engineering and drug-delivery applications, well-characterized biomaterials with controllable degradation behavior are desirable (Rydholm et al., 2005).

The thiol-ene photopolymerizations can also provide a facile method to encapsulate proteins and maintain their bioactivity. McCall and Anseth (2012) characterized the differences in recovery of bioactive proteins when exposed to similar photoinitiation conditions during thiol-ene versus acrylatepolymerizations. Following exposure to chain polymerization of acrylates, lysozyme bioactivity was approximately 50%; after step-growth thiol-ene reaction, lysozyme retained nearly 100% of its prereaction activity. Bioactive protein recovery was enhanced 1000-fold in the presence of a thiol-ene reaction, relative to recovery from solutions containing identical primary radical concentrations, but without the thiol-ene components. When the cytokine TGFβ was encapsulated in PEG hydrogels formed via the thiol-ene reaction, full protein bioactivity was preserved. Photopolymerization reactions that provide rapid gelation at low radical concentrations are highly desirable for applications that seek to encapsulate sensitive payloads, such as proteins or cells. Results of the study indicated that thiol-ene click reactions are capable of proceeding rapidly at low initiator concentrations with little to no impact on *in situ* protein bioactivity (McCall and Anseth, 2012).

8.5 Conclusions

This chapter provides various insights into the properties, techniques for activation, and the medical applications of thiol-ene/acrylate SMPs. The properties of these materials depend on their composition and chemical structure. Acrylate incorporation in the thiol-ene matrix increases the rubbery modulus of the system. The glass transition of the final matrices can be adjusted by altering the composition of the system. Finally, the presence of the ene monomer along with acrylates in the ternary system provides a potential additional route for fine-tuning network physical properties.

References

Bowman, C.N., Cramer, N.B., Nair D.P., Shandas, R., 2011. Thiol-vinyl and thiol-yne systems for shape memory polymers. Patent EP 2278938 A2.

Campos, L.M., Killops, K.L., Sakai, R., Paulusse, J.M.J., Damiron, D., Drockenmuller, E., Messmore, B.W., Hawker, C.J., 2008. Development of thermal and photochemical strategies for thiol-ene click polymer functionalization. Macromolecules 41, 7063–7070. http://dx.doi.org/10.1021/ma801630n.

Connal, L.A., Kinnane, C.R., Zelikin, A.N., Caruso, F., 2009. Stabilization and functionalization of polymer multilayers and capsules via thiol-ene click chemistry. Chem. Mater. 21, 576–578. http://dx.doi.org/10.1021/cm803011w.

Cramer, N.B., Bowman, C.N., 2001. Kinetics of thiol-ene and thiol-acrylate photopolymerizations with real-time Fourier transform infrared. J. Polym. Sci. A Polym. Chem. 39 (19), 3311–3319. http://dx.doi.org/10.1002/pola.1314.

David, R.L.A., Kornfield, J.A., 2008. Facile, efficient routes to diverse protected thiols and to their deprotection and addition to create functional polymers by thiol-ene coupling. Macromolecules 41, 1151–1161. http://dx.doi.org/10.1021/ma0718393.

Fox, T.G., Loshaek, S., 1955. Influence of molecular weight and degree of crosslinking on the specific volume and glass temperature of polymers. J. Polym. Sci. 15, 371–390. http://dx.doi.org/10.1002/pol.

Gall, K., Yakacki, C.M., Liu, Y.P., Shandas, R., Willett, N., Anseth, K.S., 2005. Thermomechanics of the shape memory effect in polymers for biomedical applications. J. Biomed. Mater. Res. A 73A (3), 339–348. http://dx.doi.org/10.1002/jbm.a.30296.

Gress, A., Volkel, A., Schlaad, H., 2007. Thio-click modification of poly[2-(3-butenyl)-2-oxazoline]. Macromolecules 40, 7928–7933. http://dx.doi.org/10.1021/ma071357r.

Harada, A., Li, J., Kamachi, M., 1992. The molecular necklace: a rotaxane containing many threaded α-cyclodextrins. Nature 356, 325–327. http://dx.doi.org/10.1038/356325a0.

Hoyle, C.E., Lee, T.Y., Roper, T., 2004. Thio-enes: chemistry of the past with promise for the future. J. Polym. Sci. A Polym. Chem. 42 (21), 5301–5338. http://dx.doi.org/10.1002/pola.20366.

Jacobine, A.F., 1993. Thiol-ene photopolymers. In: Fouassier, J.P., Rabek, J.F. (Eds.), Radiation Curing in Polymer Science and Technology, Volume III: Polymerisation Mechanisms. Elsevier Science Publishers, New York, pp. 219–268.

Jacobine, A.F., Glaser, D.M., Grabek, P.J., Mancini, D., Masterson, M., Nakos, S.T., Rakas, M.A., Woods, J.G., 1992. Photocrosslinked norbornene-thiol copolymers: synthesis, mechanical properties, and cure studies. J. Appl. Polym. Sci. 45 (3), 471–485. http://dx.doi.org/10.1002/app.1992.070450312.

Johnson, P.M., Stansbury, J.W., Bowman, C.N.J., 2008. High throughput kinetic analysis of acrylate and thiol-ene photopolymerization using temperature and temperature and exposure time gradients. J. Polym. Sci. A Polym. Chem. 46, 1502–1509. http://dx.doi.org/10.1002/pola.22491.

Kannurpatti, A.R., Anseth, J.W., Bowman, C.N., 1998. A study of the evolution of mechanical properties and structural heterogeneity of polymer networks formed by photopolymerizations of multifunctional (meth)acrylates. Polymer 39 (12), 2507–2513.

Kasprzak, S., Martin, B., Raj, T., Gall, K., 2009. Synthesis and thermomechanical behavior of (qua)ternarythiol-ene(/acrylate) copolymers. Polymer 50 (23), 5549–5558. http://dx.doi.org/10.1016/j.

Kharasch, M.S., Read, A.T., Mayo, F.R., 1938. The peroxide effect in the addition of reagents to unsaturated compounds. Xvi. The addition of thio-glycolic acid to styrene and isobutylene. Chem. Ind. (London) (57), 752–773.

Killops, K.L., Campos, L.M., Hawker, C.J., 2008. Robust, efficient, and orthogonal synthesis of dendrimers via thiol-ene "click" chemistry. J. Am. Chem. Soc. 130, 5062–5064. http://dx.doi.org/10.1021/ja8006325.

Lendlein, A., Kelch, S., 2002. Shape memory polymers. Angew. Chem. Int. Ed. 41, 2034–2057. http://dx.doi.org/10.1002/1521-3773(20020617).

Lu, H., Carioscia, J.A., Stansbury, J.W., Bowman, C.N., 2005. Investigations of step-growth thiol-ene polymerizations for novel dental restoratives. Dent. Mater. 21 (12), 1129–1136.

McCall, J., Anseth, K., 2012. Thiol-ene photopolymerizations provide a facile method to encapsulate proteins and maintain their bioactivity. Biomacromolecules 13, 2410–2417. http://dx.doi.org/10.1021/bm300671s.

Mellott, M., Searcy, K., Pishko, M., 2001. Release of protein from highly cross-linked hydrogels of poly(ethylene glycol) diacrylate fabricated by UV polymerization. Biomaterials 22, 929–941.

Nair, D.P., Cramer, N.B., Scott, T.F., Bowman, C.N., Shandas, R., 2010. Photopolymerized thiol-ene systems as shape memory polymers. Polymer 51 (19), 4383–4389. http://dx.doi.org/10.1016/j.

O'Brien, A.K., Cramer, N.B., Bowman, C.N., 2006. Oxygen inhibition in thiol-acrylate photopolymerizations. J. Polym. Sci. A Polym. Chem. 44 (6), 2007–2014. http://dx.doi.org/10.1002/pola.21304.

Ortega, A.M., Kasprzak, S.E., Yakacki, C.M., Diani, J., Greenberg, A.R., Gall, K., 2008. Structure–property relationships in photopolymerizable polymer networks: effect of composition on the crosslinked structure and resulting thermomechanical properties of a (meth) acrylate-based system. J. Appl. Polym. Sci. 110, 1559–1572. http://dx.doi.org/10.1002/app.28732.

Polizzotti, B.D., Fairbanks, B.D., Anseth, K.S., 2008. Three-dimensional biochemical patterning of click-based composite hydrogels via thiolene photopolymerization. Biomacromolecules 9, 1084–1087. http://dx.doi.org/10.1021/bm7012636.

Posner, T., 1905. Beiträge zur Kenntniss der ungesättigten Verbindungen. II. Ueber die Addition von Mercaptanen an ungesättigte Kohlenwasserstoffe. Ber. Dtsch. Chem. Ges. 38, 646–657.

Quick, D., Macdonald, K., Anseth, K., 2004. Delivering DNA from photocrosslinked, surface-eroding polyanhydrides. J. Control. Release 97, 333–343. http://dx.doi.org/10.1016/j.

Rissing, C., Son, D.Y., 2009. Application of thiol-ene chemistry to the preparation of carbosilane-thioether dendrimers. Organometallics 28, 3167–3172. http://dx.doi.org/10.1021/om9001395.

Rydholm, A., Bowmana, C., Anseth, K., 2005. Degradable thiol-acrylate photopolymers: polymerization and degradation behavior of an in situ forming biomaterial. Biomaterials 26, 4495–4506. http://dx.doi.org/10.1016/j.

Safranski, D.L., Gall, K., 2008. Effect of chemical structure and crosslinking density on the thermo-mechanical properties and toughness of (meth)acrylate shape memory polymer networks. Polymer 49 (20), 4446–4455. http://dx.doi.org/10.1016/j.

Sawhney, A.S., Pathak, C.P., Hubbell, J.A., 1993. Bioerodible hydrogels based on photopolymerized poly(ethylene glycol)-co-poly(alpha-hydroxy acid) diacrylate macromers. Macromolecules 26 (4), 581–587. http://dx.doi.org/10.1021/ma00056a005.

Senyurt, A.F., Wei, H., Hoyle, C.E., Piland, S.G., Gould, T.E., 2007. Ternary thiol-ene/acrylate photopolymers: effect of acrylate structure on mechanical properties. Macromolecules 40, 4901–4909. http://dx.doi.org/10.1021/ma062534b.

Shih, H., Lin, C.-C., 2013. Visible-light-mediated thiol-ene hydrogelation using eosin-Y as the only photoinitiator. Macromol. Rapid Commun. 34 (3), 269–273. http://dx.doi.org/10.1002/marc.

Sokolowski, W., Metcalfe, A., Hayashi, R., Yahia, L'.H., Raymond, J., 2007. Medical applications of shape memory polymers. Biomed. Mater. 2, S23–S27. http://dx.doi.org/10.1088/1748-6041/2/1/S04.

Treloar, L.R.G., 1958. The Physics of Rubber Elasticity, second ed. Oxford University Press, London.

Uekama, K., Hirayama, F., Irie, T., 1998. Cyclodextrin drug carrier systems. Chem. Rev. 98, 2045–2076. http://dx.doi.org/10.1021/cr970025p.

West, J.L., Hubbell, J.A., 1995. Photopolymerized hydrogel materials for drug-delivery applications. React. Polym. 25 (2–3), 139–147.

Xiao, H., Zhou, D., Liu, S., Qi, R., Zheng, Y., Huang, Y., Jing, X., 2011. Delivery of active DACH-Pt anticancer species by biodegradable amphiphilic polymers using thiol-ene radical addition. Macromol. Biosci. 12 (3), 367–373. http://dx.doi.org/10.1002/mabi.

Zhang, Q., Li, G.-Z., Becer, C.R., Haddleton, D.M., 2012. Cyclodextrin-centred star polymers synthesized via a combination of thiol-ene click and ring opening polymerization. Chem. Commun. 48, 8063–8065. http://dx.doi.org/10.1039/C2CC33742H.

Polyurethane shape-memory polymers for biomedical applications

9

Y.Q. Fu[1], *W.M. Huang*[2], *J.K. Luo*[3], *H. Lu*[4]
[1]Northumbria University, Newcastle upon Tyne, United Kingdom; [2]Nanyang Technological University, Singapore; [3]University of Bolton, Bolton, United Kingdom; [4]Harbin Institute of Technology, Harbin, China

9.1 Introduction

Polyurethanes (PUs) are a group of polymer materials with long and tangled linear polymer chains showing shape-memory effect (SME) (Kim et al., 1996; Huang et al., 2010b; Leng and Du, 2010). Shape-memory polyurethane (SMPU) is basically composed of soft and hard segments; thermodynamic immiscibility between these two segments leads to phase separation, which makes SMPU an excellent candidate for a shape-memory material (Huang et al., 2010b; Huang et al., 2012). In a relaxed state after fabrication of the SMPU, partially separated soft and hard segments co-exist in the polymer (Lendlein and Kelch, 2002, 2005; Behl and Lendlein, 2007; Huang et al., 2012). Hard segments act as pivot points for shape recovery, whereas soft segments are responsible for absorbing external stress applied on the SMPU. At temperatures below glass transition temperature, T_g, the soft segments do not have enough kinetic energy to achieve good mobility; thus, SMPUs are relatively difficult to be deformed in the glass state. Above T_g, SMPU transforms from a glass state to a rubber state and becomes easily deformed (see Figure 9.1, Yang, 2007). Under an external stress, the soft and hard segments reorient themselves in the direction of external force, becoming stretched (Lendlein and Kelch, 2002; Behl and Lendlein, 2007). By cooling SMPUs below T_g while maintaining the deformed shape with applied force, the mobility of the soft segments is restricted so that the deformation is maintained after removal of the constraints, as shown in Figure 9.1 (Yang, 2007). Upon re-heating above T_g, the soft segments obtain enough mobility to return to their original curled shape, resulting in the shape recovery of the SMPU.

Compared with other types of shape-memory polymers (SMPs), PU-based SMPs have many advantages, including easy processing, low cost of materials and fabrication, large recovery strains up to 1000%, wide, adjustable shape-recovery temperature range, excellent chemical properties, and biocompatibility for most SMPUs (Liang et al., 1997; Wei et al., 1998; Zdrahala and Zdrahala, 1999; Metcalfe et al., 2003; Leng and Du, 2010). The properties of SMPU, such as elasticity, crystallization temperature range, melting point, and thermal and deformation behavior, can be

Shape Memory Polymers for Biomedical Applications. http://dx.doi.org/10.1016/B978-0-85709-698-2.00009-X

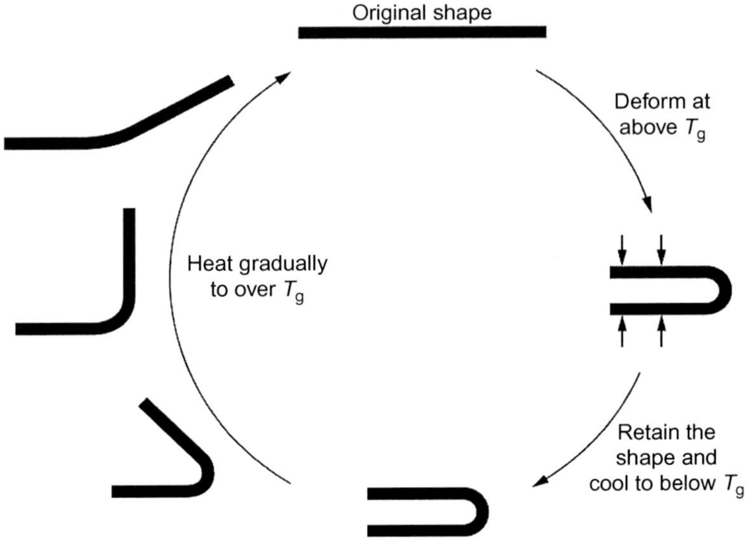

Figure 9.1 Illustration of shape-memory effect (Zhao et al., 2011).

easily tailored by changing the ratio of hard and soft segments (Leng and Du, 2010; Zhao et al., 2011).

Based on the nature of cross-linking, SMPUs can be divided into two main categories (see Figure 9.2) (Monkman, 2000a; Leng and Du, 2010; Huang et al., 2012). The first is physically cross-linked SMPUs, or thermoplastic SMPUs. Thermoplastic SMPUs are flexible and can be reshaped, as their hard segment network structures consist of long sequences of weak bonds (see Figure 9.2a). Due to their flexibility and easy reshaping, thermoplastic SMPUs are the most commonly used SMPUs for many applications (Jeong et al., 2000; Leng and Du, 2010). The second is chemically cross-linked SMPUs, or thermoset SMPUs (see Figure 9.2b), which possess a higher modulus in comparison with thermoplastic SMPUs. They lack thermal plasticity and are difficult to process, thus making them difficult for recycling and reprocessing (Huang et al., 2012).

The polyurethane SMP invented by Hayashi (1990) is currently the most studied polyurethane SMP (Tobushi et al., 1996). Mitsubishi Heavy Industries (MHI) has done extensive research on the SMPU since 1980s (Wei et al., 1998; Merlin, 2008). The T_g values of the MHI SMPUs have a wide temperature range from −30 to 65 °C, which can be applied in many commercial uses, including kitchen tools, textiles, automotive components, biomedical devices, etc. Hu's group has synthesized the SMPUs, which are mainly for textile applications (Hu et al., 2003; Zhuo et al., 2008; Chen et al., 2007a,b; Zhu et al., 2006). Work on the enhancement and triggering mechanisms of the SMPUs PU foam has been proposed and investigated by Sokolowski et al. (2007). Electrospun SMPU nanofibers have also been made (Zhuo et al., 2008). To enhance the strength of polyurethane SMPU, various fillers, such as metals, silica

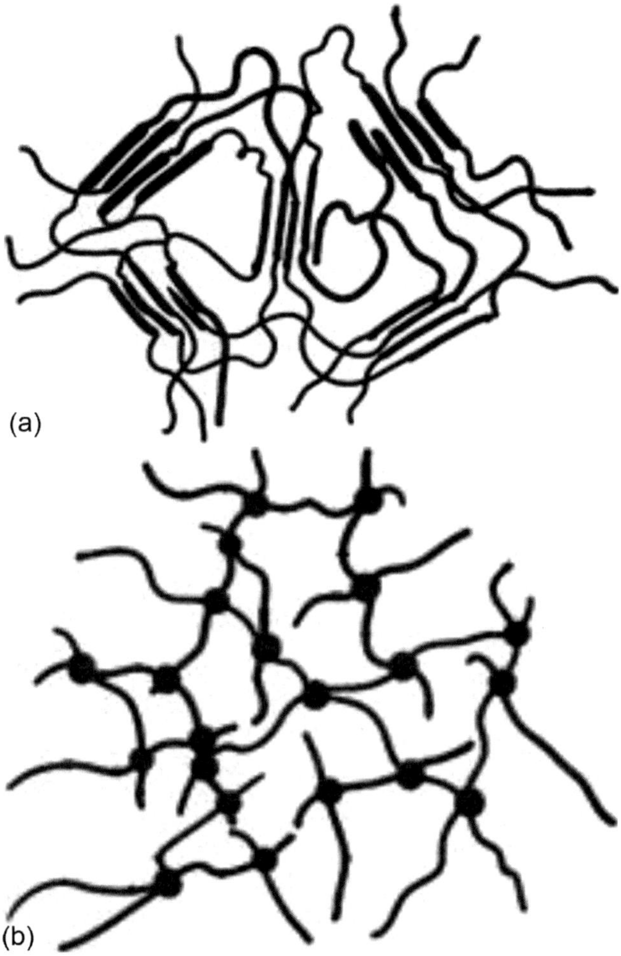

Figure 9.2 Physically (a) and chemically (b) cross-linked SMPUs.

particles, clay, carbon nanofibers (CNFs), carbon nanoparticles (CNPs), carbon nanotubes (CNTs), and graphene, have been added to PU, forming the SMP composites (Gunes et al., 2008; Cao and Jana, 2007). Although the shape recovery of SMPUs is intrinsically a thermally induced process, it can also be triggered optically, electrically, magnetically, or electromagnetically, with the addition of various functional fillers or nanoparticles (Sahoo et al., 2010; Gunes et al., 2009; Cho et al., 2005; Jung and Cho, 2010; Razzaq et al., 2007a,b).

SMPUs have been developed rapidly in recent years for medical device applications because they possess some unique properties: biocompatibility, easy to adjust transition temperatures around human body temperature (Ahmad et al., 2011), low cost, and easy synthesis procedures. Recently, reprocessability and reusability have been studied by Ahmad et al. (2012a). Various shape-memory stimuli methods other than heat, such as water, electric, light, or magnetic actuation, and magnetic field have broadened their potential medical applications significantly (Sokolowski et al., 2007; Huang et al., 2012). Some successful biomedical applications include the vascular stent (Baer et al., 2007), SMP wire for thrombus removal, deployable biomedical devices, SMP wires for suture, etc. (Small et al., 2010).

In this chapter, an overview of the properties of PU will be presented, followed by various shape-memory triggering methods. The medical applications of the SMPUs will be discussed in detail.

9.2 Properties of shape-memory polyurethane (SMPU)

9.2.1 *Microstructure*

PUs are made of long tangled polymer chains consisting of two segments: flexible, soft segments; and elastic and relatively hard segments. By selecting a proper combination and/or ratio of soft segment to hard segment, various properties such as elasticity, crystallization temperature range, and melting point can be obtained. PUs are generally produced from the reaction of molecules containing two or more isocyanate groups (—NCO) with polyol molecules containing two or more hydroxyl groups (—OH) (Huang et al., 2012). A few examples are shown in Figure 9.3. The most commonly used diisocyanates include 4,4′-diphenylmethane diisocyanate (MDI), phenylene diisocyanate (PDI), toluene diisocyanate, hexamethylene diisocyanate, and isophorone diisocyanate (IPDI) (Szycher, 1999; Bassi et al., 2003). A short chain diol, referred to as a chain extender, is normally used to produce hard segments by reacting with diisocyanate; for example, 1,4 butandiol (Ahmad et al., 2012a). Catalysis also plays an important role in the preparation of SMPUs, since it influences not only the chemical reaction rate but also the chain propagation, extension, and cross-linking (Ahmad et al., 2012a). Some commonly used catalysts include tertiary amines and organometallics. A few key factors influencing the shape-memory behaviors of SMPUs are summarized below.

9.2.1.1 *Hard segment structure*

Dependence of shape-memory behavior on hard segment content has been extensively studied (Yang et al., 2003). Lee et al. (2001) reported that SMPUs with 20 or 25 wt% of hard segment did not show shape-recovery effect because they did not have strong chemical interaction or physical cross-links due to the low content of hard segments. SMPUs with 50 wt% of hard segment content showed strong interaction among the hard segments, which resulted in a rigid structure and loss of shape-memory behavior. However, 80–95% of shape recovery was obtained for this SMPU with 30–45 wt% of hard segment content. Lowering the content of hard segments increases the hysteresis in shape-memory behavior (Lee et al., 2001, 2004). Therefore, hard segment percentage is critical in the synthesis of high-quality SMPUs. Increase in hard

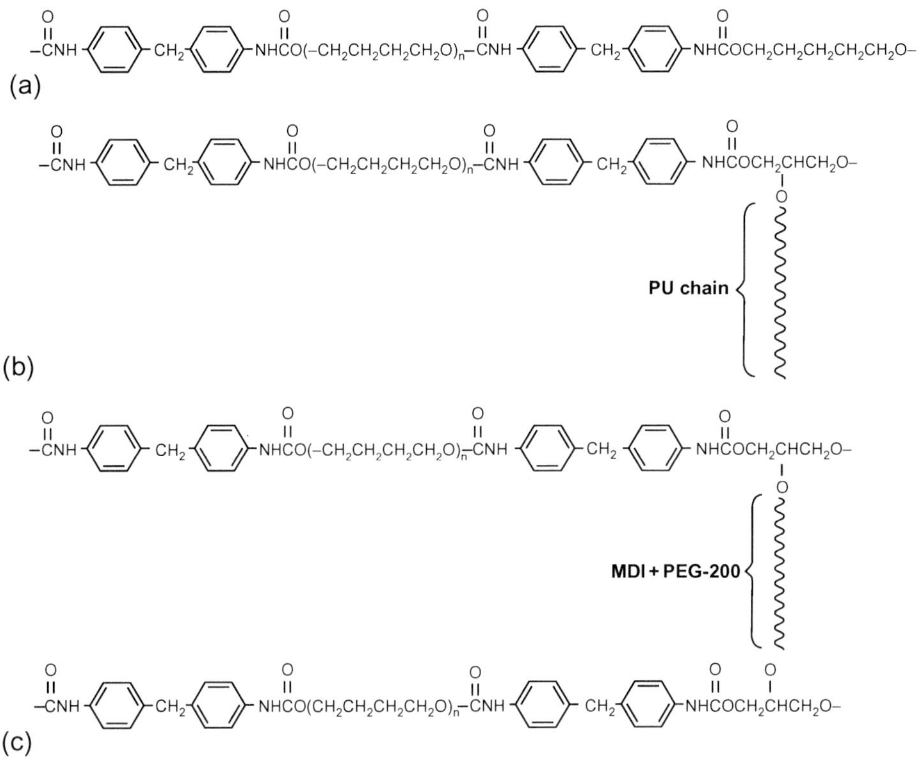

Figure 9.3 Structures of PU SMPs based on PTHF, MDI, PEG, and propanetriol with (a) linear, (b) grafted, and (c) cross-linked structure.

segment content can increase compatibility between the soft and hard segments (Huang et al., 2012). The increase in the glass transition temperature of the SMPU was also observed with the increase of hard segment content, which is attributed to the enhanced hydrogen bonding and rigidity of molecular chains (Ahmad et al., 2012b).

The effect of hard segment on the SMPU structures was studied by Yang et al. (2003). They used two different diisocyanates with different molecular structures: PDI and MDI. PDI has a planar shape, whereas MDI has a non-planar shape. PDI-based SMPUs possess superior mechanical properties over MDI-based SMPUs because of their higher crystallinity (Huang et al., 2012). The SMPUs with the PDI as the hard segment show a better shape-recovery ratio than those with MDI-based SMPUs (Yang et al., 2003). For the synthesis of medical-grade SMPUs, the MDI is often selected because of its low toxicity. Although MDI is most commonly used as the hard segment, IPDI has the advantage of producing polymers with high resistance to UV-light-related degradation, good long-term stability, and high tensile strength (Bassi et al., 2003). Hence, the combination of various diisocyanates is often used to improve the overall properties of SMPUs. For example, MDI was used to synthesis medical-grade SMPUs, while IPDI was introduced to increase the stiffness of SMPUs (Szycher, 1999; Ahmad et al., 2012a).

Addition of small monomer units in the hard segment can enhance thermo-mechanical properties of the SMPUs (Chen et al., 2007b). For example, Ding et al. (2006) found that introducing polyethylene glycol-200 (PEG-200) in hard segment (10–15%) enhanced the mechanical properties of SMPUs. An addition of PEG-200 in the SMPUs can suppress the mobility of soft segments and decrease the crystallinity of polyol and heat of fusion of SMPUs, thus enhancing the compatibility between soft and hard segments (Ding et al., 2006; Merline et al., 2008).

9.2.1.2 Soft segment structure

The long-chain polyol segments in the SMPUs are responsible for the formation of soft domains. At room temperature, the polyols can be liquid or solid, depending on their molecular weight. Long-chain polyol molecules show good flexibility and low transition temperature due to their aliphatic structure and intermolecular interactions, particularly the abundant ether bonds (Ma et al., 1997; Ahmad et al., 2012b). Consequently, the chemical structure of polyols, the reaction between the polyol and diisocyanate, and the degree of phase separation are all important for shape-memory properties of the SMPUs (Ahmad et al., 2012b). Polyols with different structures and reactivities can be used to tailor the thermo-mechanical and shape-memory properties of SMPUs (Goethals et al., 1998). Adding different types of polyols provides the SMPUs with various properties. The polyols are generally divided into two major types: polyether and polyester polyols (Chun et al., 2006). PUs based on polyether polyols are more hydrolysis-resistant than those based on polyester polyols, whereas SMPUs with polytetramethylene ether glycol have good hydrolysis and microbial resistance as well as excellent dynamic properties (Ahmad et al., 2012b). Polycaprolactone polyols have the inherent toughness and resistance of polyester and can improve the low-temperature performance of the SMPUs.

9.2.1.3 Phase separation

SMPUs typically present a micro-phase separated structure due to the thermodynamic incompatibility between the hard segment and soft segment. The micro-phase separation is thus essential for the shape-memory properties as well as for the mechanical performance, as it results in the formation of regions rich in hard segment (domains) that act as cross-linking points for the soft/switching segments (Ahmad et al., 2012b; Chen et al., 2006). Flexibility, strength, and toughness of thermoplastic PUs are dependent on the degree of phase separation of hard and soft segment domains, apart from the structure of polyols, choice of chain extenders, ratio of the hard and soft segment, the reaction process and conditions, etc. (Hu et al., 2003). Phase distribution and separation, phase composition, and micro domain size have a significant impact on the mechanical performance and shape-memory properties of SMPUs.

9.2.2 Thermo-mechanical behavior SMPU

To evaluate the mechanical and thermo-mechanical properties of SMPUs, various methods have commonly applied, including tensile tests, dynamic mechanical/thermal analysis, shape-recovery test, stability tests, etc. (Huang et al., 2006). Uniaxial tensile tests are the mostly frequently used method to investigate the behavior of the polyurethane SMP under uniaxial tension.

9.2.2.1 Stress–strain–temperature relationship

The stress–strain–temperature (σ–δ–T) relationship of SMPUs has been widely studied (Lendlein and Kelch, 2002; Huang et al., 2012). There are four steps for testing the thermo-mechanical properties of the PU-based SMPs (Tobushi et al., 1992, 2001).

(1) At a high temperature T_h ($>T_g$), the SMP specimen is loaded to a pre-determined maximum strain (ε_m) at a constant strain rate.
(2) The SMP sample is held at ε_m and cooled to a low temperature T_l ($<T_g$).
(3) After full unloading, only a very small amount of elastic strain is recovered.
(4) The free-standing sample is heated from T_l to T_h at a constant heating rate. The pre-strain is almost fully recovered with only a very small amount of strain left at T_h.

A typical stress–strain curve of the SMPU at room temperature is illustrated in Figure 9.4a; ε_t, ε_h, and ε_i denote the elastic strain, total instant recovery strain upon unloading, free recovery strain during holding (without any external load), and final residual strain, respectively (Yang, 2007). In the deformation of the SMPU, the maximum strain ε_m can be defined as:

$$\varepsilon_m = \varepsilon_t + \varepsilon_h + \varepsilon_i \tag{9.1}$$

Figure 9.4b presents one example of the strain *vs.* stress relationships of the SMPU upon loading to different maximum strains, ε_m, namely, 20%, 50%, and 100%, followed by unloading to zero stress with a loading strain rate of 10^{-3}/s (Yang et al., 2004, 2005; Yang, 2007). Upon unloading, recovery is largely attributed to elastic recovery, in particular at the early unloading stages in the small maximum strain cases.

Tensile tests were also carried out at four different strain rates at $T_g + 15$ °C following the above procedure, as shown in Figure 9.5 (Yang, 2007; Huang et al., 2012). The residual strain (ε_i) is a very small portion of maximum strain (ε_m) and decreases continuously upon further holding of the loads. Result reveals that a higher strain rate results in more instant recovery strain. It is known that, if loading time is short, the strain energy in a polymer can be stored by quick mechanical deformation at a temperature above T_g. A significant amount of strain may be recovered, but only gradually with the elapse of time. Clearly, the strain recovery is highly dependent on the strain rate. With the increase of strain rate, the elastic strain ε_t becomes smaller while ε_h increases. Since ε_i is mainly ascribed to the viscous flow of a material that is highly dependent on the strain rate, ε_i increases with the strain rate (Huang et al., 2012).

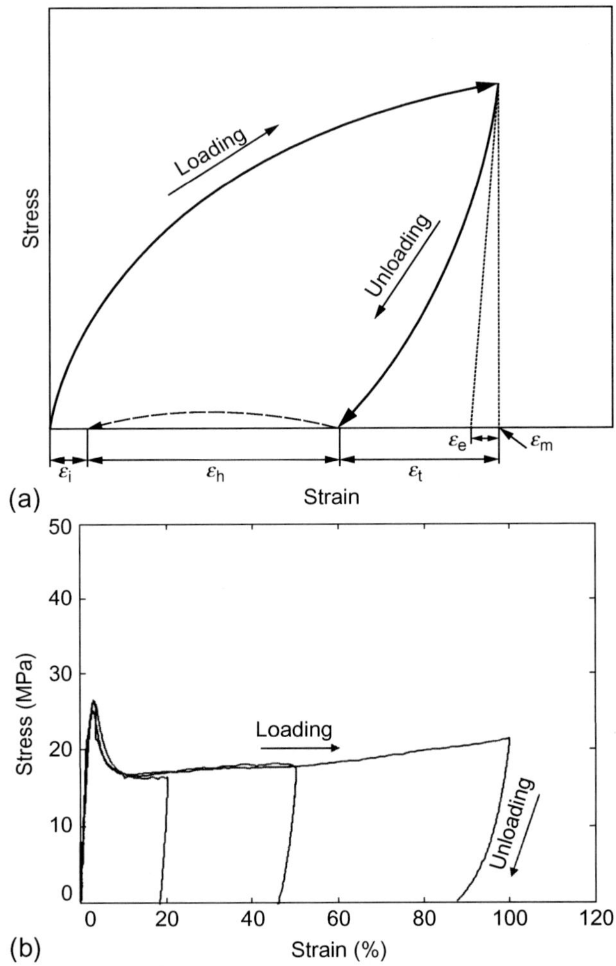

Figure 9.4 (a) Example of loading/unloading uniaxial tensile test; (b) strain versus stress relationships of SMP in loading/unloading to different maximum strains, namely, 20%, 50%, and 100%, followed by unloading to zero stress with a loading rate of 10^{-3} s (Yang et al., 2007).

The dependence of strain recovery upon the maximum pre-strain was investigated using standard tensile tests (Huang et al., 2012). The samples were loaded to different maximum strains and then unloaded to zero stress at a strain rate of 10^{-2}/s and at T_g+5 °C. The maximum pre-strains were from 50% to 600% at a 50% interval; the relationships of stress versus strain are plotted in Figure 9.6 (Yang, 2007; Huang et al., 2012). The SMP samples experienced obvious "creeping" in the strain range from 100% to 300%, followed by hardening due to reorientation and crystallization. Generally speaking, the recovery ratio decreases with the increase of maximum strain, whereas the decrease rate is more significant at a maximum strain above 200% and negligible at a maximum strain range from 100% to 200% (Huang et al., 2012).

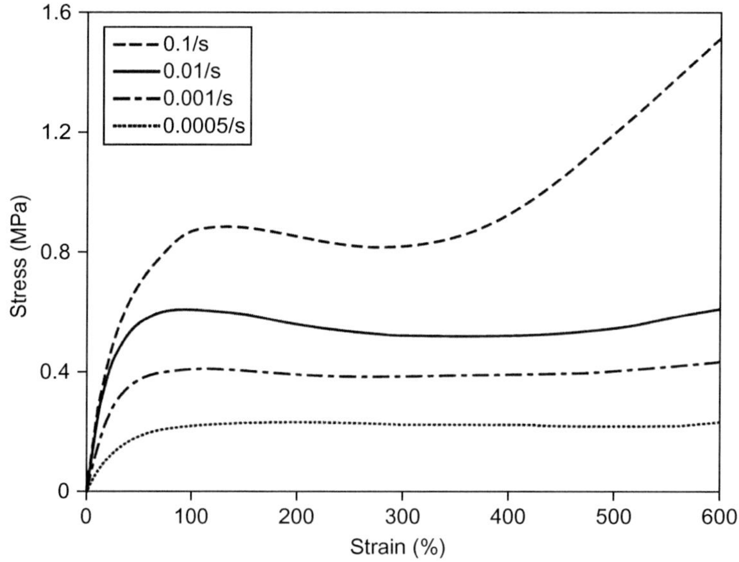

Figure 9.5 Strain-versus-stress relationships of polyurethane SMP MM3520 at $T_g + 15$ °C. From Yang et al. (2007).

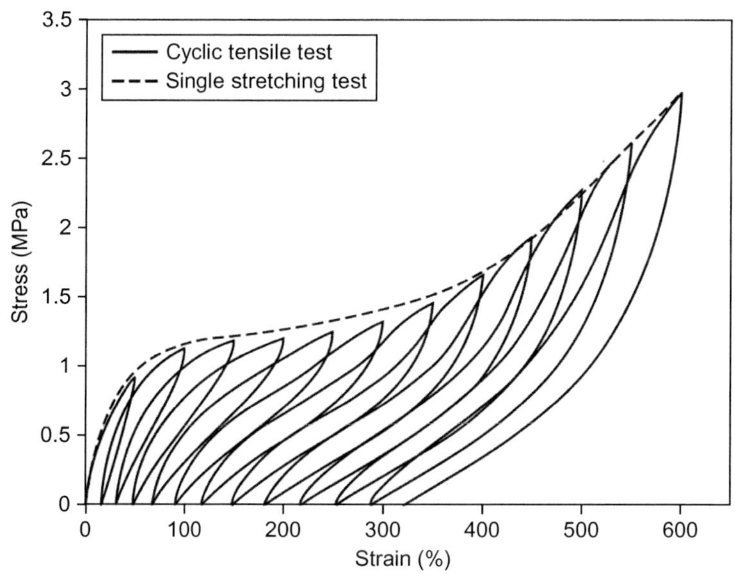

Figure 9.6 Results of cyclic tensile test and single stretching test at a constant strain rate of 0.01^{-1} s at T_g+5 °C.
From Yang (2007).

The decrease in the total instant recovery ratio can be attributed to reorientation and crystallization of the SMPUs, and the sudden decrease in the recovery ratio may be a result of decoupling in the imperfect crystalline part of the polymer in the first a few cycles (Tobushi et al., 1996).

9.2.2.2 Shape recovery tests

Recovery stress and recoverable strain are all essential in engineering applications of the SMPUs. The shape recovery of the SMPUs at different conditions was systematically studied (Huang et al., 2012). The SMPU wires were uniaxially stretched at 50 °C with a 100 N load cell to three different maximum strains, 10%, 20%, and 50%. The wires were then rapidly cooled to room temperature in 3 min with their maximum strain held, followed by unloading to zero stress. Subsequently, the pre-strained wires were heated at a constant rate of 2 °C/min. For all the pre-strained wires in the free recovery test, the recovery ratio (ratio of measured recovery strain to pre-strain; 10%, 20%, or 50%) was applied as a measure of the recovery. Figure 9.7 presents the evolution of the recovery stress and recovery ratio against temperature (Yang, 2007; Huang et al., 2012). In Figure 9.7a, the recovery stress reaches a peak at ~30 °C and then falls continuously upon further heating, in particular, at temperatures over 40 °C. The recovery stress almost vanishes at 60 °C. A larger pre-strain results in a larger recovery stress. Upon heating to 60 °C, the recovery (without constraint) was ~100%, as shown in Figure 9.7b (Yang, 2007; Huang et al., 2012).

The shape recovery ability of the SMPU is highly dependent on strain rate, temperature, and maximum strain (Huang et al., 2012). For a higher strain recovery, a higher strain rate is preferred during loading. Furthermore, it is reported that the SMPU is needed to deform at a temperature ranging from T_g+5 °C to T_g+10 °C for more recoverable strain, especially for a larger recoverable strain rate. Since severe hardening at over 200% strain results in some irreversible strain, the polyurethane SMP should be used at a strain below 200% (Huang et al., 2012). The stability of shape-recovery properties of SMP is also highly dependent on the cycle number. Upon cycling, the total instant recoverable strain deteriorates, and the stress corresponding to the maximum strain decreases (Huang et al., 2012).

9.2.2.3 Multi-shape-memory effect and temperature-memory effect

Traditionally, shape recovery of the SMPUs means its shape changes from a temporary shape directly to the original shape. Under special processing of the SMPUs or some special SMPs, shape recovery can be achieved in a step-by-step manner through one or a few intermediate shapes, which is often called multi-SME (Bellin et al., 2006, 2007; Xie et al., 2009; Pretsch, 2010). For example, by immersing different parts of polyurethane SMP wire into water for different durations, a gradient transition temperature can be achieved because of the significant influence of moisture on the glass transition temperature in the SMPU (Yang et al., 2007; Huang et al., 2005); an example is shown in Figure 9.8. If two types of soft segments inside the

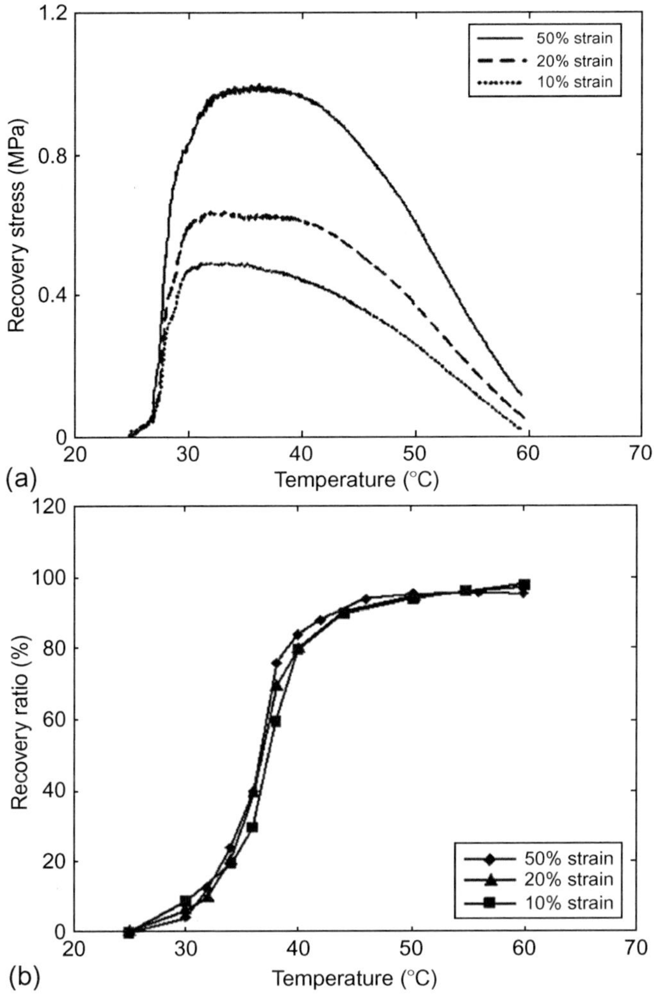

Figure 9.7 Recovery upon heating. (a) Recovery stress as a function of temperature. (b) Shape recovery ratio as a function of temperature.
From Yang (2007).

SMPU are sensitive to different types of stimuli, the triple-SME can be achieved by using different stimuli independently (Behl and Lendlein, 2010; Xie, 2010; Huang et al., 2011). Theoretically, it is possible to use only one soft-segment for the triple-SME by utilizing the glass transition and melting of these two commonly observed transitions in thermoplastic polymers (Huang et al., 2010b). Unlike most metals and their alloys, the multiple SME transition of some polymers occurs over a wide temperature range (Miaudet et al., 2007; Xie, 2010) that serves as a series of sub-transitions to achieve the multi-SME (Xie, 2010).

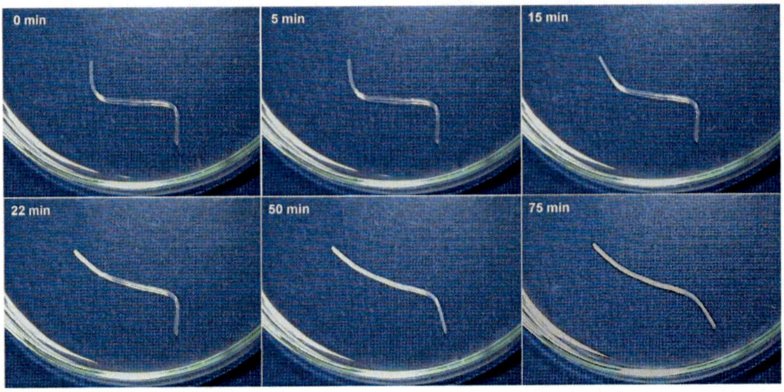

Figure 9.8 The multi-SME in thermo/moisture-responsive PU SMP upon immersing into room temperature water (moisture-responsive).
Reproduced from Huang et al. (2005), with permission.

Temperature memory effect (TME) is another related phenomenon in SMPs occurring during thermal cycling or mechanical cycling (Liu et al., 2005). The previous temperature of interruption is memorized and utilized in a later heating process. Miaudet et al. (2007) reported that in the constrained recovery test of a shape-memory nanocomposite with a broad glass transition temperature range, the maximum recovery stress occurred at the temperature at which the material was pre-deformed to the temporary shape. Huang et al. (2012) systematically studied the TME in SMPs and concluded that the TME is actually not a surprising phenomenon, but a natural response from polymers (Sun and Huang, 2010a,b; Sun et al., 2010).

9.3 Techniques for activating SME

Shape recovery of SMPUs is normally a thermally induced process; however, they can also be triggered optically, electrically, magnetically, or electromagnetically, and so on, with/without adding various functional fillers (Miaudet et al., 2007; Monkman, 2000b; Zhao et al., 2011).

9.3.1 Thermal triggering

The most common method for shape recovery in SMPUs is thermally induced (e.g., Behl and Lendlein, 2007). The SMPUs can be subjected to large deformations at an elevated temperature above their glass transition temperature T_g. Cooling the deformed sample to a temperature below T_g under constraints fixes the deformed shape of the sample. The original shape of the SMPUs will be recovered if the material is heated back to a temperature above T_g without constraints (Xu et al., 2009, 2010; Kim et al., 2010; Huang et al., 2010b).

For SMPU, the SME originates from either a glass transition temperature or melting temperature. Therefore, thermally actuated SMPs must be heated above their characteristic transition temperatures to induce the shape changes. For the SMPUs with transition temperatures close to body temperature, actuation can be accomplished simply by placing the SMP into the body and allowing heat transfer from the adjacent fluid or tissue to induce actuation. However, in some cases, a higher transition temperature would be desired, thus more mechanical rigidity can be maintained in the SMPU (i.e., higher elastic modulus) at body temperature for a precise control of actuation (Leng and Du, 2010).

9.3.2 Electric triggering

SMPU is normally considered as a non-conductive material because of its extremely low electrical conductivity (in the order of 10^{-10}–10^{-15} S/m) (Sahoo et al., 2005). Conductive SMPU can be made by dispersing conductive particles into the non-conductive SMP matrix (Leng et al., 2007; Liu et al., 2009). The fillers used for the conducting SMPs include CNTs (Cho et al., 2005; Paik et al., 2006), CNPs (Yang et al., 2005), conductive fiber (Leng et al., 2007), and metal particles, such as Au or Ni (Schmidt, 2006; Leng et al., 2007, 2008b). At a low concentration of conducting particles, conduction is mainly dominated by hopping conduction among the fillers; thus, its conductivity appears close to those of the bulk PUs, namely insulators (Xu et al., 2010). The SMP composite becomes conductive when the filler concentration is increased to a critical value, or the percolation threshold, which forms the electron bridge within the substrate by the filler and its dispersion state.

Nanosized carbon black (CB) or CNPs have been widely used for electrically conductive nanocomposites (Yang et al., 2005; Leng et al., 2008a; Meng and Hu, 2009; Koerner et al., 2004). The electrical conductivity of shape-memory PU filled with 30% CB is about 1–10^{-1} S/cm (Liu et al., 2009). However, Paik et al. (2006) found that CB is not so effective in improving the mechanical strength and shape-recovery stress of SMPs. Gunes and Jana (2008) prepared PU/CB composites by melt mixing and found that the crystallinity soft segment decreased due to the constraining effect of CBs on the mobility of the soft segment during crystallization. Figure 9.9 shows one example of electric actuation of CNP doped SMPU (Yang, 2007; Huang et al., 2012). The SMP composite was hot-pressed into a plate shape with a thickness of 2.0 mm and then cut into a "n" shape for demonstrating the SME upon heating by passing an electrical current through it. The sample can be easily bent at 60 °C, which is above T_g. Figure 9.9a shows the infrared images of the sample heated by an electrical current for 45 s (Yang, 2007; Huang et al., 2012). After switching off the electrical power and cooling back to 22 °C room temperature with the deformed shape held still, the bent shape was formed. When reheated above T_g by passing an electrical current, the sample recovered its original shape, as shown in Figure 9.9b (Yang, 2007; Huang et al., 2012).

CNFs are not only commonly used for reinforcement applications, but also as electrical conductive fillers as well as catalyst support (Gall et al., 2000, 2004). The temperature and strain have significant influences on the electrical resistivity

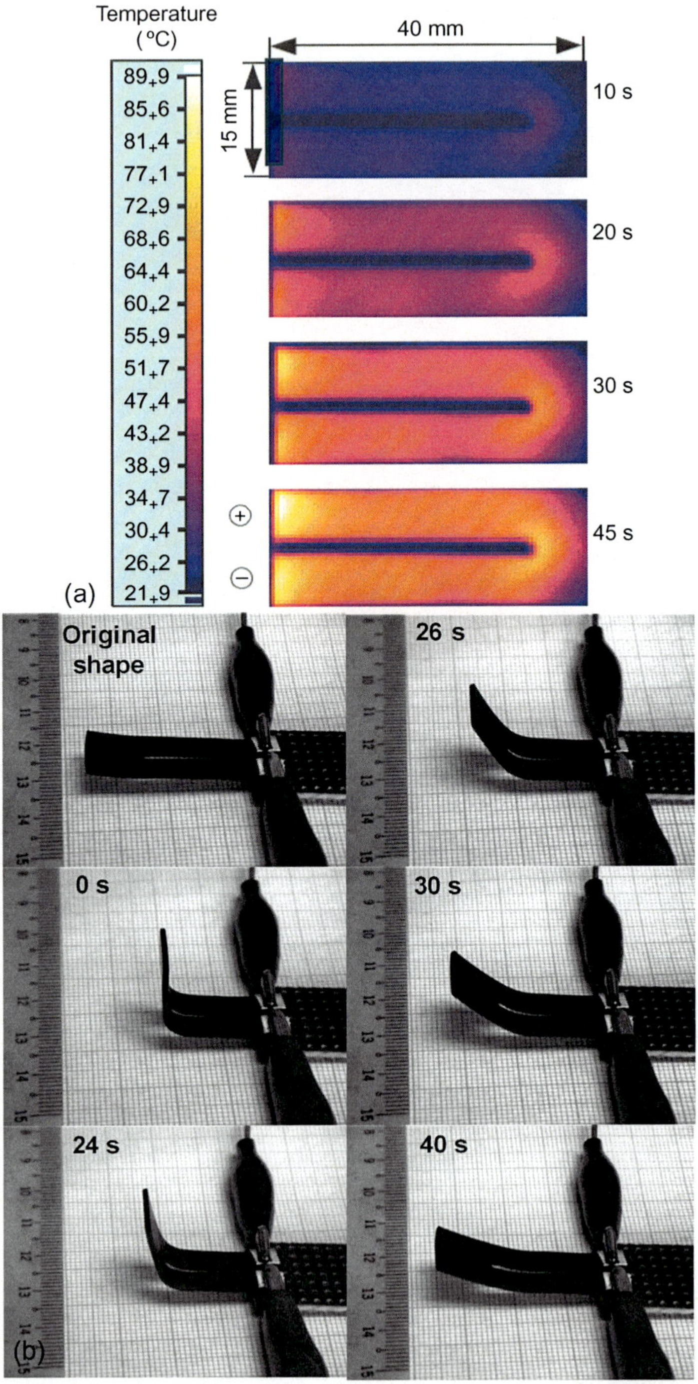

Figure 9.9 Shape-memory effect in conductive SMP carbon nanoparticles. (a) Temperature distribution taken by an infrared camera. (b) Shape-recovery upon passing an electrical current (Yang et al., 2005).

of the CNF-filled SMPs. Gunes et al. (2009) studied the relationship between electrical resistivity and sample temperature of SMPUs filled with CNFs, oxidized-CNFs, and CBs. It was found that CNF- and CB-filled SMPUs showed a positive temperature coefficient of resistivity (Gunes et al., 2009).

CNTs have been extensively studied in recent years as a replacement for the CNPs (Koerner et al., 2004). A SMPU composite incorporating 5 wt% CNTs can have an electrical conductivity of 10^{-3} S/cm (Cho et al., 2005). Paik et al. (2006) prepared PU with CNTs, and the electrical conductivity was about 2.5×10^{-3} S/cm. Because CNTs have tremendously large aspect ratios (100–10,000), many researchers have observed exceptionally low electrical percolation thresholds for CNT-based nanocomposites (Sandler et al., 2003; Bryning et al., 2005). Depending on the matrix, processing technique, and nanotube type, percolation thresholds ranging from 0.001 wt% to more than 10 wt% have been reported (Sandler et al., 2003; Choi et al., 2006). The large dispersion of the percolation threshold for electrical conductive SMPU-CNT nanocomposites is believed to be caused by processing methods used, which may result in different status of disentanglement of CNT agglomerates, uniform spatial distribution of individual CNTs, degree of alignment, dispersion, alignment, aspect ratio, and degree of surface modification of CNTs (Sahoo et al., 2010).

9.3.3 Magnetic triggering

SMPUs doped with ferromagnetic and ferrite particles, such as Ni, or Fe, FeO_x, $MgZnO_x$, and $NiZnFeO_x$, can be inductively heated by magnetic field (Kumar et al., 2010; Small et al., 2009). The electromagnetic energy from the external high frequency electromagnetic field can be transformed to heat if these ferromagnetic particles have been added inside the SMPUs (Spinks et al., 2006; Ahir and Terentjev, 2005; Ahir et al., 2006). Schmidt (2006) and Yakacki et al. (2009) used magnetic fields to remotely actuate SMP composites by incorporating iron (II,III) oxide nanoparticles into thermoplastics and thermoset SMPs (Schmidt, 2006; Razzaq et al., 2007a,b). To improve the particle dispersion in the matrix, the iron (III) oxide nanoparticles were coated with silica (Weigel et al., 2009). By selecting a ferromagnetic particle material with a Curie temperature within a safe medical limit, overheating can be avoided. Selective heating of specific device areas is also possible, and remote actuation can be realized by an externally applied magnetic field (Meng and Hu, 2009; Zhang et al., 2007). Medical devices, such as expandable stents and intravascular microactuators of SMP nanocomposites, have been demonstrated with magnetic field actuation (Buckley et al., 2006).

9.3.4 Water and solution triggering

Shape recovery of the SMPU can be induced by moisture or water that has a significant effect on the glass transition (Haung et al., 2010a; Huang, 2010). When immersed in water, water molecules diffuse into the SMPU samples and act as a plasticizer, leading to the reduction of transition temperature and resulting in shape

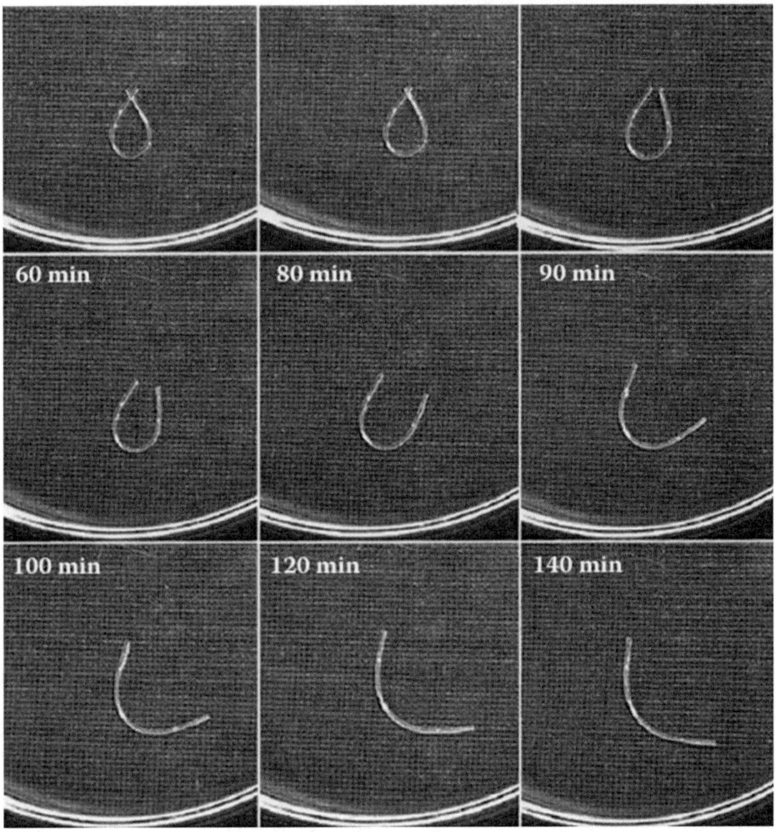

Figure 9.10 Water-driven recovery of an SMPU wire.
Reprinted from Huang et al. (2005), with permission.

recovery, as shown in Figure 9.10 (Huang et al., 2005). In the SMPUs and their composites, T_g is decreased from transition temperature to or below ambient temperature after immersion into water. The decrease of the T_g depends on the moisture uptake, which indirectly depends on the immersion time (Huang et al., 2005; Yang et al., 2004, 2006).

The SMPUs can also respond to the solution (such as solvent) by a mechanism in which the solution molecule has a plasticizing effect on polymeric materials, thus increasing the flexibility of the macromolecule chains of the SMPU (Lv et al., 2008a). These two effects reduce the transition temperature of materials until shape recovery occurs (Lv et al., 2008b). There is an interaction between the polymeric macromolecule and the micromolecule of absorbed solution, and the hydrogen bonding enlarges the flexibility of polymeric chains. In brief, water, moisture, and solution-driven SMP provide alternative triggering approaches for SMEs, and so thermo-heating becomes unnecessary (Leng and Du, 2010).

9.3.5 Light triggering

Visible or infrared (IR) light-induced SME in SMPUs can be realized by incorporating reversible photoreactive molecule switches into the SMPUs (Jiang et al., 2006); for example, cinnamic acid or cinnamylidene acetic acid moieties (Lendlein et al., 2005). Upon irradiation with light, a (2+2) cycloaddition reaction occurs between two of these light-sensitive moieties, and in sequence, a cyclobutane-ring and in this way covalent cross-links form. Irradiation with a different wavelength results in cleavage of the newly formed bonds, which causes the light induced actuation effects.

Doping with 6 wt% chemical functionalized multi-walled carbon nanotubes by grafting dodecylamine chains, the photosensitivity of oxotitanium phthalocyanine (TiOPc) is fivefold higher than that of un-doped TiOPc when exposed to 570 nm wavelength (Huang et al., 2012). The idea of resonant absorption of light by nanoparticles has been applied to other systems for biomedical applications, such as drug release. The resonant frequency could shift from deep UV-light to near IR-light; smaller nanoparticles can absorb shorter wavelength light, whereas larger nanoparticles can absorb longer wavelength light (Huang et al., 2012). Au–Au_2S nanoparticles of ~20 nm consisting of Au_2S dielectric core encapsulated by a thin gold shell are reported to have absorption peak near-IR light and demonstrated a controlled drug release (Ren and Chow, 2003). The light absorption efficiency is strongly dependent on the size, shape, and concentration of the nanoparticles.

Irradiation using infrared light with wide emission spectra causes unique heating effect to the SMPU, which can be noncontact. The capability of absorbing infrared light is determined by molecule (or atom) constitution of materials, as infrared light is absorbed in the form of molecule (or atom) resonance vibration (Leng and Du, 2010; Huang et al., 2012). SMP/CB nanocomposites have showed strong (above 6%) continuum absorption in the range from 400 to 4000 cm^{-1} (Leng and Du, 2010). The existence of CB particles increases the capability to absorb infrared light for the SMP/CB composite remarkably (Leng and Du, 2010). When SMP and SMP/CB nanocomposites are exposed to infrared light, most of the emitted energy is transmitted by the SMP, which is semi-transparent, whereas most of the emitted infrared light is absorbed by the CB, since it is black and opaque, thus causing the heating effect (Leng and Du, 2010; Huang et al., 2012).

9.4 Medical applications of SMPU

PU-based SMPs have excellent biocompatibility, verified from standard cytotoxicity and mutagenicity tests (Gall et al., 2004; Small et al., 2009). The T_g of the SMPUs can be tailored for shape restoration/self-deployment of various clinical devices. Various shape-memory stimuli methods other than heat, such as alternating magnetic field or light, have broadened their applications substantially and extended their applications to noncontact operations (Huang et al., 2012).

Because of their good biocompatibility, there are many potential medical applications using the SMPUs (Fare et al., 2005; Sokolowski et al., 2007; Metcalfe et al., 2003). Key examples proposed for medical applications include:

- Thermoset SMPU actuators for treating ischemic stroke (Metzger et al., 2002)
- SMP microfluidic reservoirs (Gall et al., 2004)
- Intravascular thrombectomy to remove blood clots; infrared diode laser activated (Metzger et al., 2005)
- Thrombus removal activated by laser light (Small et al., 2005)
- Self-deployable SMP neuronal electrodes (Sharp et al., 2006)
- Vascular stent deployed *in vitro* by laser heating (Baer et al., 2007)
- SMP dialysis needle adapters for reducing hemodynamic stress in arteriovenous grafts (Ortega et al., 2007)
- Deployable biomedical devices for minimally invasive surgery (MIS) (Baer et al., 2007)
- SMPUs in cardiovascular implants (Sokolowski et al., 2007; Jung et al., 2010a,b)
- SMPs for bondages (Ahmad et al., 2012a,b,c)
- SMPs for ocular implants (Huang et al., 2012)
- SMPs for cell manipulation (Huang et al., 2012)

MIS is regarded as one of the most important achievements in modern medicine. The benefits compared to traditional methods include reduced operative trauma, fewer wound complications, shorter hospital stays, and accelerated recoveries (Huang et al., 2012). However, MIS is more technically demanding than conventional surgery because the surgical intervention is executed remotely via two-dimensional imaging of the operative field. As a result, a surgeon faces the loss of tactile feedback, restricted maneuverability, and less efficient control of major bleeding. Shape-memory materials provide good solutions to many problems in the MIS arena (Yahia, 2000; Yoneyama and Miyazaki, 2009; Huang et al., 2012). Stainless steel and shape-memory alloys have been the dominant materials for these applications; however, there are several drawbacks associated with the use of metallic stents: stiffness, compliance mismatch with the arterial wall, and the high cost of fabrication (Miyazaki et al., 2009). Therefore, SMPs, especially SMPUs, have more potential applications to replace the SMAs.

9.4.1 Sutures

A challenge in endoscopic surgery is to tie a knot with instruments and sutures to close an incision or open lumen, and sutures are commonly used during medical operations. MIS procedures generally allow only limited space for tying knots to secure sutures in place, and surgeons must tie knots remotely through very small holes. SMP has been applied in wound closure, and the suture can be applied loosely in its temporary shape under elongated stress (Huang et al., 2012). When the temperature is raised above T_g, the suture will shrink and then tighten the knot, in which case it will apply an optimum force. Since its maximum recovery stress is safe for human body tissues, damage caused by over-tightening is no longer a serious issue. Figure 9.11 reveals that upon

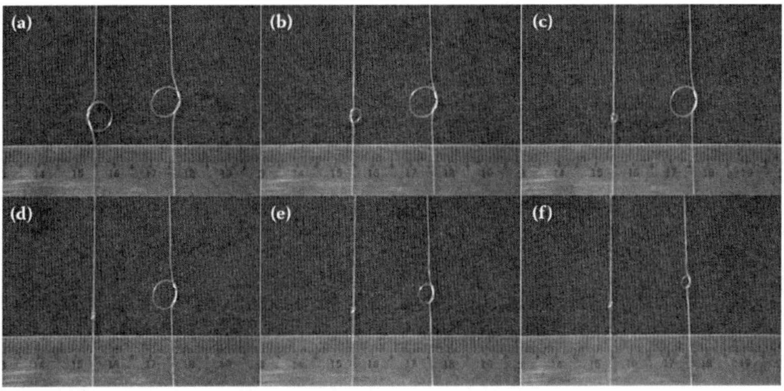

Figure 9.11 Self-tightening of two knots of SMP wires (MM3520) by immersion in room temperature water. The left piece was pre-immersed in water to reduce its T_g (Sun and Huang, 2010b).

immersion into room temperature water (about 22 °C), a polyurethane SMP knot tightens gradually (Sun and Huang, 2010a,b; Huang et al., 2012). Similarly, without heating, a knot can self-unravel and a suture can automatically tighten upon immersion into room temperature water. The sutures can also be biodegradable and show gradual mass loss during degradation (Lendlein and Kelch, 2005). For example, the hydrolyzable ester bonds are introduced into the polymers so that they would cleave under physiological conditions (Behl and Lendlein, 2007). If the SMP is biodegradable, sutures will self-degrade and disappear after time and even in a controllable manner (Lendlein and Kelch, 2005).

9.4.2 Stents

Vascular stents are small tubular scaffolds widely used in the treatment of arterial stenosis (narrowing of the vessel) to prevent acute vessel closure and late restenosis in a variety of vessels such as coronary arteries (Chen et al., 2007a, 2009). The increased flexibility, compliance, and relatively simple drug-embedding capability of SMPUs could overcome the problems encountered with current metallic vascular stents (Baer et al., 2007); for example, braided stents (Kim et al., 2010), solid-tube stents (Wache et al., 2003; Chen et al., 2007a,b; Yakacki et al., 2007), and even foam stents (Sokolowski et al., 2007). Other recent developments include drug-eluting stents and biodegradable stents (Chen et al., 2009; Wischke et al., 2010; Jung et al., 2010a,b; Wischke and Lendlein, 2010). The triggering mechanisms for the stents can be Joule heating or local laser heating (Maitland et al., 2002; Metzger et al., 2005; Baer et al., 2007; Huang et al., 2010a,b, 2012; Sun and Huang, 2010a,b).

Wache et al. (2003) conducted a feasibility study and a preliminary development on a polymer vascular stent with SMPs as a drug-delivery system. The use of the SMP stent

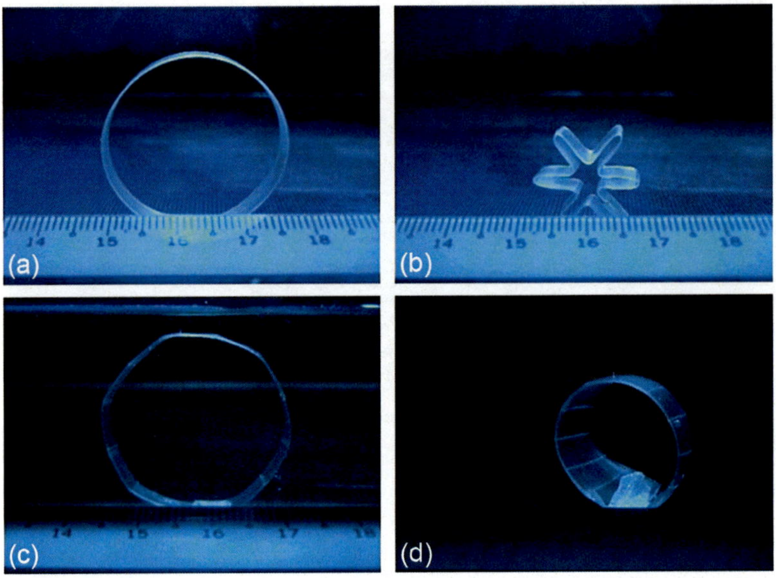

Figure 9.12 Retraction of a PU SMP stent in water. (a) After pre-stretching; (b) after folding; (c) after deployment in water; (d) after retraction in water.
Reproduced with permission from Yang et al. (2006).

as a drug-delivery system leads to significant reduction of restenosis and thrombosis. In bladder and prostate cancer treatments, retractable stents are preferred, but current conventional methods are mechanical dilations, endoscopic incision, or laser vaporization. Their success rates are low, and patients must undergo repeated treatments. A removable stent is a better option because it does not require a highly specialized reconstructive bladder neck repair procedure and is replaced annually. A retractable stents have been proposed to utilize the thermo- and moisture-responsive qualities of SMPUs (Huang et al., 2007). As shown in Figure 9.12, a SMP thin-wall tube was pre-expanded at high temperatures and then cooled back to room temperature (Yang et al., 2006). Subsequently, it was mechanically deformed into a star shape. After immersion into room temperature water, it mechanically expanded back into its circular shape. Since this SMP is also moisture-responsive, it shrinks after a time. As its diameter reduces, the stent can be easily removed (Huang et al., 2010a,b, 2012).

9.4.3 Cell and drug manipulation

Targeted drug release to specified cells at molecular level is currently an attractive topic in medical research (Han et al., 2010; Hartl and Hayer-Hartl, 2009). The thermo/moisture-responsiveness in polyurethane SMP sheds light on the possibility of realizing micro/nanodevices for surgery/operation at the cell level. As illustrated in Figure 9.13 (Sun and Huang, 2010b), a micro vehicle made of SMP is stretched and then inserted into a living cell. Upon absorbing moisture inside the cell, the

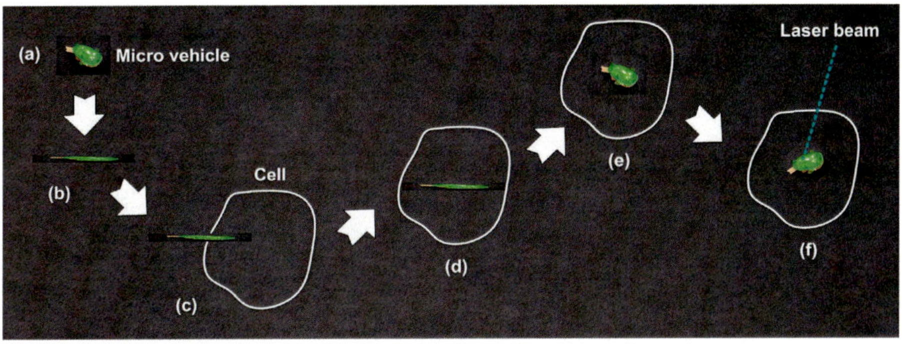

Figure 9.13 Delivery of a micro vehicle into a living cell for inside operation under a laser beam (illustration). (a) The original shape of a micro vehicle; (b) the shape of vehicle after reshaping; (c) inserting the deformed vehicle into a cell; (d) the vehicle fully inside the cell; (e) shape recovery of the vehicle; (f) in operation of the vehicle powered by a laser beam from outside. Reproduced from Sun and Huang (2010b).

SMP recovers its original shape. As the recovery strain in solid or porous SMPs is on an order of hundred percent, it becomes achievable to make cell- or sub-cell-sized machines using the thermo/moisture-responsive SMP and then deliver the machines into living cells for operation controlled by an outside laser beam (Johnson et al., 2007; Huang et al., 2010b).

9.4.4 Bandages

A venous leg ulcer is a common illness in developed countries (Fletcher et al., 1997). In this disease, the lower leg deteriorates because of reduced physical activity and poor blood circulation; the illness often affects the elderly. For patients with venous disease, application of gradient external compression can help minimize or reverse vascular change by forcing blood from the interstitial spaces back into the vascular and lymphatic compartments, hence leading to effective treatment (Ahmad et al., 2012c). Although there are various types of commercial bandages available for venous ulcer treatment, most have good elasticity but produce low compression forces.

Because pre-stretched thermal-responsive SMP strips will generate various shrinking forces upon heat stimulation, bandages made up of a number of SMP strips may generate distributed pressure and can be used for venous leg treatment (Ahmad et al., 2012a,b,c). An SMP actuator-based bandage has been proposed by Ahmad et al. (2012a,b,c) for leg ulcer treatments, as shown in Figure 9.14; they are made of a number of SMP strips with different strains with gradient pressure distribution. SMPUs have a suitable transition temperature range of 40–50 °C, have a low recovery stress (0.05–0.1 MPa), and are flexible. Therefore, these SMPUs are potentially useful in the proposed bandages. Thermal-responsive SMP strips are attached to fabrics that will be part of the underlay padding of the bandage, and the SMP strips are pre-stretched to fixed lengths or strains. In its fully developed form, the SMP bandage can be wrapped on the venous leg and held in position by Velcro fasteners or other similar means.

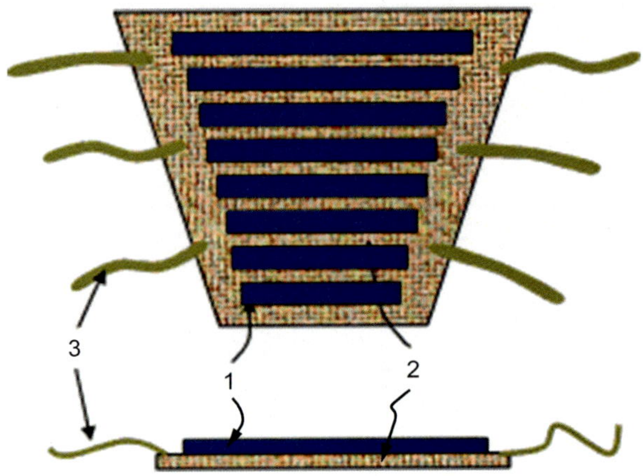

Figure 9.14 Design of the proposed SMP bandages, which can be applied/removed from a limb like a normal bandage once activated. 1, SMP strips; 2, Fabric; 3, Fasteners.

Upon application of an external heat using a normal hair dryer or a hot towel, the SMP stripes will shrink and partially return to their original shapes, providing a predefined force or pressure distribution acting on the venous leg for treatment. If the pressure drops during use, pressure readjustment can be easily achieved by using a hair dryer or a hot towel to warm up the SMP bandage, locally or as a whole. This can be done by the patient at home; without the need for a trained nurse/doctor, treatment is significantly simplified (Ahmad et al., 2012a,b,c).

9.4.5 Other applications

PU-based SMPs have potential as artificial muscles for a prosthesis if they can develop relatively large forces (1–3 MPa) and are able to shrink or elongate (Yahia, 2000; Metzger et al., 2002, 2005). SMP materials can be used to manufacture catheters that remain stiff externally for accurate manipulation by the physician, but become softer and more comfortable inside the human body. With a soft catheter, there will be fewer arterial wall injuries than with the conventional rigid catheter. They will also be easier to manipulate and apply into tortuous vessels.

A blood clot may cause an ischemic stroke, depriving the brain of oxygen and often resulting in permanent disability. As an alternative to conventional clot-dissolving drug treatment, a laser-activated device for the mechanical removal of blood clots has been proposed (Small et al., 2005). The deformed SMPU straight rods could be inserted by MIS into the vascular occlusion. The microactuator, which is mounted on the end of an optical fiber, is then transformed into its pre-deformed corkscrew shape by laser heating. Once deployed into the corkscrew shape, the microactuator is retracted from the captured thrombus, enabling the mechanical removal of the thrombus (Small et al., 2009).

Maitland et al. (2002) reported thermally activated SMP-based mechanical clot extraction devices to treat ischemic stroke. These devices were designed to be delivered through a catheter and penetrate the clot in a narrow form and then actuate into a clot-grabbing form for extraction. After doping the SMP with dye, laser-absorbing photothermal actuation of corkscrew-shaped and umbrella-shaped devices have been demonstrated, which can be actuated using a diode laser operating at a wavelength of 810 nm into the SMP device. Metzger et al. (2002, 2005) further demonstrated that the SMP corkscrew device could hold a blood clot against vascular physiological forces.

Mitral valve insufficiency occurs when the mitral valve does not close properly, resulting in the regurgitation of blood from the left ventricle to the left atrium (flow reversal). Valve repair, as opposed to replacement, is the preferred method of treatment; SMPU would be a good candidate (Enriquez-Sarano et al., 1995). SMPs can also be applied for minimally invasive tissue engineering. Tissues can be grown on SMP scaffolds and potentially delivered into the body using minimally invasive techniques and implanted to initiate repair or reconstruction of tissues or organs (Small et al., 2009). Biodegradable SMPs could be applied in pharyngeal mucosa reconstruction, bone regeneration, and organ repair (Small et al., 2009).

9.5 Summary and future trends

PU-based SMPs are smart materials with the unique characteristic of remembering their original shapes upon stimulation. They have been widely used in engineering, space exploration, and particularly in medical devices. Although SMPUs possess low mechanical strength and recovery stress compared to shape-memory alloys, their unique properties, such as high-shape recovery ratio, low recover stress, and flexibility, make them significant for various applications. SMPUs have many excellent properties: they are easy to manufacture, have a strong resistance to organic solvents and aqueous solutions, offer good, long-term stability against sunlight exposure, and have excellent and consistent elastic properties as well as biocompatibility. The multiple-responsive shape-memory feature of SMPUs further enables them to be used as a potential candidate for many biomedical devices, in particular MIS.

Properties of SMPUs can be tailored by varying the molecular weight of polyol, hard segment content, chain extender, or even moisture. Low recovery stress, modulus, and stiffness in SMPs are the main obstacles for their wide application. Incorporation of metals, nanofillers, clays, and tubes into PU matrices not only enhance the mechanical properties and recovery stress of SMPs, but also produce multifunctional composites. Shape recovery of SMPUs is normally a thermally induced process; however, they can also be triggered optically, electrically, magnetically, or electromagnetically, or by water or moisture, by adding various functional fillers. Various shape-memory stimuli methods other than heat, such as alternating magnetic field or light, have broadened their applications substantially and extended their applications to noncontact operations. The SMPUs have been proposed for many biomedical applications, including thermoset SMPU actuators for treating ischemic stroke, thrombus removal activated by laser light, self-deployable SMP neuronal electrodes, vascular stent, suture in microsurgery, ocular implants, bondages, cell manipulation, and cell therapy.

References

Ahir, S.V., Terentjev, E.M., 2005. Photomechanical actuation in polymer–nanotube composites. Nat. Mater. 4, 491–495.

Ahir, S.V., Tajbakhsh, A.R., Terentjev, E.M., 2006. Self-assembled shape-memory fibre of triblock liquid–crystal polymers. Adv. Funct. Mater. 16, 556–560.

Ahmad, M., Luo, J.K., Xu, B., Purnawali, H., King, P.J., Chalker, P., Fu, Y.Q., Huang, W.M., Miraftab, M., 2011. Synthesis and characterization of polyurethane-based shape memory polymers for tailored T_g around body temperature for medical applications. Macromol. Chem. Phys. 202, 592–602.

Ahmad, M., Luo, J.K., Miraftab, M., 2012a. Feasibility study of polyurethane shape-memory polymer actuators for pressure bandage application. Sci. Technol. Adv. Mater. 13, 015006.

Ahmad, M., Xu, B., Purnawali, H., Fu, Y.Q., Huang, W.M., Miraftab, M., Luo, J.K., 2012b. High performance shape memory polyurethane synthesized with high molecular weight polyols as soft segment. Appl. Sci. 2, 535–548.

Ahmad, M., Luo, J.K., Purnawali, H., Huang, W.M., King, P.J., Chalker, P.R., Miraftab, M., 2012c. Making shape memory polymers reprocessable and reusable by a simple chemical method. J. Mater. Chem. 20 (2012), 3442–3448.

Baer, G.M., Wilson, T.S., Benett, W.J., et al., 2007. Fabrication and in vitro deployment of a laser activated shape memory polymer vascular stent. BioMed. Eng. Online 6, 43.

Bassi, M., Tonelli, C., Di, A.M., 2003. Glass transition behavior of a microphase segregated polyurethane based on PFPE and IPDI. A calorimetric study. Macromolecules 36, 8015.

Behl, M., Lendlein, A., 2007. Shape-memory polymers. Mater. Today 10, 20–28.

Behl, M., Lendlein, A., 2010. Triple-shape polymers. J. Mater. Chem. 20, 3335–3345.

Bellin, I., Kelch, S., Langer, R., et al., 2006. Polymeric triple-shape materials. Proc. Natl. Acad. Sci. U. S. A. 103, 18043–18047.

Bellin, I., Kelch, S., Lendlein, A., 2007. Dual-shape properties of triple-shape polymer networks with crystallizable network segments and grafted side chains. J. Mater. Chem. 17, 2885–2891.

Bryning, M.B., Islam, M.F., Kikkawa, J.M., Yodh, A.G., 2005. Very low conductivity threshold in bulk isotropic single-walled carbon nanotube–epoxy composites. Adv. Mater. 17, 1186–1191.

Buckley, P.R., McKinley, G.H., Wilson, T.S., Small, W., et al., 2006. Inductively heated shape memory polymer for the magnetic actuation of medical devices. IEEE Trans. Biomed. Eng. 53, 2075–2083.

Cao, F., Jana, S.C., 2007. Nanoclay-tethered shape memory polyurethane nanocomposites. Polymer 48, 3790–3800.

Chen, S.J., Cao, Q., Jing, B., Cai, Y.L., Liu, P.S., Hu, J.L., 2006. Effect of microphase-separation promoters on the shape-memory behavior of polyurethane. J. Appl. Polym. Sci. 102, 5224.

Chen, M., Tsai, H., Chang, Y., et al., 2007a. Rapidly self-expandable polymeric stents with a shape-memory property. Biomacromolecules 8, 2274–2780.

Chen, S.J.J., Hu, L., Liu, Y.Q., Liem, H.M., Zhu, Y., Liu, Y.J., 2007b. Effect of SSL and HSC on morphology and properties of PHA based SMPU synthesized by bulk polymerization method. J. Polym. Sci. Pt. B-Polym. Phys. 45, 444–454.

Chen, M., Chang, Y., Liu, C., et al., 2009. The characteristics and *in vivo* suppression of neointimal formation with sirolimus-eluting polymeric stents. Biomaterials 30, 79–88.

Cho, J.W., Kim, J.W., Jung, Y.C., Goo, N.S., 2005. Electroactive shape-memory polyurethane composites incorporating carbon nanotubes. Macromol. Rapid Commun. 26, 412–416.

Choi, N.Y., Kelch, S., Lendlein, A., 2006. Synthesis, shape-memory functionality and hydrolytical degradation studies on polymer networks from poly(rac-lactide)-*b*-poly(propylene oxide)-*b*-poly(rac-lactide) dimethacrylates. Adv. Eng. Mater. 8, 439–445.
Chun, B.C., Cho, T.K., Chung, Y.C., 2006. Enhanced mechanical and shape memory properties of polyurethane block copolymers chain-extended by ethylene diamine. J. Eur. Polym. 42, 3367.
Ding, X.M., Hu, J.L., Tao, X.M., Hu, C.P., 2006. Preparation of temperature sensitive polyurethanes for smart textiles. J. Tex. Res. 76, 406.
El-Feninat, F., Laroche, G., Fiset, M., Mantovani, D., 2002. Shape memory materials for biomedical applications. Adv. Eng. Mater. 4, 91–104.
Enriquez-Sarano, M., Tajik, A.J., Bailey, K.R., Seward, J.B., 1993. Color flow imaging compared with quantitative Doppler assessment of severity of mitral regurgitation: influence of eccentricity of jet and mechanism of regurgitation. J. Am. Coll. Cardiol. 21, 1211–1219.
Fare, S., Valtulina, V., Petrini, P., Alessandrini, E., Pietrocola, G., Tanzi, M.C., Speziale, P., Visai, L., 2005. In vitro interaction of human fibroblasts and platelets with a shape-memory polyurethane. J. Biomed. Mater. Res. A 73A, 1–11.
Fletcher, A., Cullum, N., Sherdon, T.A., 1997. A systematic review of compression treatment for venous leg ulcers. J. Br. Med. 315, 576.
Gall, K., Mikulas, M., Munshi, N.A., Beavers, F., Tupper, M., 2000. Carbon fiber reinforced shape memory polymer composites. J. Intell. Materials Syst. Struct. 11, 877–886.
Gall, K., Kreiner, P., Turner, D., et al., 2004. Shape-memory polymer for microelectromechanical systems. J. Microelectromechanical Syst. 13, 472–483.
Goethals, E.J., Reyntjens, W., Lievens, S., 1998. Poly(vinyl ethers) as building blocks for new materials. Macromol. Symp. 132, 57–64.
Gunes, I.S., Jana, S.C., 2008. Shape memory polymers and their nanocomposites: a review of science and technology of new multifunctional materials. J. Nanosci. Nanotechnol. 8, 1616–1637.
Gunes, I.S., Cao, F., Jana, S.C., 2008. Evaluation of nanoparticulate fillers for development of shape memory polyurethane nanocomposites. Polymer 49, 2223–2234.
Gunes, I.S., Jimenez, G.A., Jana, S.C., 2009. Carbonaceous fillers for shape memory actuation of polyurethane composites by resistive heating. Carbon 47, 981–997.
Han, D., Pal, S., Liu, Y., et al., 2010. Folding and cutting DNA into reconfigurable topological nanostructures. Nat. Nanotechnol. 5, 712–717.
Hartl, F.U., Hayer-Hartl, M., 2009. Converging concepts of protein folding *in vitro* and *in vivo*. Nat. Struct. Mol. Biol. 16, 574–581.
Hayashi, S., 1990. Technical report on preliminary investigation of shape memory polymers. Mitsubishi Heavy Industries, Research and Development Center, Nagoya, Japan.
Hu, J.L., Zeng, Y.M., Yan, H.J., 2003. Influence of processing conditions on the microstructure and properties of shape memory polyurethane membranes. Text. Res. J. 73, 172.
Huang, W.M., 2010. Thermo-moisture responsive polyurethane shape memory polymer for biomedical devices. Open Med. Dev. J. 2, 11–19.
Huang, W.M., Yang, B., An, L., et al., 2005. Water-driven programmable polyurethane shape memory polymer: demonstration and mechanism. Appl. Phys. Lett. 86, 114105.
Huang, W.M., Lee, C.W., Teo, H.P., 2006. Thermomechanical behavior of a polyurethane shape memory polymer foam. J. Intell. Mater. Syst. Struct. 17, 753–760.
Huang, W.M., Yang, B., Liu, N., Phee, S.J., 2007. Water-responsive programmable shape memory polymer devices. Int. Conf. Smart Mater. Nanotechnol. Eng. 6423, 64231–64237.
Huang, W.M., Yang, B., Zhao, Y., Ding, Z., 2010a. Thermo-moisture responsive polyurethane shape-memory polymer and composites: a review. J. Mater. Chem. 20, 3367–3381.
Huang, W.M., Ding, Z., Wang, C.C., et al., 2010b. Shape memory materials. Mater. Today 13, 44–51.

Huang, W.M., Yang, B., Fu, Y.Q., 2012. Polyurethane Shape Memory Polymers. CRC Press, Boca Raton, FL, USA, 33487-2742.

Jeong, H.M., Lee, S.Y., Kim, B.K., 2000. Shape memory polyurethane containing amorphous reversible phase. J. Mater. Sci. 35, 1579–1583.

Jiang, H.Y., Kelch, S., Lendlein, A., 2006. Polymers move in response to light. Adv. Mater. 18, 1471–1475.

Johnson, C.P., Tang, H., Carag, C., et al., 2007. Forced unfolding of protein within cells. Science 317, 663–666.

Jung, Y.C., Cho, J.W., 2010. Application of shape memory polyurethane in orthodontic. J. Mater. Sci. Mater. Med. 21, 2881–2886.

Jung, F., Wischke, C., Lendlein, A., 2010a. Degradable, multifunctional cardiovascular implants: challenges and hurdles. MRS Bull. 35, 607–613.

Jung, Y.C., Yoo, H.J., Kim, Y.A., Cho, J.W., Endo, M., 2010b. Electroactive shape memory performance of polyurethane composite having homogeneously dispersed and covalently cross-linked carbon nanotubes. Carbon 48, 1598–1603.

Kim, B.K., Lee, S.Y., Xu, M., 1996. Polyurethanes having shape memory effect. Polymer 37, 5781–5793.

Kim, J.H., Kang, T.J., Yu, W., 2010. Simulation of mechanical behavior of temperature-responsive braided stents made of shape memory polyurethanes. J. Biomech. 43, 632–643.

Koerner, H., Price, G., Pearce, N.A., Alexander, M., Vaia, R., 2004. Remotely actuated polymer nanocomposites—stress-recovery of carbon-nanotube-filled thermoplastic elastomers. Nat. Mater. 3, 115–120.

Kumar, U.N., Kratz, K., Wagermaier, W., et al., 2010. Non-contact actuation of triple-shape effect in multiphase polymer network nanocomposites in alternating magnetic field. J. Mater. Chem. 20, 3404–3415.

Lee, B.S., Chun, B.C., Chung, Y.C., Sul, K.I., Cho, J.W., 2001. Structure and thermomechanical properties of polyurethane block copolymers with shape memory effect. Macromolecules 34, 6431.

Lee, S.H., Kim, J.W., Kim, B.K., 2004. Shape memory polyurethanes having crosslinks in soft and hard segments. Smart Mater. Struct. 13, 1345–1350.

Lendlein, A., Kelch, S., 2002. Shape-memory polymers. Angew. Chem. Int. Ed. 41, 2034–2057.

Lendlein, A., Kelch, S., 2005. Degradable, multifunctional polymeric biomaterials with shape-memory. In: Van der Biest, O., et al. (Ed.), In: Functionally Graded Materials VIII, vol. 219. Technology Transition Publications, Leuven, Belgium, pp. 492–493.

Lendlein, A., Jiang, H., Junger, O., Langer, R., 2005. Light-induced shape-memory polymers. Nature 434, 879–882.

Leng, J.S., Du, S.Y., 2010. Shape-Memory Polymers and Multifunctional Composites. CRC Press, Boca Raton, FL.

Leng, J., Lv, H., Liu, Y., Du, S., 2007. Electroactivate shape-memory polymer filled with nano-carbon particles and short carbon fibers. Appl. Phys. Lett. 91, 144105.

Leng, J.S., Huang, W.M., Lan, X., Liu, Y.J., Liu, N., Phee, S.Y., Du, S.Y., 2008a. Significantly reducing electrical resistivity by forming conductive Ni chains in a polyurethane shape-memory polymer/carbon-black composite. Appl. Phys. Lett. 92, 204101.

Leng, J.S., Lan, X., Huang, W.M., Liu, Y.J., Liu, N., Phee, S.Y., Du, S.Y., et al., 2008b. Electrical conductivity of shape memory polymer embedded with micro Ni chains. Appl. Phys. Lett. 92, 014104.

Liang, C., Rogers, C.A., Malafeew, E., 1997. Investigation of shape memory polymers and their hybrid composites. J. Intel. Mat. Syst. Str. 8, 380–386.

Liu, G.Q., Ding, X.B., Cao, Y.P., et al., 2005. Novel shape-memory polymer with two transition temperatures. Macromol. Rapid Commun. 26, 649–652.
Liu, Y., Lv, H., Lan, X., Leng, J., Du, S., 2009. Review of electro-active shape-memory polymer composite. Compos. Sci. Technol. 69, 2064.
Lv, H.B., Leng, J.S., Liu, Y.J., Du, S.Y., 2008a. Shape-memory polymer in response to solution. Adv. Eng. Mater. 10, 592–595.
Lv, H.B., Liu, Y.J., Zhang, D., Leng, J.S., Du, S., 2008b. Solution-responsive shape-memory polymer driven by forming hydrogen bonding. Adv. Mater. Res. 47–50, 258–261.
Ma, Z.L., Zhao, W.G., Liu, Y.F., Shi, J.R., 1997. Intumescent polyurethane coatings with reduced flammability based on spirocyclic phosphate-containing polyols. J. Appl. Polym. Sci. 66, 471–475.
Maitland, D.J., Metzger, M.F., Schumann, D., et al., 2002. Photothermal properties of shape memory polymer micro-actuators for treating stroke. Lasers Surg. Med. 30, 1–11.
Meng, Q.H., Hu, J.L., 2009. A review of shape memory polymer composites and blends. Composites A 40, 1661.
Merlin, M., 2008. Using NiTi shape memory alloy wires for the geometry active control in a cooling fan. Adv. Geomater. Struct. 1, 51–61.
Merline, J.D.C., Nair, P.R., Gouri, C., Bandyopadhyay, G.G., Ninan, K.N., 2008. Polyether polyurethanes: synthesis, characterization, and thermoresponsive shape memory properties. J. Appl. Polym. Sci. 107, 4082–4092.
Metcalfe, A., Desfaits, A.C., Salazkin, I., Yahia, L., Sokolowski, W.M., Raymond, J., 2003. Cold hibernated elastic memory foams for endovascular interventions. Biomaterials 24, 491–497.
Metzger, M.F., Wilson, T.S., Schumann, D., et al., 2002. Mechanical properties of mechanical actuator for treating ischemic stroke. Biomed. Microdevices 4, 89–96.
Metzger, M.F., Wilson, T.S., Maitland, D.J., 2005. Laser-activated shape memory polymer microactuator for thrombus removal following ischemic stroke: preliminary *in vitro* analysis. IEEE J. Selected Top. Quantum Electron. 11, 892–900.
Miaudet, P., Derre, A., Maugey, M., et al., 2007. Shape and temperature memory of nanocomposites with broadened glass transition. Science 318, 1294–1296.
Miyazaki, S., Fu, Y.Q., Huang, W.M., 2009. Thin Film Shape Memory Alloys: Fundamentals and Device Applications. Cambridge University Press, Cambridge.
Monkman, G.J., 2000a. Advances in shape memory polymer actuation. Mech. Mater. 10, 489.
Monkman, G.J., 2000b. Advances in shape memory actuation. Mechatronics 10, 489–498.
Ortega, J., Maitland, D.J., Wilson, T.S., Tsai, W., Savas, O., Saloner, D., 2007. Vascular dynamics of a shape memory polymer foam aneurysm treatment technique. Annu. Biomed. Eng. 35, 1870–1884.
Paik, I.H., Goo, N.S., Jung, Y.C., Cho, J.W., 2006. Development and application of conducting shape memory polyurethane actuators. Smart Mater. Struct. 15, 1476–1482.
Pretsch, T., 2010. Triple-shape properties of a thermoresponsive poly(ester urethane). Smart Mater. Struct. 19, 015006.
Razzaq, M.Y., Anhalt, M., Frormann, L., Weidenfeller, B., 2007a. Thermal, electrical and magnetic studies of magnetite filled polyurethane shape memory polymers. Mater. Sci. Eng. A 444, 227–235.
Razzaq, M.Y., Anhalt, M., Frormann, L., Weidenfeller, B., 2007b. Mechanical spectroscopy of magnetite filled polyurethane shape memory polymers. Mater. Sci. Eng. A 471, 57–62.
Ren, L., Chow, G.M., 2003. Synthesis of NIR-sensitive Au–Au_2S nanocolloids for drug delivery. Mat. Sci. Eng. C 23, 113.
Sahoo, N.G., Jung, Y.C., Goo, N.S., Cho, J.W., 2005. Conducting shape memory polyurethane-polypyrrole composites for an electroactive actuator. Macromol. Mater. Eng. 290, 1049–1055.

Sahoo, N.G., Rana, S., Cho, J.W., Li, L., Chan, S.H., 2010. Polymer nanocomposites based on functionalized carbon nanotubes. Prog. Polym. Sci. 35, 837–867.

Sandler, J.K.W., Kirk, J.E., Kinloch, I.A., Shaffer, M.S.P., Windle, A.H., 2003. Ultra-low electrical percolation threshold in carbon-nanotube-epoxy composites. Polymer 44, 5893–5899.

Schmidt, A.M., 2006. Electromagnetic activation of shape memory polymer networks containing magnetic nanoparticles. Macromol. Rapid Commun. 27, 1168–1172.

Sharp, A.A., Panchawagh, H.V., Ortega, A., et al., 2006. Toward a self-deploying shape memory polymer neuronal electrode. J. Neural Eng. 3, L23–L30.

Small, W., Wilson, T.S., Benett, W.J., Loge, J.M., Maitland, D.J., 2005. Laser activated shape memory polymer intravascular thrombectomy device. Opt. Express 13, 8204–8213.

Small IV, W., Singhal, P., Wilson, T.S., Maitland, D.J., 2010. Biomedical applications of thermally activated shape memory polymers. J. Mater. Chem. 20 (18), 3356–3366.

Sokolowski, W., Metcalfe, A., Hayashi, S., et al., 2007. Medical applications of shape memory polymers. Biomed. Mater. 2, S23–S27.

Spinks, G.M., Mottaghitalab, V., Bahrami-Saniani, M., Whitten, P.G., Wallace, G.G., 2006. Carbon-nanotube-reinforced polyaniline fibers for high-strength artificial muscles. Adv. Mater. 18, 637.

Sun, L., Huang, W.M., 2010a. Mechanisms of the multi-shape memory effect and temperature memory effect in shape memory polymers. Soft Matter 6, 4403–4406.

Sun, L., Huang, W.M., 2010b. Thermo/moisture responsive shape-memory polymer for possible surgery/operation inside living cells in future. Mater. Design 31, 2684–2689.

Sun, L., Huang, W.M., Cheah, J.Y., 2010. The temperature memory effect and the influence of thermo-mechanical cycling in shape memory alloys. Smart Mater. Struct. 19, 055005.

Szycher, M., 1999. Szycher's Handbook of Polyurethanes. CRC Press, Boca Raton.

Tobushi, H., Hayashi, S., Kojima, S., 1992. Mechanical properties of shape memory polymer of polyurethane series: basic characteristics of stress-strain-temperature relationship. JSME Int. J. Ser. 1 (35), 296–302.

Tobushi, H., Hara, H., Yamada, E., et al., 1996. Thermomechanical properties in a thin film of shape memory polymer of polyurethane series. Smart Mater. Struct. 5, 483–491.

Tobushi, H., Okumura, K., Hayashi, S., Ito, N., 2001. Thermomechanical constitutive model of shape memory polymer. Mech. Mater. 33, 545–554.

Wache, H.M., Tartakowska, D.J., Hentrich, A., et al., 2003. Development of polymer stent with shape memory effect as a drug delivery system. J. Mater. Sci. Mater. Med. 14, 109–112.

Wei, Z.G., Sandstroröm, R., Miyazaki, S., 1998. Shape-memory materials and hybrid composites for smart systems: Part I Shape-memory materials. J. Mater. Sci. 33, 3743–3762.

Weigel, T., Mohr, R., Lendlein, A., 2009. Investigation of parameters to achieve temperatures required to initiate the shape-memory effect of magnetic nanocomposites by inductive heating. Smart Mater. Struct. 18, 025011.

Wischke, C., Lendlein, A., 2010. Shape-memory polymers as drug carriers - a multifunctional system. Pharm. Res. 27, 527–529.

Wischke, C., Beffe, A.T., Lendlein, A., 2010. Controlled drug release from biodegradable shape-memory polymers. Adv. Polym. Sci. 226, 177–205.

Xie, T., 2010. Tunable polymer multi-shape memory effect. Nature 464, 267–270.

Xie, T., Xiao, X.C., Cheng, Y.T., 2009. Revealing triple-shape memory effect by polymer bilayers. Macromol. Rapid Commun. 30, 1823–1827.

Xu, B., Huang, W.M., Pei, Y.T., et al., 2009. Mechanical properties of attapulgite clay-reinforced polyurethane shape memory nanocomposites. Eur. Polym. J. 45, 1904–1911.

Xu, B.Y.Q.Fu., Ahmad, M., Luo, J.K., Huang, W.M., Kraft, A., Reuben, R., Pei, Y.T., Chen, Z. G., Th, J., De Hosson, M., 2010. Thermo-mechanical properties of polystyrene-based shape memory nanocomposites. J. Mater. Chem. 20, 3442–3448.

Yahia, L., 2000. Shape memory implants. In: Yakacki, C.M., Shandas, R., Lanning, C., et al. (Eds.), Unconstrained Recovery Characterization. Springer, Heidelberg.

Yakacki, C.M., Shandas, R., Lanning, C., Rech, B., Eckstein, A., Gall, K., 2007. Unconstrained recovery characterization of shape-memory polymer networks for cardiovascular applications. Biomaterials 28, 2255–2263.

Yakacki, C.M., Satarkar, N.S., Gall, K., Likos, R., Hilt, J.Z., 2009. Shape-memory polymer networks with Fe_3O_4 nanoparticles for remote activation. J. Appl. Polym. Sci. 112, 3166–3176.

Yang, B., 2007, Characterisation of polyurethane shape memory polymers. PhD Thesis, Nanyang Technological University, Singapore.

Yang, J.H., Chun, B.C., Chung, Y., Cho, J.H., 2003. Comparison of thermal/mechanical properties and shape memory effect of polyurethane block-copolymers with planar or bent shape of hard segment. Polymer 44, 3251.

Yang, B., Huang, W.M., Li, C., Lee, C.M., Li, L., 2004. On the effects of moisture in a polyurethane shape memory polymer. Smart Mater. Struct. 13, 191–195.

Yang, B., Huang, W.M., Li, C., Li, L., Chor, J.H., 2005. Qualitative separation of the effects of carbon nanopowder and moisture on the glass transition temperature of polyurethane shape memory polymer. Scr. Mater. 53, 105–107.

Yang, B., Huang, W.M., Li, C., Li, L., 2006. Effects of moisture on the thermomechanical properties of a polyurethane shape memory polymer. Polymer 47, 1348–1356.

Yang, F., Wornyo, E., Gall, K., King, W.P., 2007. Nanoscale indent formation in shape memory polymers using a heated probe tip. Nanotechnology. 18, 285302.

Yoneyama, T., Miyazaki, S., 2009. Shape Memory Alloys for Biomedical Applications. Woodhead Publishing Limited, Cambridge, UK.

Zhang, C.S., Ni, Q.Q., Fu, S.Y., Kurashiki, K., 2007. Electromagnetic interference shielding effect of nanocomposites with carbon nanotube and shape memory polymer. Compos. Sci. Technol. 67, 2973–2980.

Zhao, Y., Huang, W.M., Fu, Y.Q., 2011. Formation of micro/nano-scale wrinkling patterns atop shape memory polymers. J. Micromech. Microeng. 21, 067007.

Zhu, Y., Hu, J.L., Yeung, L.Y., Liu, Y., Ji, F.L., Yeung, K.W., 2006. Development of shape memory polyurethane fiber with complete shape recoverability. Smart Mater. Struct. 15, 1385–1394.

Zhuo, H.T., Hu, J.L., Chen, S.J., 2008. Electrospun polyurethane nanofibres having shape memory effect. Mater. Lett. 62, 2074–2076.

Zdrahala, R.J., Zdrahala, I.J., 1999. Biomedical applications of polyurethanes: a review of past promises, present realities, and a vibrant future. J. Biomater. Appl. 14, 67–90.

Polylactic acid (PLA)-based shape-memory materials for biomedical applications

10

J. Xu, J. Song
University of Massachusetts Medical School, Worcester, MA, USA

10.1 Introduction

10.1.1 The shape-memory effect in polymers

The shape-memory effect is not a "new" phenomenon or property. In his classical book *Principles of Polymer Chemistry*, Flory (1953) cited the experimental description recorded in 1806 by the English natural and experimental philosopher John Gough:

> *If a thong of Caoutchouc (a kind of nature rubber) be stretched, in water warmer than itself, it retains its elasticity unimpaired; on the contrary, if the experiment be made in water colder than itself, it loses part of its retractile power, being unable to recover its former figure; but let the thong be placed in hot water, while it remains extended for want of spring, and the heat will immediately make it contract briskly.*

Such an experiment is essentially the same as how we demonstrate that a polymer possesses shape-memory properties today (Lendlein and Kelch, 2002).

Rather than being an intrinsic materials property, the shape-memory effect results from the chemical composition and network structure of a polymer and its appropriate processing and programming. The driving force behind a polymer recovering to its "memorized" shape is the recoiling tendency of strained polymeric chains to the lower-energy random-coiled state (Xu and Song, 2010). As long as polymeric chains could be stretched without complete relaxation, there would be some recovering tendency from the chains that should result in some extent of shape recovery. Such a scenario is relatively easy to realize in most polymeric materials. In fact, the shape-memory effect has been observed in almost all kinds of polymers, both chemical cross-linked and physically cross-linked (Lendlein and Kelch, 2002). Depending on the specific chemical composition, network structure, and processing methods, however, the efficiency of their shape-memory behaviors vary.

The industrial applications of the shape-memory effect of polymers date back to 1950s, when chemist Paul Cook, the founder of Raychem Corporation, invented heat shrink tubing from radiation cross-linked polyethylene (Cook, 1990). However, the biomedical applications of shape-memory polymers (SMPs) remained largely

Shape Memory Polymers for Biomedical Applications. http://dx.doi.org/10.1016/B978-0-85709-698-2.00010-6

unexplored until the publication of a series of landmark papers by Lendlein, Langer, and colleagues in the early 2000s (Lendlein et al., 2001; Lendlein and Kelch, 2002; Lendlein and Langer, 2002). Since then, there has been an explosion of (renewed) interests from both academia and industry exploring a wide range of applications, including biomedical applications, of SMPs, with >100 SMP-related papers and patents published annually. Recent progress on the development and applications of SMPs has been extensively reviewed by Lendlein's group (Lendlein and Kelch, 2002; Behl and Lendlein, 2007a,b; Behl et al., 2010), Mather's group (Liu et al., 2007; Mather et al., 2009), Sokolowski's group (Sokolowski et al., 2007; Sokolowski and Tan, 2007), and many others (Dietsch and Tong, 2007; Rousseau, 2008; Meng and Hu, 2009; Ionov, 2010) since 2001. Today, the most challenging aspect and thus the focus of SMP research is no longer to identify/demonstrate shape-memory property in different materials, but to address key limitations for their practical applications, for instance, for biomedical uses.

This chapter focuses on SMPs incorporating lactic acid-based polymers as major network components. Following the introduction of the synthesis and basic properties of polylactic acid (PLA), we discuss the basic requirement for exhibiting shape-memory properties and review the history and progress on PLA-based SMPs and the mechanisms of shape-recovery activations. We conclude the chapter with a brief discussion on the limitations of current PLA-based SMPs for biomedical applications and suggest some future directions. We adopt the terminologies defined in our previous review (Xu and Song, 2011) to describe the shape-memory properties here.

10.1.2 History and general properties of lactic acid-based polymers

PLA, the homopolymer of lactic acid, has been known for more than 80 years. It was initially prepared by Wallace Carothers in 1932 by heating lactic acid under vacuum. Such a manufacturing technique was further refined and patented by Dupont in 1954. Lactic acid, first identified in sour milk in 1780 by Carl Wilhelm Scheele (Benninga, 1990), could be produced by either chemical synthesis or fermentation of carbohydrates. Optically pure chiral lactic acid, however, is difficult to obtain by chemical synthesis, which usually gives a racemic mixture of L- and D-stereoisomer that is difficult to separate. By contrast, the fermentation method produces chiral lactic acid inexpensively in a ratio of 99.5% of L-isomer to 0.5% of D-isomer (Wee et al., 2006).

The PLA manufactured by the early polymerization techniques had low molecular weights and poor mechanical properties and thus did not gain enough industrial interest. The breakthrough ring-opening polymerization (ROP) of lactides developed by Cargill around the 1990s (Gruber and O'Brien, 2005) changed this situation. In this patented ROP technique, low-molecular-weight PLA prepolymer was first prepared by a continuous condensation reaction of aqueous lactic acid. The prepolymer was next converted into lactide via intramolecular cyclization using tin catalyst. The molten lactide mixture was then subjected to vacuum distillation and purified into optically pure chiral lactide monomers and used for ROP to produce high-molecular-weight PLA. The whole process eliminated the use of costly and environmentally unfriendly solvents, and the lactide monomer could be recovered after the polymerization. The advances in catalysts and the ROP process improvements have further decreased the production cost of the lactide monomers and the PLA. The breakthrough led to the formation of NatureWorks (originally Cargill Dow LLC) in 1998, which is still operating the first and largest commercial PLA manufacturing plant today. Mitsui Chemicals (Japan) recently commercialized an azeotropic dehydration process using a high-boiling-point solvent to obtain high-molecular-weight PLA directly from lactic acid, but this method still faces the typical challenges associated with the polycondensation process in terms of cost (e.g., requiring a large reactor for solvent evaporation and solvent recovery), increased color, and racemization (Gruber and O'Brien, 2005; Garlotta, 2002). The ROP method using lactides as the monomer, capable of achieving higher molecular weight and narrower molecular weight distribution, is still the most adopted method in both laboratory research and industrial manufacturing (Kricheldorf, 2004; Biela et al., 2006; Coulembier et al., 2006; Gupta and Kumar, 2007).

PLA is generally considered a thermoplastic material with high elastic modulus, high tensile strength, and low elongation at break. Compared with other commercial thermoplastics, PLA is relatively brittle with low impact strength; it has poor processing characteristics, including vulnerability to hydrolysis and low crystallization rate. Since lactic acid could exist in two forms, D-lactic acid and L-lactic acid, the dimeric cyclic lactide could exist in three chiral-configurations (diastereomers): L-lactide, D,L-lactide, and D-lactide. D,L-Lactide has a higher melting point (116–119 °C) than L-lactide, D-lactide (94–96 °C), or meso-lactide (nonchiral; 43–47 °C) (Ahmed and Varshney, 2011; Inkinen et al., 2011). The stereochemical structure and the physical properties of PLA can be readily modified by varying the monomer stereochemistry, monomer feed ratios, and the polymerization conditions. Isotactic PLA, including poly(D-lactide) (PDLA) and poly(L-lactide) (PLLA), is a highly crystalline material, while poly(D,L-lactide) (PDLLA) is amorphous. PLLA is the more extensively studied due to the relative ease of obtaining optically pure L-lactide. Pure PLLA, with a crystallinity of about 37%, has a glass transition temperature (T_g) of 60–65 °C, a melting temperature (T_m) of 173–178 °C, an elastic modulus of 3–4 GPa, and a tensile strength of 50–70 MPa with an elongation at break of 2–10% (Ahmed and Varshney, 2011). The incorporation of D-lactide in PLA results in a material that gradually changes from semicrystalline into amorphous (when the D-lactide content is greater than 15%). Amorphous PLA generally has a lower elastic modulus and tensile strength and a slightly higher elongation at break. Besides chemical compositions, the molecular weight and manufacturing process of PLA also greatly affect its microstructures and mechanical properties (Garlotta, 2002).

The affordability of the starting materials along with the high tensile strength and elastic modulus, the hydrolytic and enzymatic degradability, and the nontoxic degradation products of the polymers make lactic acid-based polymers attractive for biomedical applications in addition to commodity thermoplastics. In the past three decades, lactic acid-based polymers have been used for applications ranging from food packaging materials (Ahmed and Varshney, 2011) to drug-delivery carriers (Langer and Tirrell, 2004; Cameron and Shaver, 2011), surgical implants, and tissue engineering scaffolds (Middleton and Tipton, 2000). Accordingly, numerous strategies, including stereo-complexation (Tsuji and Ikada, 1999), copolymerization (Grijpma and Pennings, 1994), and blending (Hongzhi and Jinwen, 2012), have been explored to endow PLA with tailored properties (e.g., shape-memory property) for specific applications (e.g., biomedical uses).

10.2 Lactic acid-based shape-memory polymers (SMPs)

10.2.1 Basic structure requirement of lactic acid-based SMPs for biomedical applications

Shape-memory properties have been observed in many polymers, including chemically cross-linked thermosets and physically cross-linked thermoplastics. The common structural feature of all SMP networks is the presence of shape-fixing and shape-switching parts. The shape-fixing parts are the structural domains or net-points in an SMP network that maintains dimensional stability during deformation and recovery. They could be chemically cross-linked or formed through physical entanglement/crystallization of polymer chains driven by strong noncovalent interactions (e.g., hydrogen bonding, van der Waals, π–π stacking, electrostatic attractions). The shape-switching parts are the long polymeric chains between the shape-fixing parts that are stretched during deformation (temporary shape programming) to store elastic energy and are responsible for the elastic recoiling during the shape recovery upon stimulation.

Since both physical entanglement and the crystallization of long PLA can act as the net-points, all high-molecular-weight PLA, including PLLA, PDLA, PDLLA, and their stereo-complexes, should theoretically have shape-memory ability. In reality, however, the observation of the shape-memory effect in PLA is often limited to small deformations due to their tendency to break when the programming stains exceed 10%. This drawback limits the potential for programming strained temporary shapes (e.g., for minimally invasive surgical delivery) that are drastically different from the relaxed permanent configurations (e.g., conforming to a complex tissue defect configuration) for biomedical uses.

For biomedical applications, it is also highly desirable to have the transition temperature of an SMP slightly above body temperature to ensure stable shape fixing in a minimally invasive configuration during surgical delivery and to safely trigger the shape recovery to a preprogrammed configuration. The glass transition temperature (T_g) of PLA around 60 °C thus limits its direct use *in vivo* due to concerns over potential tissue damage that such a high triggering temperature may incur. Ideally, the *in vivo* degradation profile of PLA-based SMP tissue scaffolds or medical implants should also be tuned to match its intended function *in vivo*.

Accordingly, much of the work on biomedical uses of SMPs with high-molecular-weight PLA as major network components is to increase their toughness and decrease their T_gs without deteriorating shape-memory efficiency. Meanwhile, lactic acid is incorporated into the network chains of other nondegradable SMPs to improve their degradation profile for potential use as resorbable SMP implants.

10.2.2 History and recent progress on PLA-based SMPs

The first PLA-based SMP was disclosed in a patent by Langer, Lendlein, and colleagues at MIT (Langer et al., 2000). They disclosed the preparation of low-molecular-weight poly(lactide-*co*-glycolide)diol (PLGA, Mn ~ 2000 g/mol) by copolymerization of glycolide with L,L-lactide with ethylene glycol as an initiator. The copolymer diol was further used with oligo(*p*-dioxanone)diol (ODX) to prepare multiblock polyester-urethane. PLGA diol and ODX, the soft and hard segments in the obtained polyester-urethane, respectively, functioned as the shape-switching and shape-fixing parts of the SMP network. In their following report published in the journal *Science* (Lendlein and Langer, 2002), it was pointed out that the degradation of L-lactide-based polyesters led to a nonlinear mass loss with a sudden release of acidic degradation products that can potentially elicit strong inflammatory responses.

Following this landmark work exploring multiblock degradable SMPs for biomedical applications and the subsequent review by Lendlein and Kelch (2002), a lot of patents and publications on degradable SMPs were filed and published. A large portion of these work adopted the multiblock polymer concept, where high-molecular-weight polymers consisting of discrete blocks with different transition temperatures acted as shape-fixing and shape-switching parts during the shape-memory programming, respectively. Most of these materials reported excellent shape-memory properties with shape-fixing and shape-recovery ratios over 90% at low deformations.

Most of the work from Lendlein's group on SMPs containing lactic acid in the network chains used low-molecular-weight oligomers prepared by copolymerization of lactide and other monomers (Langer et al., 2000; Lendlein and Langer, 2002; Bertmer et al., 2005a,b; Choi et al., 2006; Choi and Lendlein, 2007; Kelch et al., 2008; Lendlein et al., 2009; Wischke et al., 2009; Neffe et al., 2010; Pierce et al., 2011). These SMPs were prepared as either semicrystalline, high-molecular weight, linear polyesterurethanes through chain extension of oligomeric diols with difunctional extenders, or chemically cross-linked by reacting multifunctional oligomers with cross-linkers.

To overcome the unfavorable degradation profiles associated with semicrystalline SMPs and to obtain a more homogenous network, Lendlein and colleagues reported an amorphous lactic acid-based SMP in 2005 (Alteheld et al., 2005). Specifically, they chemically cross-linked 3- and 4-arm oligo[(*rac*-lactide)-*co*-glycolide] (M_n: 1000–10,000) with aliphatic diisocyanate. The obtained amorphous cross-linked polyester-urethanes were transparent, and exhibited excellent shape-memory properties and more favorable bulk-degradation profiles. However, this series of SMPs exhibited relatively high T_gs between 48 and 66 °C. In a following study (Lendlein et al., 2009), they tuned the T_g closer to body temperature by cross-linking 4-arm oligocopolyesters incorporating *p*-dioxanone, diglycolide, or ε-caprolactone with *rac*-lactide. T_gs ranging from 14 to 56 °C were achieved by altering comonomer types and ratios without compromising the elastic properties of the polymer network. A broad range of hydrolytic degradation rates were also obtained accordingly.

Using a parallel strategy, Lendlein and colleagues also prepared photo-cross-linked oligo(L-lactide-*ran*-glycolide) dimethacrylate as another amorphous SMP system (Bertmer et al., 2005a,b). The shape-memory properties of these photo-cross-linked SMPs were studied by solid-state ^{13}C NMR, which showed nearly complete shape recovery similar to those observed with the amorphous polyesterurethane systems. The polymer networks obtained were also transparent in appearance and hydrolytically degradable (Choi and Lendlein, 2007). As in the amorphous urethane-cross-linked SMPs, the crosslinking density in these SMPs could also be controlled by the molecular weight of the oligo(L-lactide-*ran*-glycolide), and their mechanical properties at the elastic state above T_g increased with decreasing molecular weight of the oligomers. However, the T_gs for this series of SMPs were independent of the M_n of the oligomer and were all about 55 °C. Compared with the urethane cross-linked amorphous network, the photo-cross-linked oligo(L-lactide-*ran*-glycolide) dimethacrylate were also relatively brittle at their glassy state below T_g, with an elongation at break (ε_B) of only 43%, and more difficult to handle during shape-memory programming.

To improve the glassy state elasticity of the above photo-cross-linked SMPs, the strategy of incorporating another amorphous elastic phase with a T_g lower than that of the cross-linked SMP was explored in two subsequent studies. In the first study, the oligo(L-lactide-*ran*-glycolide) dimethacrylate was replaced with an ABA triblock macrodimethacrylate based on poly(*rac*-lactide)-*b*-poly(propylene oxide)-*b*-poly(*rac*-lactide) where both the poly(propylene oxide) and the poly(*rac*-lactide) blocks were long enough to form separate phases (Choi et al., 2006). Upon photo-polymerization, phase-separated, amorphous, and degradable block copolymer networks were obtained. Besides a lower T_g at ~ -45 °C corresponding to the poly (propylene oxide) block, a second T_g varying from 11 to 43 °C, corresponding to a mixed phase of poly(propylene oxide) and poly(*rac*-lactide) blocks, was obtained depending on the poly(*rac*-lactide) block length. The materials' elasticity at the glassy state was significantly improved with the elongation at break (ε_B) ranging from 70% to 210% depending on the poly(*rac*-lactide) block length. This represents a major improvement over the ε_B of 43% for the SMPs prepared from the photo-cross-linked oligo(L-lactide-*ran*-glycolide) dimethacrylate. This cross-linked network also retained good shape-memory properties, with a high shape-fixing ratio (92–96%) and shape-recovery ratio (87% to over 99%).

In the other subsequent study, a second amorphous phase with a low glass transition temperature ($T_{g,l}$) was incorporated by copolymerization of oligo(L-lactide-*ran*-glycolide) dimethacrylate with acrylate monomers (Kelch et al., 2008). In such a design, poly[(L-lactide)-*ran*-glycolide] segments formed the phase with the higher glass transition temperature ($T_{g,h}$), while the polyacrylate chains formed by the photo-polymerization constituted the second amorphous phase with a lower glass transition temperature ($T_{g,l}$). In contrast to the other SMPs that usually use the phase with $T_{g,l}$ for shape-memory programming and the phase with $T_{g,h}$ for maintaining network structures, this design used $T_{g,h}$ as the shape-memory programming temperature. The phase with $T_{g,l}$, which would remain mobile as long as the temperature used to fix the temporary shape was higher than $T_{g,l}$, acted as embedded elastomeric component in this case and significantly improved the elasticity of the material at its glassy state.

However, the network structures of these SMPs were very complex, and the $T_{g,h}$ were not independent of the acrylate monomer structure or ratio as expected. Amorphous multiphase materials with good glassy state elasticity were only obtained by copolymerization with hexyl acrylate. In all other formulations examined, the incorporation of acrylate monomers into the network decreased the $T_{g,h}$, indicating the formation of a network structure with more mixed phases. In this design, a significant part of the network would not participate in the deformation; thus, its recovery stress was conceivably limited to the poly[(L-lactide)-*ran*-glycolide] segments. Unfortunately, no shape-recovery stress data were available to confirm this speculation.

A more practical and economic way to modulate polymer properties than copolymer synthesis is the physical blending of polymers. Mather's group studied the shape-memory properties of the blend of poly(vinyl acetate) (PVAc) and PLA (Liu and Mather, 2003). Their goal was to create semicrystalline thermoplastic SMPs with two miscible commercial polymer components. In this study, they blended high-molecular weight PVAc (M_n=500,000 g/mol; T_g=35 °C) with PLA containing 92% L-isomer and 8% D-isomer (M_n not reported; T_g=56 °C, T_m=165 °C) to obtain a semicrystalline thermoplastic. The polymers showed complete miscibility at all blending ratios examined with a single T_g. The observed T_g-versus-polymer blend composition curves showed a slight positive deviation from the Fox equation, indicating strong interactions between the two polymers. The degree of crystallinity of the blend decreased monotonically with increasing PVAc fraction, while the crystalline lamellae size remained unchanged. The PVAc/PLA blends exhibited typical thermal-mechanical properties for semicrystalline thermoplastics. For instance, they exhibited relatively high modulus at the glassy state; their modulus sharply decreased when temperature reached around the T_g and then plateaued until the temperature approached the T_m. The shape-memory properties of the 30:70 PLA/PVAc blend was demonstrated by a bending test, which typically exerts low strains. The bended sample, with a 0.5-mm thickness, quickly recovered to its original shape in less than 10 s. No quantitative thermal mechanical properties or shape-memory properties were reported.

Recently, a PLA/biodegradable polyamide elastomer (PAE) blend exhibiting shape-memory capability upon high deformation was reported by Zhang et al. (2009). The blend was prepared by melt mixing commercial PLA (M_n=1.0 × 10^5 g/mol) with PEBAX 2533 (Atofina Chemicals Corporation, France), a commercial copolymer of polyamide-12 (M_w=530, 22 wt%) and polytetramethyleneoxide (M_w=2000, 78 wt%). The PAE was dispersed in the PLA matrix uniformly with good interfacial adhesions between the two phases, and the size of the PAE domains was on the order of submicrometers. Two distinct T_gs were observed, and they shifted towards each other as the blend ratio of the minor component PAE increased, indicating that PAE and PLA were partially miscible in the blend. The storage modulus at room temperature (glassy state) for the PAE/PLA blend gradually decreased with increasing PAE content. Unlike the brittle neat PLA, which had a tensile strength of 46.8 MPa with an elongation at break of only 5.1% and displayed no yield point during strain test, all PLA/PAE blends showed typical yielding behavior upon tensile loading, and the elongation at break increased while storage modulus and tensile strength decreased with increasing PAE content. For instance, the elongation increased significantly to 161.5% for the 5% PAE blend and to 194.6% for the 10% PAE blend, while their storage modulus and tensile strength only changed slightly (e.g., 48.1 and 40.9 MPa for the 5% and 10% PAE content, respectively). The role of PAE in this blend is likely as a plasticizer, which reduced the interactions between PLA chains and the T_g accordingly. The temporary shape of this blend could be formed at room temperature.

Wang et al. recently reported the preparation of an SMP blend from two immiscible lactide-containing polyesters, poly(L-lactide-*co*-ε-caprolactone) (PLLCA, $M_w = 182{,}806$, PDI $= 1.58$, LA:CL = 77:23) and poly(L-lactide-*co*-glycolide) (PLLGA, $M_w = 344{,}605$, PDI = 2.20, LA:GA = 85:15) (Wang et al., 2010). Both polyesters exhibited shape-memory properties by themselves. All the blends showed phase separations owing to the immiscibility of PLLCA and PLLGA. The PLLGA phase transformed from a droplet-like dispersed morphology in lower content blends to a continuous phase at higher contents. Both the mechanical properties and shape-memory properties of the blends transitioned from PLLCA-dominated properties to PLLGA-dominated properties with increasing PLLGA contents. Detailed thermal mechanical characterizations of the blends were not reported.

Researchers are also exploring shape-memory properties in high-molecular-weight copolymers of lactide as alternatives to the chemically cross-linked systems or those based on prepolymer extensions. The advantages of such an approach include relatively easy preparation and more predictable T_g (controlled by co-monomer feeding ratio). However, success is limited in terms of achieving improved shape-memory properties or thermal mechanical properties (Min et al., 2007; Lu et al., 2008; Dong et al., 2010; Yang et al., 2010), probably due to the difficulty in controlling the shape-fixing and shape-switching parts by direct copolymerization of different monomers. Most of the studies using this approach gained some improvements on one property at the cost of another. It has been difficult to establish a reliable network-structure–shape-memory property relationship for this approach based on limited data.

Most SMP networks reviewed above have either amorphous lactic acid-containing polymeric chains in a chemical cross-linked network or semicrystalline lactic acid-containing segments in a physical cross-linked network. In 2009, Mather's group reported an interesting "double cross-linked" lactic-acid containing system (Knight et al., 2009). It is a network chemically cross-linked by photo-initiated Michael addition between a tetrathiol and the acrylate end-capped, POSS-centered, PLGA diol (POSS-PLGA). The covalent C–S linkages and the POSS netpoints can both be considered as cross-links of the resulting network. Crystallization of the POSS moieties within an amorphous PLGA matrix was found in both the POSS-centered PLGA diol and the cross-linked network. The POSS content in the POSS-PLGA diol and the network was dictated by the molecular weight of the PLGA. The cross-linked network exhibited a quite constant T_g (~37 °C), while the crystallinity and T_m increased with increasing POSS content (or decreasing PGLA molecular weight). The inclusion of the POSS in the PLGA backbone also increased the tensile modulus both above and below the T_g. As expected, this double-cross-linked network showed two thermal transitions and two apparent rubbery plateaus in the modulus-temperature curve.

Thus, either T_g or T_m could be chosen as the transition temperature (T_{trans}) for shape-memory programming. When using T_g as the T_{trans}, the sample was elongated at 60 °C, fixed at 25 °C, unloaded, and then heated to 60 °C to trigger recovery. When using T_m as the T_{trans}, the sample was elongated at 120 °C, fixed at 60 °C for 5 min, unloaded, and then heated to 120 °C to trigger recovery. However, the shape-memory properties in neither scenario were ideal. When T_g was used as the T_{trans}, the sample showed good shape-fixing ratio (>99%) but poor recovery ratio of ~27% in the first and subsequent shape-memory cycles. When T_m was used as the T_{trans}, the sample showed poor shape-fixing ratio of ~55%, although nearly 100% strain recovery. Longer annealing during the shape-fixing step was able to improve the shape-fixing ratio to 82.4%. The crystallization of POSS in PLGA backbone also slowed down hydrolytic degradation of the network (likely by slowing water diffusion) compared to the POSS-free cross-linked network and also helped maintain the temporary shape of the material during its degradation in buffer.

About the same time, we also developed a POSS-enhanced, PLA-based SMP network tailored for *in vivo* biomedical applications (Xu and Song, 2010). Unlike the POSS-PLGA diol in Mather's system, where its main function was to promote physical interaction of polymer chains (e.g., crystallization), we designed star-branched POSS-$(PLA_n)_8$ macromers, with eight identical PLA arms ($n = 10$, 20, or 40) grafted from the octahydroxylated POSS core, as the basic building block of an urethane-cross-linked amorphous SMP network. We hypothesized that such a chemically cross-linked network will have multiple benefits: (1) the chemical cross-linking of all reactive ends of the star-branched macromer via urethane linkages could lead to the formation of a homogenous network with minimized plastic deformations that are often observed with un-tethered polymer chains in physically cross-linked SMPs, thereby narrowing glass transitions and improving shape-recovery efficiency. In principle, when all polymer chains freeze below T_{trans} and are uniformly activated above T_{trans} in a homogenous network like this, complete shape fixing and efficient shape recovery can be accomplished within a narrow T_{trans} window; (2) the properties of the urethane-tethered polymeric chains between the POSS netpoints could be altered during controlled macromer synthesis, thereby enabling systemic tuning of the T_{trans} and the degradation profile, among other properties, of the SMP for tailored biomedical applications; (3) the rigid POSS nanoparticles could act as a strengthening filler to improve the recovery stress in addition to serving as netpoints in the cross-linked network. A control SMP network (Org-SMP) cross-linked from a less bulky and more flexible all-organic octa-hydroxylated macromer (Org-$(PLA_n)_8$) ($n = 10$, 20, or 40) was also prepared to facilitate a comparative study of the role of the core structure of the macromer on the thermal mechanical/shape-memory properties of the SMP network.

Quantitative characterizations of the thermal mechanical property and shape-memory property of these SMP networks supported our hypotheses. The POSS-SMP networks all exhibited an extremely narrow glass transition range, with peak widths at the half peak height (WHPH) less than 10 °C, accompanied by sharp storage modulus changes of up to 3 orders of magnitude around the glass transitions. By contrast, most conventional SMP networks exhibit wide glass transitions (WHPH > 20 °C) with no more than 2 orders of magnitude modulus change around the T_{trans}. Such a narrow glass transition endowed POSS-SMPs with excellent shape fixing at body temperature, which was slightly below their T_gs, and instant recovery at a safe triggering temperature slightly above their T_gs. Indeed, we showed that all POSS-SMPs exhibited stable temporary shape fixing at room temperature for over 1 year, instant and complete recovery around 50 °C, and over 2-GPa storage modulus at body temperature. Moreover, the POSS cores exerted unique impact on the T_g. In contrast to Org-SMPs where the T_gs decreased with the increase of PLA chain length as a result of lower density of the urethane crosslinks, the T_gs of POSS-SMPs increased from 42.8 °C with shorter PLA arm length ($n = 10$) to 48.4 °C with longer PLA arm length ($n = 40$). The storage modulus of POSS-SMPs and Org-SMPs at the rubbery state both decreased with the increase of PLA arm length, consistent with the expected lower densities of POSS netpoints at longer inter-netpoint chain lengths. Finally, like most PLA-containing SMPs, these POSS-SMPs were also degradable, with their *in vitro* and *in vivo* degradation rates increased with decreasing PLA lengths. In a subsequent study using a rat subcutaneous implantation model, we further demonstrated that the POSS-SMPs were minimally immunogenic compared to PLA controls (Filion et al., 2011). Although this system exhibited multiple features desirable for *in vivo* applications, it still suffers from the common limitations of most thermosets, such as less convenient fabrication (compared to thermoplastics) and relatively low maximum strains (<200%).

To combine the advantages of thermosets and thermoplastics, Inoue et al. prepared a PLA-based SMP with thermo-reversible chemical cross-links by Diels–Alder reaction between furanyl-terminated 4-arm or 6-arm PLA and difunctional or trifunctional maleimide cross-linker (Yamashiro et al., 2008; Inoue et al., 2009). This SMP network exhibited shape-memory properties as good as those accomplished by urethane-cross-linking. The thermo-reversible cross-links in this SMP allowed it to be remolded into new shapes with retained shape-memory properties when heated to >160 °C. Unfortunately, the mechanical properties of these SMPs were inferior to those of the base PLA materials due to the relatively low cross-linking efficiency (e.g., only two-thirds of the furans or maleimides were reacted). This deficiency may be overcome by adopting more reactive thermo-reversible cross-links, increasing the density of the reactive handles within the network, and/or employing strategies to reduce the viscosity during the cross-linking.

10.2.3 Mechanisms for activating the shape-memory effect in PLA-based materials

The shape-memory effect is not an intrinsic property of polymeric materials. It results from the chemical composition and network structure of a polymer and its appropriate processing and programming. It requires the coexistence of net-point parts and reversible switching parts, which are responsible for maintaining the material's dimensional stability and the reversible response to thermal stimulus, respectively. The intrinsic mechanism for shape-memory behavior in polymers is the reversible freezing and activation of polymeric chain motion in the switching parts below and above T_{trans}, respectively. Thus, theoretically, any polymer network possessing these two structural components could be programmed to exhibit the shape-memory effect. Nowadays, nearly all major classes of polymers including polyurethanes, epoxys, polyolefins, and polyesters have been reported to exhibit shape-memory properties (Behl et al., 2010; Lendlein and Kelch, 2002; Behl and Lendlein, 2007b; Mather et al., 2009; Liu et al., 2007).

The driving force for shape recovery in SMPs is the recoiling of polymeric chains from a strained configuration (temporary state) to a less-ordered, lower-energy configuration ("memorized" permanent state), namely, the entropy elasticity. Shape-recovery from a temporary shape can be initiated by external stimuli such as heat, magnetic field, electric field, moisture, or light. Here, we categorize the shape recovery of SMPs into the following three triggering mechanisms and discuss the latest progress based on how the network structure is changed during shape recovery.

10.2.3.1 Heat-driven shape recovery

In this shape-recovery triggering mechanism, the frozen glassy network chains become elastic when the surrounding temperature is raised above the critical temperature (T_g or T_m). The shape recovery of most reported SMPs is triggered by this mechanism, in which the polymer chain motion is activated by either direct external heat from the environment or by heat generated by embedded fillers in response to magnetic, electric, and light actuations. Although direct heating is most commonly utilized to trigger shape recovery of SMPs, it is not always feasible for their *in vivo* applications due to concerns over excessive heat-induced tissue damage. The search for efficient indirect heating has thus become an important task for the biomedical applications of SMPs.

Heating electro-active SMP by electricity to induce shape recovery was first reported in 2004 (Koerner et al., 2004). Many electro-active SMPs have been developed by incorporating conductive fillers such as carbon black, carbon nanotubes (CNTs), carbon fibers, polypyrrole, or conductive metal particles within the SMP network. However, the shape recovery of these SMPs induced by the electric field are usually not as efficient as those induced by direct heating, mainly due to the inadequate conductivity of the nonpercolating conductive network formed by discrete fillers. The use of nonwoven carbon nanofibers (CNFs) as a predefined conductive network for SMPs fabrication could address this challenge (Luo and Mather, 2010). For instance, an epoxy-based SMP matrix incorporating CNFs fully recovered its original shape in less than 2 s upon induction by alternating electric fields. Because of the better thermal conductivity of CNFs than the polymer matrix, the SMP/CNF nanocomposite in fact recovered faster than the control SMP without CNFs under conventional heating. Moreover, the incorporation of CNFs had little effect on the T_g of the epoxy-based SMP, but significantly improved its storage modulus at the elastic state above T_g, which could be useful for improving the recovery stress. Unfortunately, a compromised tensile strain of the composite SMP was observed with the incorporation of CNFs.

Taking advantage of the heat generated by embedded magnetic particles in alternating magnetic fields, magnetic SMP composites were also developed (Mohr et al., 2006). Silica-coated iron(III) oxide nanoparticles were incorporated into two thermoplastic SMP matrices, a polyetherurethane with a T_g of 74 °C (used as T_{trans}), and a biodegradable multiblock copolymer of hard poly(*p*-dioxanone) segments and soft poly(ε-caprolactone) segments where the T_m of the soft segment was used as T_{trans}. Magnetically and thermally induced shape recovery efficiencies of these SMPs were comparable. The maximum temperature and the time required to reach T_{trans} by alternating magnetic fields were a function of the strength and frequency of the alternating magnetic fields applied.

The heat energy required to trigger shape recovery of SMPs could be gathered from multiple sources. Lendlein, Kumar, and colleagues recently demonstrated the feasibility of combining alternating magnetic fields with conventional heating to reach T_{trans} of dual-shaped and multiple-shaped SMPs (Kumar et al., 2011). The combination of multiple heating sources can overcome the limitations of the single source.

Whereas earlier designs of SMP composites responsive to indirect heating mainly utilized a single type of fillers homogenously embedded within the SMP matrices, a recently reported indirect heating mechanism utilized multiple types of fillers (He et al., 2011). Sophisticated shape-memory programming could be realized by stepwise, selective activation of these fillers. For instance, iron oxide (Fe_3O_4) nanoparticles and CNTs emit induced heat by two very different radiofrequencies (RFs), 296 kHz and 13.56 MHz, respectively. These nanofillers can be embedded into different regions of a polymer composite, enabling independent heating (thus recovery) of each region by remote actuation at the selected RF.

The surface plasmon resonance (SPR)-generated photothermal effect of gold nanoparticles or nanorods was recently explored as another shape-recovery triggering mechanism (Hribar et al., 2009). Gold nanorod was encapsulated in an amorphous and biodegradable SMP network prepared by photopolyemrization of tert-butyl acrylate and poly(β-amino esters) (PBAEs) diacrylate. Significant and rapid heating was accomplished in the SMP containing Au nanorods upon exposure to near infrared (NIR) light at 770 nm, and the intensity and efficiency of the induced heating was dependent upon both the concentration of the Au nanorods and the NIR light intensity. For example, the SMP network with a high concentration of Au nanorods was heated to 50 °C (above the T_g) when exposed to 0.3 W of the NIR light for 60 s and activated the shape recovery. Moreover, the incorporation of the Au nanorods did not increase the cytotoxicity of the material.

Zhang et al. applied this shape-recovery induction strategy with a biodegradable semicrystalline SMP using T_m as the T_{trans} (Zhang et al., 2012). They prepared a series of polyurethane/gold nanoparticle (AuNPs) composites by cross-linking 8-arm branched poly(ε-caprolactone), poly(ε-caprolactone) coated AuNPs with hexamethylene diisocyanate. The final materials are a semicrystalline chemically cross-linked network. With a 0.57-W/cm^2 laser irradiation, the local temperature rose by as high as 25 °C and induced the shape recovery of the SMP while the environment temperature remained far lower in the T_{trans}. The extent of the local temperature increase could be tuned by the laser power. Further, a spatially selective shape recovery was realized by exposures of different parts of the nanocomposite film to separate lasers. Multiple intermediate shapes between the temporary and permanent shapes were obtained by terminating the laser irradiation at various times, a feature not readily accomplished by conventional heating.

These temporally and spatially controlled, light-triggered (particularly by NIR light that are known for deep-tissue penetration depths) shape recoveries are very attractive for SMPs with relatively high T_{trans} for *in vivo* biomedical applications. They may reduce the need for fine-tuning the T_{trans}, which has proven to be challenging without sacrificing other desired properties of the SMP. This method also provides a simple way to afford conventional two-way SMPs with multi-staged shape recoveries. To the best of our knowledge, lactic-acid containing SMPs using such a light-driven triggering mechanism have not been reported yet, but are worth exploring given the significant advantages for *in vivo* applications.

10.2.3.2 "Plasticizing effect"-triggered shape recovery

Besides heating SMPs above T_{trans} to trigger the recoiling of the polymer chains, another possibility for triggering shape recovery is to decrease the T_{trans} dynamically by environmental factors. In this mechanism, interactions between the SMP and external environmental factors (other than heat) result in changes of the physical structure of the SMP network. An example of this is water-induced shape memory, where a reduced T_{trans} resulting from the plasticizing effect of water led to the shape recovery.

Yang et al. from Singapore were the first to report this so-called "water-responsive shape-memory effect" (Huang et al., 2005, 2010; Yang et al., 2006). Their work was inspired by their serendipitous observation that a prefolded polyurethane SMP 3520 thin film (from Mitsubishi Heavy Industry, $T_g = 35$ °C) recovered its original shape and became rubber-like after a 1-month exposure in air at room temperature (~22 °C). Subsequent investigations revealed that the moisture absorbed onto the SMPs had weakened the hydrogen bonding between the polymer chains and caused the decrease of its T_g by 10–13 °C, thus the "premature" shape recovery at room temperature. Following this discovery, water-driven shape recovery was applied to several other SMP systems (Chen et al., 2012; Zhu et al., 2012; Pierce et al., 2011; Paakinaho et al., 2012), and the more universal concept of using "plasticizing effect" imposed by environmental factors for triggering shape recovery was explored in the context of solvent-induced shape-memory effect (Du and Zhang, 2010).

Water-driven shape recovery was also reported for lactic acid-containing SMPs (Pierce et al., 2011). For example, the T_gs of the previously discussed chemically cross-linked amorphous biodegradable SMPs based on poly[(*rac*-lactide)-*co*-glycolide] star-shaped macrotriol or macrotetrols (developed by Lendlein and colleagues) were lowered from 55 to 66 °C to below body temperature upon the uptake of water. The programmed samples kept their temporary shape at room temperature in water or at 37 °C under dry conditions, but underwent shape recovery at 37 °C water.

The plasticizing effect of water was also recently observed in amorphous SMPs based on high molecular weight linear PDLLA (Paakinaho et al., 2012). PDLLA and sterilized PDLLA (by γ-irradiation with a minimum radiation dose of 25 kGy) were compared for the water-driven shape-memory properties. Upon the diffusion of a small amount of water (1 wt%) into the material, the T_g significantly decreased by 10–13 °C. The samples programmed with a temporary shape and kept in 37 °C aqueous buffer (pH 7.4) underwent shape recovery after 10 weeks (the shape-recovery ratio of 94% for non-γ-irradiated samples and 97% for γ-irradiated samples). Meanwhile, the temporarily shaped samples kept in the dry state at 37 °C or in the same aqueous buffer at 21 °C showed negligible shape recovery. The γ-irradiated samples showed twice as fast shape recovery but similar shape recovery ratio as the nonirradiated sample when stored in aqueous buffer at 37 °C, confirming that the plasticizing effect of water directly correlated with the ease of water diffusion through the polymer network.

Shape recovery response induced by water, however, is relatively slow (e.g., taking hours) since the decrease of T_g is dependent on the diffusion of water within the polymer network, the rate and extent of which is often limited in PLA- or other hydrophobic polymer-based SMPs. The incomplete/partial penetration of water within a 3-D SMP network also means that the hydration-induced recovery stress also tends to be small. As water is more readily absorbed on a sample surface than an interior, in practice, thin wires or films rather than bulk 3-D materials are more suitable for moisture-induced shape recovery.

10.2.3.3 Shape recovery induced by chemical structure changes

Since changes in chemical structures of SMP network can decrease T_{trans}, it is possible that such a change can also trigger the shape recovery of the SMP. Currently, chemical structure change-triggered shape recovery was only demonstrated with photo-responsive SMPs upon light activation. Liquid crystalline elastomers or cross-linked networks containing azobenzene groups are the most explored. The *trans–cis* photo-isomerization of azobenzene can lead to nematic-to-isotropic (N–I) phase transition of the network chains, inducing a macroscopic network contraction with a contraction strain of 10–25% (Li et al., 2003). Recently, Wu et al. demonstrated NIR-induced shape deformation and recovery with azotolane-containing cross-linked liquid-crystal polymers that were surface-coated with upconversion nanophosphors (Wu et al., 2011). The lower-energy NIR light has deeper tissue penetration depth than UV and is a more desirable and safer light source for *in vivo* applications. Combining the upconversion of NIR irradiation to local UV emission enabled by the nanophosphor and the conventional UV-sensitive functional groups embedded within the polymer network, NIR-triggered shape recovery may be implemented with photo-sensitive SMPs *in vivo*. Given that the light-induced liquid crystal phase transition and macroscopic deformation are reversible, two-directional shape-memory behavior may be programmed using this strategy.

Another type of light-induced, chemical structure change-driven shape recovery was earlier demonstrated by Lendlein et al. (2005) with a network polymerized from *n*-butylacrylate, hydroxyethyl methacrylate, ethyleneglycol-1-acrylate-2-cinnamic acid, and poly(propylene glycol)-dimethacrylate. The reversible [2+2] cycloaddition reaction enabled by cinnamic acid under different wavelengths of UV irradiation allowed for the modulation of the network cross-linking density for shape fixing (cycloaddition enabled by irradiation at >260 nm) and recovery (e.g., shorter wavelength irradiation at <260 nm reversed the cycloaddition of cinnamic acid). Compared with conventional SMPs, these photo-responsive SMPs showed a comparable shape-recovery ratio. However, the shape-fixing ratio of such a system was much lower (~50%), likely due to the inadequate [2+2] cycloaddition efficiency during the fixing upon irradiation with longer wavelength light (>260 nm). Overall, chemical structure change-driven shape recovery remains relatively unexplored in the design of SMPs for biomedical applications.

10.3 New directions and future perspectives

The "intelligent" shape-memory effect of SMPs has inspired the design of many prototype systems for a wide range of biomedical applications, including self-folding devices (Randall et al., 2012), microactuators for treating stroke (Maitland et al., 2002), cardiovascular stents (Yakacki et al., 2007), self-tightening sutures (Lendlein and Kelch, 2005), and minimally invasive/self-fitting tissue engineering scaffolds (Neuss et al., 2009; Bencherif et al., 2012). The focus of SMP research today is no longer to identify/demonstrate the shape-memory effect in new polymer systems. Instead, overcoming the limitations of existing SMPs for tailored practical applications such as biomedical uses has become increasingly important.

Although many reports in the literature claim excellent shape-memory properties for a wide range of polymer networks, it is difficult to compare these properties across different systems due to the difficulty in implementing standard conditions and methods for quantitative shape-memory characterizations. Shape-memory properties are dependent upon not only sample chemical compositions and network structures, but also their processing and programming. Systematic investigations on the relationship between shape-memory properties and all these underlying factors are still lacking (Rousseau and Xie, 2010; Gall et al., 2004; Yakacki et al., 2008a,b, 2011). More work is needed in this aspect.

The relatively small recovery stresses (<10 MPa), low recovery speed for large-dimension samples, and the limitation to one-way memory are a few common limitations shared by many SMP networks. These limitations are yet to be satisfactorily addressed. For degradable SMPs designed for *in vivo* applications (e.g., PLA-based SMPs), additional challenges in programming suitable degradation profiles and minimizing the immunogenicity of their degradation products need to be met. Although some SMPs exhibited properties attractive for potential *in vivo* applications, little has been done to demonstrate the feasibility of their *in vivo* applications using clinically relevant animal models, whether in terms of their minimally invasive surgical delivery, short-term safety of the triggered shape recovery, or their long-term safety. Work in this area is critical in enabling the clinical translation of these exciting materials, and lessons learned from the much-needed *in vivo* studies are also essential in designing higher-performance SMPs.

With the development of new ROP catalysts (Majerska and Duda, 2004; Dove et al., 2005; Pratt et al., 2006; Chuma et al., 2008; Yu et al., 2012), better understanding of the polymerization kinetics of lactides and other cyclic monomers (Nomura et al., 2010), and more matured techniques for the preparation of well-defined functional prepolymers (Braunecker and Matyjaszewski, 2007) and the formation of controlled network (Lovell et al., 2001; Nair et al,., 2012a,b), PLA-based SMP network with well-defined properties could be more readily prepared (Li et al., 2011, 2012; Ho et al., 2012; Sarazin et al., 2011). These enabling tools can accelerate our understanding of the structure–performance relationship of SMPs. To accelerate the commercialization of SMP-based smart medical implants, a multi-disciplinary approach to simultaneously improve polymer network design, implement smarter and more clinically relevant activation mechanism, and engineer multiple SMPs into an integrated device will have to be taken.

10.4 Further information

Major industrial leaders in lactic acid/lactide and PLA manufacturing:

- http://www.purac.com/purac-biomaterials
- http://www.natureworksllc.com/About-NatureWorks

Manufacturers specializing in SMPs:

- Cornerstone Research Group Inc. USA—http://www.crgrp.com/corporate/case-studies/smp-commercialization
- SMP Technologies, Japan—http://www.smptechno.com/index_en.html

References

Ahmed, J., Varshney, S.K., 2011. Polylactides-chemistry, properties and green packaging technology: a review. Int. J. Food Prop. 14, 37–58.

Alteheld, A., Feng, Y.K., Kelch, S., Lendlein, A., 2005. Biodegradable, amorphous copolyester-urethane networks having shape-memory properties. Angew. Chem. Int. Ed. 44, 1188–1192.

Behl, M., Lendlein, A., 2007a. Actively moving polymers. Soft Matter 3, 58–67.

Behl, M., Lendlein, A., 2007b. Shape-memory polymers. Mater. Today 10, 20–28.

Behl, M., Razzaq, M.Y., Lendlein, A., 2010. Multifunctional shape-memory polymers. Adv. Mater. 22, 3388–3410.

Bencherif, S.A., Sands, R.W., Bhatta, D., Arany, P., Verbeke, C.S., Edwards, D.A., Mooney, D. J., 2012. Injectable preformed scaffolds with shape-memory properties. Proc. Natl. Acad. Sci. U. S. A. 109, 19590–19595.

Benninga, H., 1990. A History of Lactic Acid Making: A Chapter in the History of Biotechnology. Chemists and Chemistry Series, vol. 11. Kluwer Academic Publishers, The Netherlands. ISBN 978-0-7923-0625-2.

Bertmer, M., Buda, A., Blomenkamp-Hofges, I., Kelch, S., Lendlein, A., 2005a. Biodegradable shape-memory polymer networks: characterization with solid-state NMR. Macromolecules 38, 3793–3799.

Bertmer, M., Buda, A., Blomenkamp-Hofges, I., Kelch, S., Lendlein, A., 2005b. Solid-state NMR characterization of biodegradable shape-memory polymer networks. Macromol. Symp. 230, 110–115.

Biela, T., Kowalski, A., Libiszowski, J., Duda, A., Penczek, S., 2006. Progress in polymerization of cyclic esters: mechanisms and synthetic applications. Macromol. Symp. 240, 47–55.

Braunecker, W.A., Matyjaszewski, K., 2007. Controlled/living radical polymerization: features, developments, and perspectives. Prog. Polym. Sci. 32, 93–146.

Cameron, D.J.A., Shaver, M.P., 2011. Aliphatic polyester polymer stars: synthesis, properties and applications in biomedicine and nanotechnology. Chem. Soc. Rev. 40, 1761–1776.

Chen, S.J., Hu, J.L., Chen, S.G., 2012. Studies of the moisture-sensitive shape memory effect of pyridine-containing polyurethanes. Polym. Int. 61, 314–320.

Choi, N.Y., Lendlein, A., 2007. Degradable shape-memory polymer networks from oligo [(L-lactide)-*ran*-glycolide]dimethacrylates. Soft Matter 3, 901–909.

Choi, N.Y., Kelch, S., Lendlein, A., 2006. Synthesis, shape-memory functionality and hydrolytical degradation studies on polymer networks from poly(*rac*-lactide)-*b*-poly(propylene oxide)-*b*-poly(*rac*-lactide) dimethacrylates. Adv. Eng. Mater. 8, 439–445.

Chuma, A., Horn, H.W., Swope, W.C., Pratt, R.C., Zhang, L., Lohmeijer, B.G.G., Wade, C.G., Waymouth, R.M., Hedrick, J.L., Rice, J.E., 2008. The reaction mechanism for the organocatalytic ring-opening polymerization of L-lactide using a guanidine-based catalyst: hydrogen-bonded or covalently bound? J. Am. Chem. Soc. 130, 6749–6754.

Cook, P., 1990. The business of innovation: an interview with Paul Cook. Interview by William Taylor. Harv. Bus. Rev. 68, 96.

Coulembier, O., Degee, P., Hedrick, J.L., Dubois, P., 2006. From controlled ring-opening polymerization to biodegradable aliphatic polyester: especially poly(beta-malic acid) derivatives. Prog. Polym. Sci. 31, 723–747.

Dietsch, B., Tong, T., 2007. A review—features and benefits of shape memory polymers (SMPs). J. Adv. Mater. 39, 3–12.

Dong, W.J., Jiang, J.S., Xie, M.R., 2010. Preparation and properties of shape memory poly (L-lactic-*co*-glycolic acid) (PLLGA). Acta Chim. Sin. 68, 2243–2249.

Dove, A.P., Pratt, R.C., Lohmeijer, B.G.G., Waymouth, R.M., Hedrick, J.L., 2005. Thiourea-based bifunctional organocatalysis: supramolecular recognition for living polymerization. J. Am. Chem. Soc. 127, 13798–13799.

Du, H.Y., Zhang, J.H., 2010. Solvent induced shape recovery of shape memory polymer based on chemically cross-linked poly(vinyl alcohol). Soft Matter 6, 3370–3376.

Filion, T.M., Xu, J., Prasad, M.L., Song, J., 2011. In vivo tissue responses to thermal-responsive shape memory polymer nanocomposites. Biomaterials 32, 985–991.

Flory, P.J., 1953. Principles of Polymer Chemistry, second ed. Cornell University Press, Ithaca, New York.

Gall, K., Dunn, M.L., Liu, Y.P., Stefanic, G., Balzar, D., 2004. Internal stress storage in shape memory polymer nanocomposites. Appl. Phys. Lett. 85, 290–292.

Garlotta, D., 2002. A literature review of poly(lactic acid). J. Polym. Environ. 9, 22.

Grijpma, D.W., Pennings, A.J., 1994. (Co)polymers of L-lactide, 2. Mechanical properties. Macromol. Chem. Phys. 195, 1649–1663.

Gruber, P., O'Brien, M., 2005. Polylactides "NatureWorks® PLA". In: Biopolymers Online. Wiley-VCH Verlag GmbH & Co. KGaA, Germany.

Gupta, A.P., Kumar, V., 2007. New emerging trends in synthetic biodegradable polymers—polylactide: a critique. Eur. Polym. J. 43, 4053–4074.

He, Z.W., Satarkar, N., Xie, T., Cheng, Y.T., Hilt, J.Z., 2011. Remote controlled multishape polymer nanocomposites with selective radiofrequency actuations. Adv. Mater. 23, 3192–3196.

Ho, R.M., Li, M.C., Lin, S.C., Wang, H.F., Lee, Y.D., Hasegawa, H., Thomas, E.L., 2012. Transfer of chirality from molecule to phase in self-assembled chiral block copolymers. J. Am. Chem. Soc. 134, 10974–10986.

Hongzhi, L., Jinwen, Z., 2012. Toughening modification of poly(lactic acid) via melt blending. In: Biobased Monomers, Polymers, and Materials, vol. 1105. American Chemical Society, Washington D.C., pp. 27–46.

Hribar, K.C., Metter, R.B., Ifkovits, J.L., Troxler, T., Burdick, J.A., 2009. Light-induced temperature transitions in biodegradable polymer and nanorod composites. Small 5, 1830–1834.

Huang, W.M., Yang, B., An, L., Li, C., Chan, Y.S., 2005. Water-driven programmable polyurethane shape memory polymer: demonstration and mechanism. Appl. Phys. Lett. 86.

Huang, W.M., Yang, B., Zhao, Y., Ding, Z., 2010. Thermo-moisture responsive polyurethane shape-memory polymer and composites: a review. J. Mater. Chem. 20, 3367–3381.

Inkinen, S., Hakkarainen, M., Albertsson, A.-C., Södergård, A., 2011. From lactic acid to poly (lactic acid) (PLA): characterization and analysis of PLA and its precursors. Biomacromolecules 12, 523–532.

Inoue, K., Yamashiro, M., Iji, M., 2009. Recyclable shape-memory polymer: poly(lactic acid) crosslinked by a thermoreversible Diels–Alder reaction. J. Appl. Polym. Sci. 112, 876–885.

Ionov, L., 2010. Actively-moving materials based on stimuli-responsive polymers. J. Mater. Chem. 20, 3382–3390.

Kelch, S., Choi, N.Y., Wang, Z.G., Lendlein, A., 2008. Amorphous, elastic AB copolymer networks from acrylates and poly[(L-lactide)-*ran*-glycolide]dimethacrylates. Adv. Eng. Mater. 10, 494–502.

Knight, P.T., Lee, K.M., Chung, T., Mather, P.T., 2009. PLGA-POSS end-linked networks with tailored degradation and shape memory behavior. Macromolecules 42, 6596–6605.

Koerner, H., Price, G., Pearce, N.A., Alexander, M., Vaia, R.A., 2004. Remotely actuated polymer nanocomposites—stress-recovery of carbon-nanotube-filled thermoplastic elastomers. Nat. Mater. 3, 115–120.

Kricheldorf, H.R., 2004. Biodegradable polymers with variable architectures via ring-expansion polymerization. J. Polym. Sci. A Polym. Chem. 42, 4723–4742.

Kumar, U.N., Kratz, K., Heuchel, M., Behl, M., Lendlein, A., 2011. Shape-memory nanocomposites with magnetically adjustable apparent switching temperatures. Adv. Mater. 23, 4157–4162.

Langer, R., Tirrell, D.A., 2004. Designing materials for biology and medicine. Nature 428, 487–492.

Langer, R., Lahann, J., Schmidt, A., Grablowitz, H., 2000. Biodegradable shape memory polymers. US Patent 6,160,084.

Lendlein, A., Kelch, S., 2002. Shape-memory polymers. Angew. Chem. Int. Ed. 41, 2034–2057.

Lendlein, A., Kelch, S., 2005. Shape-memory polymers as stimuli-sensitive implant materials. Clin. Hemorheol. Microcirc. 32, 105–116.

Lendlein, A., Langer, R., 2002. Biodegradable, elastic shape-memory polymers for potential biomedical applications. Science 296, 1673–1676.

Lendlein, A., Schmidt, A.M., Langer, R., 2001. AB-polymer networks based on oligo(epsilon-caprolactone) segments showing shape-memory properties. Proc. Natl. Acad. Sci. U. S. A. 98, 842–847.

Lendlein, A., Jiang, H.Y., Junger, O., Langer, R., 2005. Light-induced shape-memory polymers. Nature 434, 879–882.

Lendlein, A., Zotzmann, J., Feng, Y.K., Alteheld, A., Kelch, S., 2009. Controlling the switching temperature of biodegradable, amorphous, shape-memory poly(*rac*-lactide) urethane networks by incorporation of different comonomers. Biomacromolecules 10, 975–982.

Li, M.H., Keller, P., Li, B., Wang, X., Brunet, M., 2003. Light-driven side-on nematic elastomer actuators. Adv. Mater. 15, 569–572.

Li, J., Stayshich, R.M., Meyer, T.Y., 2011. Exploiting sequence to control the hydrolysis behavior of biodegradable PLGA copolymers. J. Am. Chem. Soc. 133, 6910–6913.

Li, J., Rothstein, S.N., Little, S.R., Edenborn, H.M., Meyer, T.Y., 2012. The effect of monomer order on the hydrolysis of biodegradable poly(lactic-*co*-glycolic acid) repeating sequence copolymers. J. Am. Chem. Soc. 134, 16352–16359.

Liu, C., Mather, P.T., 2003. Thermomechanical characterization of blends of poly (vinyl acetate) with semicrystalline polymers for shape memory applications. In: Proceedings of Annual Technical Conference Society of Plastics Engineers. ANTEC 2003, vol. 2. Society of Plastics Engineers, Brookfield, CT, pp. 1962–1966.

Liu, C., Qin, H., Mather, P.T., 2007. Review of progress in shape-memory polymers. J. Mater. Chem. 17, 1543–1558.

Lovell, L.G., Berchtold, K.A., Elliott, J.E., Lu, H., Bowman, C.N., 2001. Understanding the kinetics and network formation of dimethacrylate dental resins. Polym. Adv. Technol. 12, 335–345.

Lu, D.D., Zhang, X.W., Zhou, T.H., Ren, Z.L., Wang, S.F., Lei, Z.Q., 2008. Biodegradable poly (lactic acid) copolymers. Prog. Chem. 20, 339–350.

Luo, X.F., Mather, P.T., 2010. Conductive shape memory nanocomposites for high speed electrical actuation (vol 6, pg 2146, 2010). Soft Matter 6, 6210.

Maitland, D.J., Metzger, M.F., Schumann, D., Lee, A., Wilson, T.S., 2002. Photothermal properties of shape memory polymer micro-actuators for treating stroke. Lasers Surg. Med. 30, 1–11.

Majerska, K., Duda, A., 2004. Stereocontrolled polymerization of racemic lactide with chiral initiator: combining stereoelection and chiral ligand-exchange mechanism. J. Am. Chem. Soc. 126, 1026–1027.

Mather, P.T., Luo, X.F., Rousseau, I.A., 2009. Shape memory polymer research. Annu. Rev. Mater. Res. 39, 445–471.

Meng, Q.H., Hu, J.L., 2009. A review of shape memory polymer composites and blends. Compos. Part A Appl. Sci. Manuf. 40, 1661–1672.

Middleton, J.C., Tipton, A.J., 2000. Synthetic biodegradable polymers as orthopedic devices. Biomaterials 21, 2335–2346.

Min, C.C., Cui, W.J., Bei, J.Z., Wang, S.G., 2007. Effect of comonomer on thermal/mechanical and shape memory property of L-lactide-based shape-memory copolymers. Polym. Adv. Technol. 18, 299–305.

Mohr, R., Kratz, K., Weigel, T., Lucka-Gabor, M., Moneke, M., Lendlein, A., 2006. Initiation of shape-memory effect by inductive heating of magnetic nanoparticles in thermoplastic polymers. Proc. Natl. Acad. Sci. U. S. A. 103, 3540–3545.

Nair, D.P., Cramer, N.B., Gaipa, J.C., McBride, M.K., Matherly, E.M., McLeod, R.R., Shandas, R., Bowman, C.N., 2012a. Two-stage reactive polymer network forming systems. Adv. Funct. Mater. 22, 1502–1510.

Nair, D.R., Cramer, N.B., McBride, M.K., Gaipa, J.C., Shandas, R., Bowman, C.N., 2012b. Enhanced two-stage reactive polymer network forming systems. Polymer 53, 2429–2434.

Neffe, A.T., Tronci, G., Alteheld, A., Lendlein, A., 2010. Controlled change of mechanical properties during hydrolytic degradation of polyester urethane networks. Macromol. Chem. Phys. 211, 182–194.

Neuss, S., Blomenkamp, I., Stainforth, R., Boltersdorf, D., Jansen, M., Butz, N., Perez-Bouza, A., Knuchel, R., 2009. The use of a shape-memory poly(is an element of-caprolactone) dimethacrylate network as a tissue engineering scaffold. Biomaterials 30, 1697–1705.

Nomura, N., Akita, A., Ishii, R., Mizuno, M., 2010. Random copolymerization of epsilon-caprolactone with lactide using a Homosalen–Al complex. J. Am. Chem. Soc. 132, 1750–1751.

Paakinaho, K., Heino, H., Pelto, M., Hannula, M., Tormala, P., Kellomaki, M., 2012. Programmed water-induced shape-memory of bioabsorbable poly(D,L-lactide): activation and properties in physiological temperature. J. Mater. Sci. Mater. Med. 23, 613–621.

Pierce, B.F., Bellin, K., Behl, M., Lendlein, A., 2011. Demonstrating the influence of water on shape-memory polymer networks based on poly[(*rac*-lactide)-*co*-glycolide] segments in vitro. Int. J. Artif. Organs 34, 172–179.

Pratt, R.C., Lohmeijer, B.G.G., Long, D.A., Waymouth, R.M., Hedrick, J.L., 2006. Triazabicyclodecene: a simple bifunctional organocatalyst for acyl transfer and ring-opening polymerization of cyclic esters. J. Am. Chem. Soc. 128, 4556–4557.

Randall, C.L., Gultepe, E., Gracias, D.H., 2012. Self-folding devices and materials for biomedical applications. Trends Biotechnol. 30, 138–146.

Rousseau, I.A., 2008. Challenges of shape memory polymers: a review of the progress toward overcoming SMP's limitations. Polym. Eng. Sci. 48, 2075–2089.

Rousseau, I.A., Xie, T., 2010. Shape memory epoxy: composition, structure, properties and shape memory performances. J. Mater. Chem. 20, 3431–3441.

Sarazin, Y., Liu, B., Roisnel, T., Maron, L., Carpentier, J.F., 2011. Discrete, solvent-free alkaline-earth metal cations: metal center dot center dot center dot fluorine interactions and ROP catalytic activity. J. Am. Chem. Soc. 133, 9069–9087.

Sokolowski, W.M., Tan, S.C., 2007. Advanced self-deployable structures for space applications. J. Spacecr. Rockets 44, 750–754.

Sokolowski, W., Metcalfe, A., Hayashi, S., Yahia, L., Raymond, J., 2007. Medical applications of shape memory polymers. Biomed. Mater. 2, S23–S27.

Tsuji, H., Ikada, Y., 1999. Stereocomplex formation between enantiomeric poly(lactic acid)s. XI. Mechanical properties and morphology of solution-cast films. Polymer 40, 6699–6708.

Wang, L.S., Chen, H.C., Xiong, Z.C., Pang, X.B., Xiong, C.D., 2010. Novel degradable compound shape-memory-polymer blend: mechanical and shape-memory properties. Mater. Lett. 64, 284–286.

Wee, Y.J., Kim, J.N., Ryu, H.W., 2006. Biotechnological production of lactic acid and its recent applications. Food Technol. Biotechnol. 44, 10.

Wischke, C., Neffe, A.T., Steuer, S., Lendlein, A., 2009. Evaluation of a degradable shape-memory polymer network as matrix for controlled drug release. J. Control. Release 138, 243–250.

Wu, W., Yao, L., Yang, T., Yin, R., Li, F., Yu, Y., 2011. NIR-light-induced deformation of cross-linked liquid-crystal polymers using upconversion nanophosphors. J. Am. Chem. Soc. 133, 15810–15813.

Xu, J.W., Song, J., 2010. High performance shape memory polymer networks based on rigid nanoparticle cores. Proc. Natl. Acad. Sci. U. S. A. 107, 7652–7657.

Xu, J.W., Song, J., 2011. Thermal responsive shape memory polymers for biomedical applications. In: Fazel-Rezai, R. (Ed.), Biomedical Engineering—Frontiers and Challenges. InTech: http://www.intechopen.com/articles/show/title/thermal-responsive-shape-memory-polymers-for-biomedical-applications.

Yakacki, C.M., Shandas, R., Lanning, C., Rech, B., Eckstein, A., Gall, K., 2007. Unconstrained recovery characterization of shape-memory polymer networks for cardiovascular applications. Biomaterials 28, 2255–2263.

Yakacki, C.M., Shandas, R., Safranski, D., Ortega, A.M., Sassaman, K., Gall, K., 2008a. Strong, tailored, biocompatible shape-memory polymer networks. Adv. Funct. Mater. 18, 2428–2435.

Yakacki, C.M., Willis, S., Luders, C., Gall, K., 2008b. Deformation limits in shape-memory polymers. Adv. Eng. Mater. 10, 112–119.

Yakacki, C.M., Nguyen, T.D., Likos, R., Lamell, R., Guigou, D., Gall, K., 2011. Impact of shape-memory programming on mechanically-driven recovery in polymers. Polymer 52, 4947–4954.

Yamashiro, M., Inoue, K., Iji, M., 2008. Recyclable shape-memory and mechanical strength of poly(lactic acid) compounds cross-linked by thermo-reversible Diels–Alder reaction. Polym. J. 40, 657–662.

Yang, B., Huang, W.M., Li, C., Li, L., 2006. Effects of moisture on the thermomechanical properties of a polyurethane shape memory polymer. Polymer 47, 1348–1356.

Yang, J., Liu, F., Yang, L., Li, S.M., 2010. Hydrolytic and enzymatic degradation of poly (trimethylene carbonate-*co*-D,L-lactide) random copolymers with shape memory behavior. Eur. Polym. J. 46, 783–791.

Yu, I., Acosta-Ramirez, A., Mehrkhodavandi, P., 2012. Mechanism of living lactide polymerization by dinuclear indium catalysts and its impact on isoselectivity. J. Am. Chem. Soc. 134, 12758–12773.

Zhang, W., Chen, L., Zhang, Y., 2009. Surprising shape-memory effect of polylactide resulted from toughening by polyamide elastomer. Polymer 50, 1311–1315.

Zhang, H.J., Xia, H.S., Zhao, Y., 2012. Optically triggered and spatially controllable shape-memory polymer-gold nanoparticle composite materials. J. Mater. Chem. 22, 845–849.

Zhu, Y., Hu, J.L., Luo, H.S., Young, R.J., Deng, L.B., Zhang, S., Fan, Y., Ye, G.D., 2012. Rapidly switchable water-sensitive shape-memory cellulose/elastomer nano-composites. Soft Matter 8, 2509–2517.

Biodegradable shape-memory polymers for biomedical applications

11

S. Strandman, X.X. Zhu
University of Montreal, Montreal, QC, Canada

11.1 Introduction

Shape-memory polymers (SMPs) are materials capable of recovering their permanent shape from a temporary one upon the exposure to a specific stimulus, such as heating. This capability is not an intrinsic property of the material, but results from a combination of the polymer structure and its specific processing considered as polymer functionalization. Triggered responsiveness is an attractive feature for developing smart biomaterials and medical devices, including tissue engineering, orthodontic, cardiovascular, and surgical applications (Small et al., 2007). Biocompatibility, biointegration, medical safety, and often biodegradability are key considerations (Ulery et al., 2011). Also, properties such as easy processability as well as the tunability of the actuation temperature and the thermo-mechanical behavior are desirable (Lendlein et al., 2010). Ideally, the materials should show mechanical properties mimicking those of targeted tissues to avoid necrosis or abnormal growth (Lendlein and Langer, 2002; Wang et al., 2002). An important approach for reaching these goals particularly in terms of biocompatibility and biodegradability is to design SMPs based on natural polymers, such as natural polypeptides or polysaccharides, or synthetic macromolecules built from compounds naturally occurring in the human body to minimize the toxic side effects (Martina and Hutmacher, 2007; Tschan et al., 2012; Ulery et al., 2011). For example, polyanhydrides or polyesters can be made of molecules abundant in human metabolism, such as from lactic acid, glycerol, or bile acids (Barrett and Yousaf, 2009). The versatility of the starting compounds and resulting polymers allows the tailoring of the degradation and mechanical properties according to particular applications. In addition, some of these materials show tunable shape-memory properties, making them promising candidates for dynamic mechanical devices (Gautrot and Zhu, 2006a, 2008, 2009a).

This chapter introduces the most common biodegradable SMPs, including materials based on biopolymers, biomolecule-based synthetic polymers, and synthetic polymers bearing degradable linkers (Section 11.2). The methods of activating the shape-memory effect are presented with the focus on thermally activated SMPs, which are exemplified through bile acid-based shape-memory copolymers with tunable thermo-mechanical properties (Section 11.3). The biodegradability and the biomedical applications of

Shape Memory Polymers for Biomedical Applications. http://dx.doi.org/10.1016/B978-0-85709-698-2.00011-8

SMPs, particularly in medical devices, are discussed in Section 11.4 with the emphasis on the advantages and limitations of the biodegradable shape-memory systems introduced so far as well as the future perspectives of the field (Section 11.5).

11.2 Biodegradable shape-memory polymers (SMPs)

11.2.1 Background

SMPs can change their shape in a predefined way when a suitable stimulus activates the molecular switching moieties. This character results from the effect of the morphology and processing of the polymer. The material is first formed into its initial permanent shape. It is then "programmed," i.e., fixed into a temporary shape. After applying an external stimulus, the material recovers its initial permanent shape. These cycles can be repeated several times to yield different temporary shapes in subsequent cycles. Some of the everyday applications of SMPs are heat-shrinkable tubings and films for electronic wiring or packing as well as smart fabrics (Rainer et al., 1964; Arditti et al., 1971; Cho, 2010); rapid developments have been seen in fields such as aerospace engineering (Cho, 2010; Liu and Leng, 2010) and biomedicine (Small et al., 2007; Lendlein et al., 2010; Serrano et al., 2011). Due to environmental concerns, biodegradability is nowadays a desirable feature for the materials in everyday life, but it is essential in certain biomedical applications of SMPs; for example, in intelligent medical devices or implants for minimally invasive surgery, among others (Section 11.4). The advantage of biodegradable medical materials is that they do not require surgery for their removal from the body, while the shape-memory property would allow a shape change of the implant or medical device from a compressed and thus easily insertable shape to an expanded application shape (Yakacki and Gall, 2010). The degradability can be achieved by introducing hydrolyzable bonds in the polymer chain. The structures of common synthetic polymers bearing such bonds are presented in Table 11.1, with applications ranging from vaccine adjuvants and drug-delivery systems to hard tissue engineering and prosthetics (Ulery et al., 2011). Polymeric biomaterials may be degraded via chemical and enzymatic oxidation upon exposure to body fluids and tissues, via hydrolytic degradation catalyzed by acids, bases, or salts, and via enzyme-catalyzed hydrolysis reactions (Azevedo and Reis, 2005; Lyu and Untereker, 2009). Hydrolytic degradation rates (λ) can vary greatly from very hydrolytically unstable (polyphosphazenes) to hydrolytically stable (polyamides, Table 11.1). The catalytic effect of enzymes can be strong and, hence, *in vivo* degradation rates of some biomaterials may be significantly higher than those of *in vitro* experiments (Azevedo and Reis, 2005).

11.2.2 Polyesters

Probably the most important class of biodegradable materials possessing shape-memory characteristics are α-hydroxy acid-based copolyesters. Poly(L-lactide) (PLLA) and poly(DL-lactide) (PDLLA) (general structure in Table 11.1) and

Table 11.[illegible] Common synthetic [illegible] polymers, their general structures, and hydrolytic degradation rates

Polymer	Structure	Degradation rate constant λ (s^{-1})	References
Polyphosphazenes	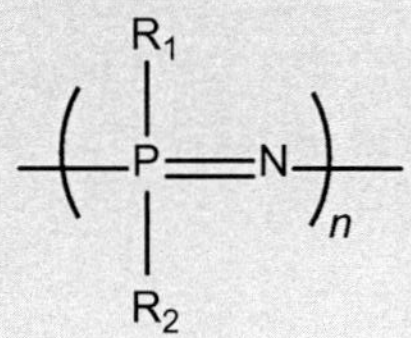	4.5×10^{-2}–1.4×10^{-7}	Ulery et al. (2011)
Polyanhydrides	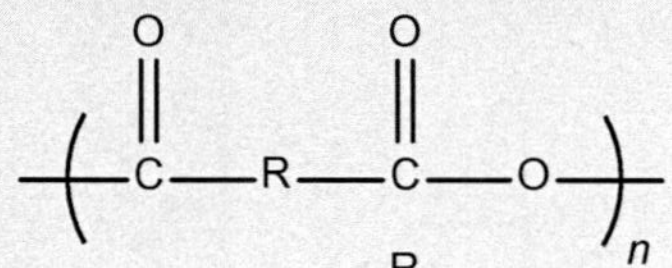	1.9×10^{-3}–9.4×10^{-7}	von Burkersroda et al. (2002) and Ulery et al. (2011)
Polyacetals	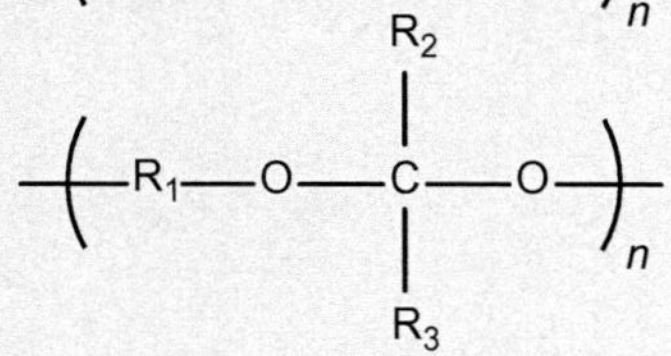	2.7×10^{-8}	von Burkersroda et al. (2002)
Poly(ortho ester)s	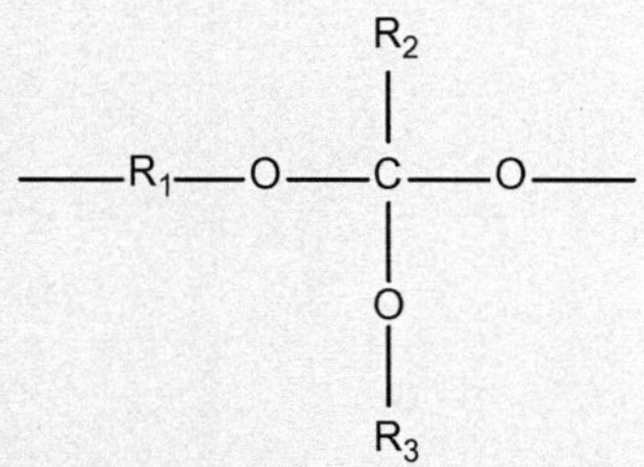	4.8×10^{-5}	von Burkersroda et al. (2002)
Polyphosphoesters	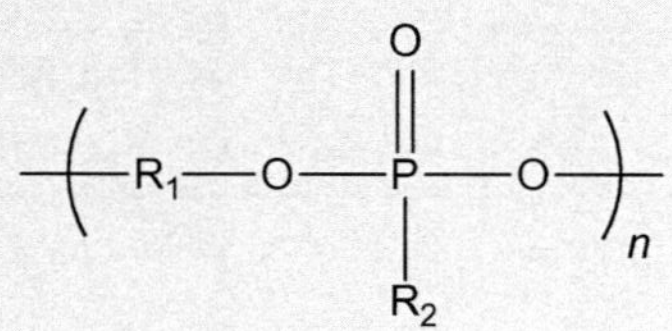	1.4×10^{-6}	Ulery et al. (2011)

Continued

Table 11.1 Continued

Polymer	Structure	Degradation rate constant λ (s^{-1})	References
Polyglycolide (polyester)	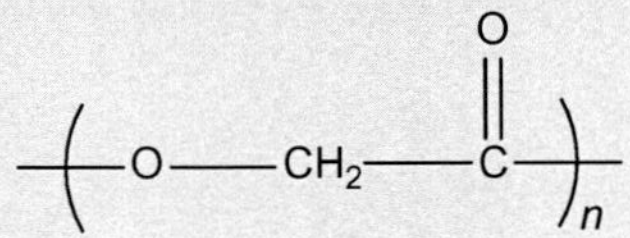	1.5×10^{-7}	Iordanskii et al. (1994)
Poly(ε-caprolactone) (polyester)	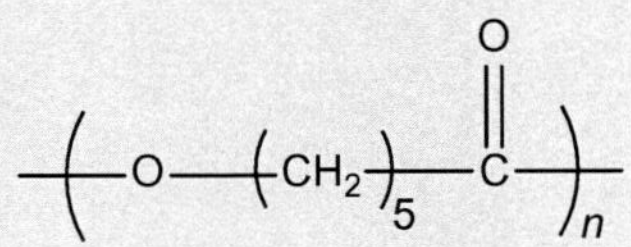	3.5×10^{-8}; 9.7×10^{-8}	Ulery et al. (2011) and von Burkersroda et al. (2002)
Polyurethanes	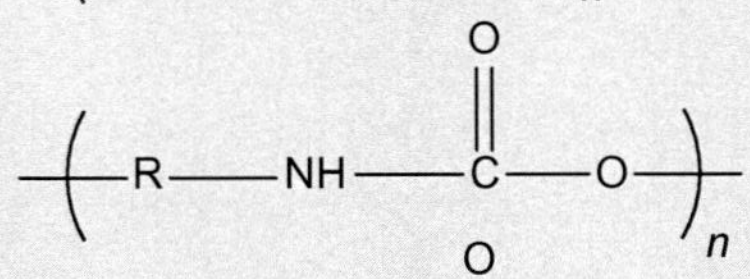	8.3×10^{-8}	Ulery et al. (2011)
Polylactide (polyester)	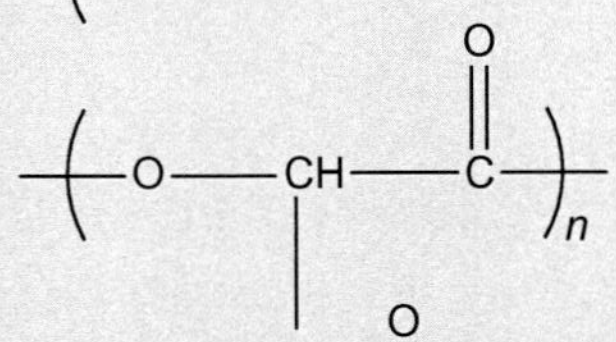	9.7×10^{-8}; 6.6×10^{-9}	Chen et al. (2011) and von Burkersroda et al. (2002)
Polycarbonates	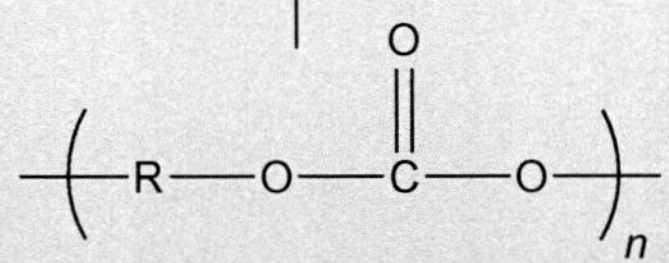	4.1×10^{-10}	Ulery et al. (2011)
Polyamides	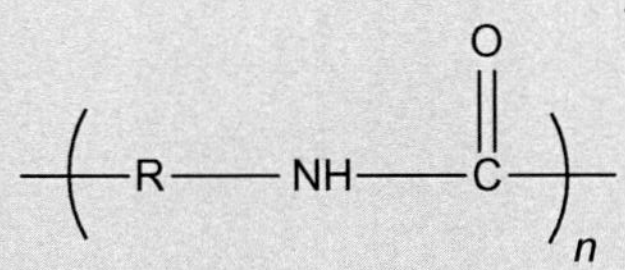	2.6×10^{-13}	von Burkersroda et al. (2002)

Adapted from Ulery et al. (2011), with permission.

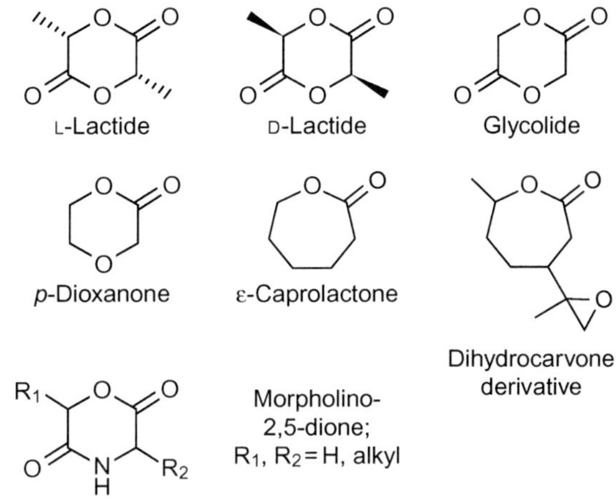

Figure 11.1 Common cyclic monomers for the synthesis of biodegradable (co)polymers.

polyglycolide (PGA) are synthesized by the ring-opening polymerization (ROP) of corresponding six-membered cyclic diesters (Figure 11.1), while poly (ε-caprolactone) (PCL, Table 11.1) is prepared from a seven-membered cyclic mono-ester (Figure 11.1). PLLA is one of the most widely used biodegradable polymers in biomedical and pharmaceutical applications, owing to its good mechanical strength, degradability, and biocompatibility (Sabir et al., 2009); however, some of its limitations are poor hydrophilicity, relatively poor processability, and high rigidity and crystallinity, similar to PCL (Feng and Guo, 2009; Sabir et al., 2009). While PGA has a glass transition temperature (T_g) close to body temperature (36–40 °C, Feng and Guo, 2009; Tsuji, 2005), the T_g values of PLLA and PDLLA are well above it (T_g = 57–60 °C and 50–54 °C, respectively, Feng and Guo, 2009). PCL is semicrystalline at room temperature with a molar-mass-dependent melting point (when M_n > 10 kDa, T_m = 64 °C) and a very low T_g at −60 °C, but it degrades more slowly than PLLA due to its hydrophobicity (Lendlein et al., 2005b). These thermal transitions play an important role in the temperature-activated shape-memory behavior (Section 11.3). A variety of materials with tailored mechanical and shape-memory properties, transition temperatures, and degradation profiles can be produced by copolymerization and crosslinking procedures. Crosslinking is often used for fixing the permanent shape of the material (Lendlein and Kelch, 2002). Uncross-linked copolyesters exhibiting shape-memory characteristics include, for example, P(LLA-*co*-GA) (Wong et al., 2007), P(LLA-*co*-CL) (Lu et al., 2008), poly(LLA-*co*-GA)-*block*-poly(*p*-dioxanone) (Lendlein and Kelch, 2002), poly(ε-caprolactone-*block*-alkylene adipate), and poly(ε-caprolactone-*block*-*p*-dioxanone) (Behl et al., 2009). Poly (*p*-dioxanone) (PPDO) is a synthetic histocompatible and biodegradable poly(ester-ether) prepared by ROP from a corresponding cyclic monomer (Figure 11.1) (Yang et al., 2002).

A wide range of biocompatible polyesters can be obtained through the polycondensation of polyols and diacids endogenous to human metabolism, resulting in cross-linked materials (Barrett and Yousaf, 2010). Shape-memory characteristics have been reported for poly(glycerol-sebacate) (Cai and Liu, 2007), poly(glycerol-dodecanoate) (Migneco et al., 2009), and poly(diol citrate)s composed of 1,8-octanediol, 1,12-dodecanediol, and 1,16-hexadecanediol as diols copolymerized with citric acid bearing one hydroxyl and three carboxylic acid groups (Serrano et al., 2011). Bio-based poly(propylene sebacate) was synthesized from 1,3-propanediol, sebacic acid, and itaconic acid produced via fermentation or extraction. The cross-linked products exhibited excellent shape-memory properties, where the applicable temperature range and shape-recovery speed were tuned by a copolymerization with diethyleneglycol to tailor the chain flexibility (Guo et al., 2011). A less common approach for natural product-derived polyesters was reported by Lowe and coworkers (2009), where dihydrocarvone found in caraway oil was oxidized to an epoxylactone (Figure 11.1) and copolymerized with ε-caprolactone to yield cross-linked SMPs.

11.2.3 Poly(ester-amide)s

Combining different types of monomers with degradable bonds provides a way of introducing both hard and soft segments into the structure to yield the shape-memory property and to tune the hydrolytic and enzymatic degradation rates of the materials (Feng et al., 2010). The SMPs may also contain non-degradable or even inorganic components as part of the polymer chain or the network, such as poly(ethylene glycol) (PEG), polypropylene glycol, or polyhedral silsesquioxane (POSS) (Venkatraman et al., 2006; Choi et al., 2006; Lee et al., 2008). Poly(ester-amide)s are commonly synthesized via various polycondensation methods, including melt, solution and bulk polycondensations, and interfacial polymerization (Rodriguez-Galan et al., 2011). As a special class of poly(ester-amides), block copolymers based on polydepsipeptides, alternating copolymers of α-hydroxy- and α-amino acids, have shown a temperature-controlled shape-memory behavior (Feng et al., 2010). A common synthetic route toward polydepsipeptides is the ROP of morpholine-2,5-diones (cyclic dimers of an α-hydroxy- and an α-amino acid, Figure 11.1), providing higher molar masses than the stepwise active ester-peptide coupling reactions (Feng and Guo, 2009). Morpholine-2,5-diones can also be copolymerized with cyclic esters, such as L-lactide or ε-caprolactone, for random-alternating copolymers or block copolymers (Feng et al., 2010). Multiblock copolymers composed of PCL and polydepsipeptide segments have shown excellent shape-memory properties and rapid hydrolytic degradation that changes the material from elastic to brittle (Feng et al., 2009).

11.2.4 Poly(ester-urethane)s and poly(urethane-urea)s

Poly(ester-urethane)s and poly(urethane-urea)s are common SMPs for biomedical applications and segmented polymers can be obtained by the synthesis of polyester macrodiols or "pre-polymers," followed by the condensation with coupling agents, such as diisocyanates and chain extenders (diols for polyurethanes, diamines for polyureas) (Zini et al., 2007; Pretsch et al., 2009). For example, a three-arm star-like PCL was reacted with a 4,4′-diisocyanate and 1,6-hexanediol, and the resulting biodegradable poly(ester-urethane) showed excellent shape-memory effects close to the body temperature (Xue et al., 2009). Shape-memory poly(urethane-urea)s based on poly (lactide-*co*-*p*-dioxanone) were synthesized by reacting the ROP-produced macrodiol copolymers first with hexamethylene diisocyanate, followed by a reaction with butanediamine. Faster degradation and lower degradation-induced acidity was observed in comparison with PDLLA (Wang et al., 2010). Other examples from a wide selection of prepolymers include aliphatic polycarbonates (Xu and Zhang, 2007), P(LA-*co*-CL) copolymers (Wang et al., 2007), and copolymers of oligo(ε-caprolactone) and oligo (depsipeptide) or oligo(pentadecalactone) (Feng et al., 2009; Behl et al., 2010).

11.2.5 Bile acid-based polymers

Bile acids (Figure 11.2) are endogenous amphiphilic steroidal acids abundant in the body and they have attracted considerable research effort due to their important role in biological processes such as solubilization of fats and fat-soluble vitamins, regulation of metabolism, inflammation, and cell proliferation (Hoffmann, 1999; Marin, 2009) and their potential applications in sensors and biomedical field (Gautrot and Zhu, 2006a,b, 2009b; Mukhopadhyay and Maitra, 2004). Their combination of rigid bent backbone, functional groups with well-controlled chemistry, and facial amphiphilicity allows designing various host–guest complexation and drug-delivery systems as well as novel functional materials (Tamminen and Kolehmainen, 2001; Zhu and Nichifor, 2002; Zhao, 2007; Zhang and Zhu, 2009). In addition, the relatively high pK_a of bile acids would suggest a moderate variation of local pH upon degradation of these materials (Fini and Roda, 1987). Bile acids can be incorporated into a polyester backbone using metathesis chemistry and ROP of large bile acid-based macrocycles (Figure 11.3), driven by entropy and an increased conformational freedom experienced by each repeating unit (Strandman et al., 2011; Xue and Mayer, 2009). This method, entropy-driven ring-opening polymerization (ED-ROP), affords high-molar-mass polymers in high yields, and the resulting amorphous materials exhibit excellent temperature-controlled shape-memory properties combined with biodegradability. In addition, the materials' stiffness, T_g, and shape-recovery temperature can be tuned

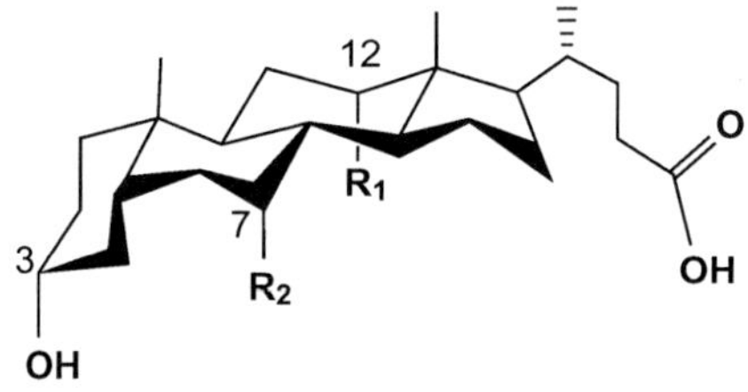

Bile acid	R_1	R_2
Cholic acid	OH	OH
Deoxycholic acid	H	OH
Chenodeoxycholic acid	OH	H
Lithocholic acid	H	H

Figure 11.2 Structures of common bile acids.

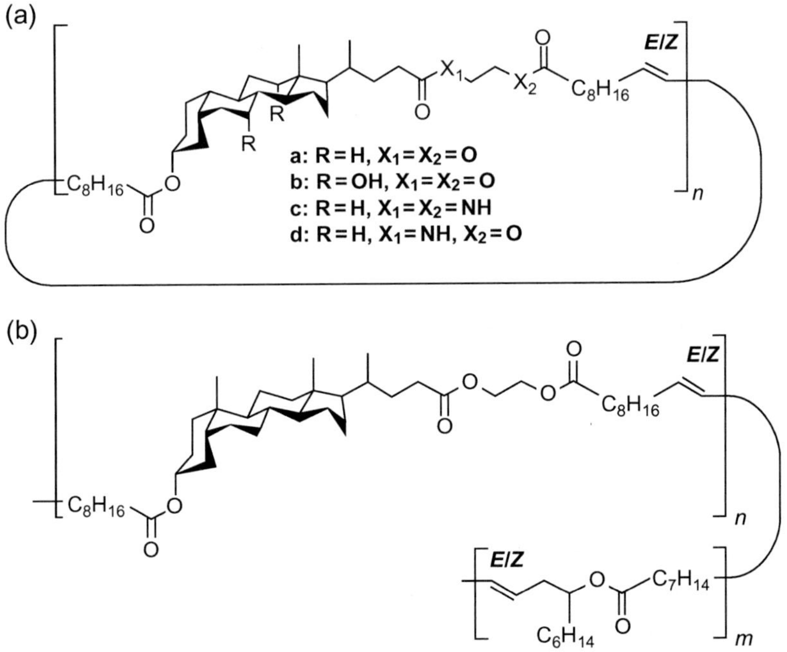

Figure 11.3 Structures of (a) selected bile acid-based macrocycles and (b) an example of lithocholate acid and ricinoleic acid-based copolymers.

by modifying the chemical structure or by copolymerizing with other macrocycles derived from natural origins, warranting a wide range of applications, particularly in the biomedical field (Gautrot and Zhu, 2006b, 2008, 2009a; Thérien-Aubin et al., 2010). The use of bile acids offers remarkable freedom of design, as their chemical structure can be altered, for instance, to improve the biocompatibility, enhance cell adhesion, or release specific factors from the materials. The shape-memory performance of bile acid-based polymers and its tailoring will be discussed in the next section.

11.2.6 Natural polysaccharide-based materials

Starch, a natural polymer with shape-memory characteristics, is an abundant and inexpensive resource for biodegradable or biocompatible materials, obtained from a wide variety of higher plants. It is composed of two polysaccharides with different intrinsic glass transition temperatures (T_g); linear amylose (20–35 wt%) and branched amylopectin (65–80 wt%) (Figure 11.4), whose ratio depends on the source plant (Mitrus et al., 2009; Liu et al., 2010). Extensive processing yields thermoplastic starch, which exhibits good shape-memory performance comparable with synthetic SMPs (Véchambre et al., 2011) and can be used to make both humidity- and temperature-responsive materials (Chaunier and Lourdin, 2009). Another natural polysaccharide, chitosan (Figure 11.4), has been successfully employed as a blended

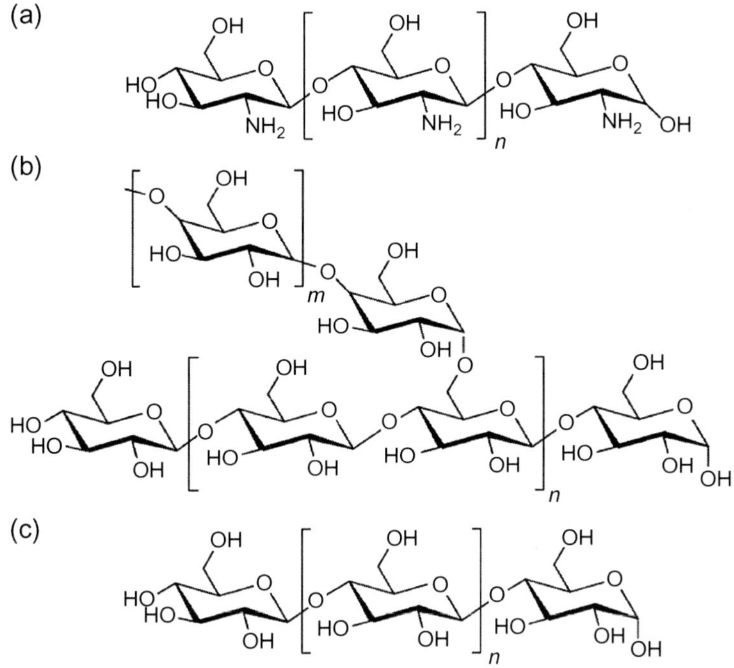

Figure 11.4 Structure of common polysaccharides used for shape-memory materials: (a) amylose, (b) amylopectin, (c) chitosan.

material cross-linked with an epoxy compound to yield biodegradable stents with hydration-controlled shape memory (Chen et al., 2007). Chitosan is a biodegradable and biocompatible linear aminopolysaccharide obtained by the deacetylation of chitin, a widespread natural polysaccharide whose major sources are the shells of crustaceans, such as crabs, shrimps, prawns, and lobsters (Kumar et al., 2004).

11.3 Activation and tailoring the shape-memory effect

11.3.1 Activating the shape-memory effect

SMPs can recover relatively large strains in response to a stimulus, which can be temperature, UV light (Lendlein et al., 2005a; Wu et al., 2011), stress (Heuwers et al., 2012), or compression (Yakacki et al., 2011). The effect of temperature can also be activated indirectly using magnetic field (Mohr et al., 2006), electric current (Cho et al., 2005), laser (Maitland et al., 2002), infrared light (Koerner et al., 2004), or ultrasound (Li et al., 2012), or through exploiting the plasticizing effect of water that can lower the transition temperatures (Huang et al., 2005; Yang et al., 2004, 2006) or dissolve selected segments of the copolymer (Jung et al., 2006). The change from a temporary shape to the original one is predefined and determined by the mechanical deformation to the temporary shape, the "programming" of the material (Behl and Lendlein, 2007b). For most SMPs investigated so far, dual-shape memory has been reported, but recently, multi-shape memory effect has also been shown. For example, a triple-shape material can change its shape from a temporary shape A to another temporary shape B, and finally to a permanent shape C (Xie, 2010; Shao et al., 2012). Multi-shape memory effect can exploit either several obviously independent transition temperatures or a broad glass transition of the material. Within a broad T_g range, multiple temporary shapes can be fixed and recovered by changing the temperature in small increments. Therefore, for example, both triple- and quadruple-shape memory effects have been shown for a same material, depending on the programming sequence (Shao et al., 2012). A broad transition temperature can be considered as an infinite number of transitions, leading to the theoretical possibility of infinite number of memorized shapes.

The suitable SMP architectures consist of netpoints determining the permanent shape and switching segments that allow the deformability. The netpoints can be of chemical (covalent cross-links) or physical (intermolecular interactions) nature. The reversible fixation of the temporary shape requires stimuli-sensitive switches that form additional reversible cross-links. These can be established by reversible chemical bonds, intermolecular interactions, or solidification of switching domains when cooled below their thermal transition temperatures, such as T_g, T_m, or liquid crystalline transition temperatures (Behl et al., 2011) Figure 11.5 demonstrates a thermally induced shape-memory effect in a polymer with the shape-memory transition temperature $T_{trans}=T_g$. Physical cross-linking through hydrogen bonding, inclusion complexation, or physical entanglement of high-molar-mass polymers has been described (Luo et al., 2008, 2010; Gautrot and Zhu, 2009a; Wang and Xie, 2010; Li et al., 2011; Shao et al., 2012). Reversible chemical bonding can be achieved by introducing photoreactive groups, such as cinnamic acid, cinnamylidene acetic acid, or cinnamamide groups undergoing photoreversible [2+2] cycloaddition reactions

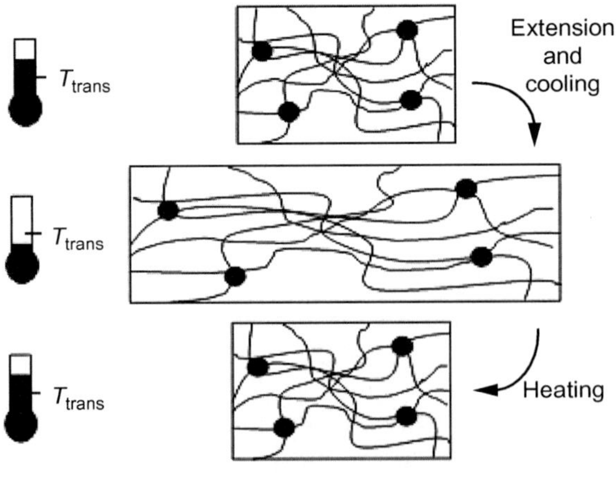

Figure 11.5 Schematic representation of the thermally induced shape-memory effect for a polymer network with $T_{trans}=T_g$. When the temperature is raised above the T_{trans} of the switching segments, these segments are flexible and the polymer can be deformed elastically. The temporary shape is fixed by cooling down below T_{trans}. If the polymer is heated up again, the permanent shape is recovered. Reprinted from Lendlein and Kelch (2002) with permission. Copyright 2012 John Wiley and Sons.

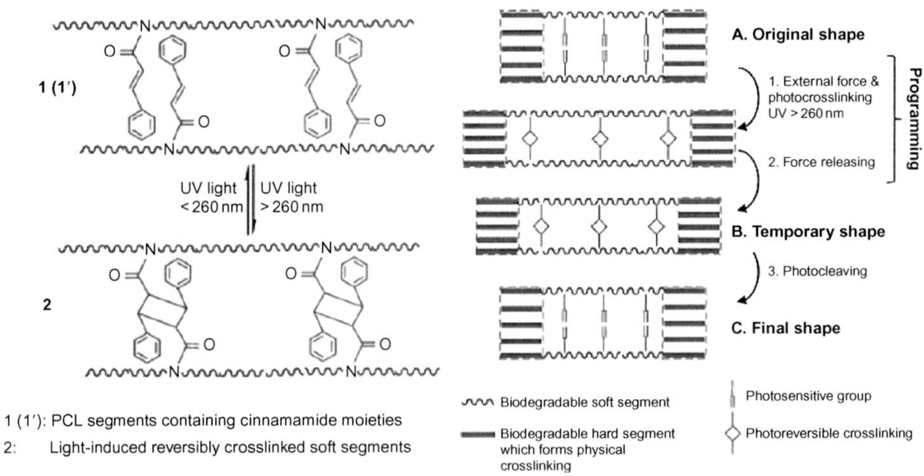

Figure 11.6 Reversible cross-linking of poly(ester-urethane)s based on PLLA and cinnamamide-derivatized-PCL segments through light-induced [2+2] cycloaddition reaction (left) and shape-memory effect of the polymers.
Reprinted from Wu et al. (2011), with permission. Copyright 2012 American Chemical Society.

when exposed to alternating wavelengths (Lendlein et al., 2005a; Wu et al., 2011), and an example of such system as well as its shape-memory effect is shown in Figure 11.6.

11.3.2 Quantifying the shape-memory effect

Cyclic thermo- or photomechanical stress- or strain-controlled tests give a full description of parameters quantifying the shape-memory effect of temperature- or light-triggered materials through the percentage of shape fixing (shape fixity ratio R_f) and the extent of shape recovery (shape recovery ratio R_r). In the case of thermal stimulus, the transition temperature is determined (Behl and Lendlein, 2007a). The shape fixity ratio R_f describes the ability of the material to fix the mechanical deformation applied during the programming process; it is equal to the amplitude ratio of the fixed deformation to the total deformation. For example, in a strain-controlled experiment, it is defined as

$$R_f(N) = \varepsilon_u(N)/\varepsilon_m \tag{11.1}$$

where $\varepsilon_u(N)$ is the strain after the relaxation (withdrawal of the tensile strength) in the Nth cycle and ε_m is the maximum strain. The shape recovery ratio R_r quantifies how well the permanent shape has been memorized by the material and is defined in a strain-controlled protocol as

$$R_r(N) = \left(\varepsilon_m - \varepsilon_p(N)\right)/\left(\varepsilon_m - \varepsilon_p(N-1)\right) \tag{11.2}$$

where ε_p is the strain after recovery (Behl and Lendlein, 2007a). Different protocols for cyclic thermo-mechanical tensile tests have been highlighted by Wagermaier and coworkers (2010). These tests are usually carried out by dynamic mechanical analyzer (DMA, or dynamic mechanical thermal analyzer, DMTA) to determine the viscoelastic properties. Examples of two cyclic thermo-mechanical testing experiments, "warm-drawing" and "cold-drawing," are shown in Figure 11.7 for bile acid-based

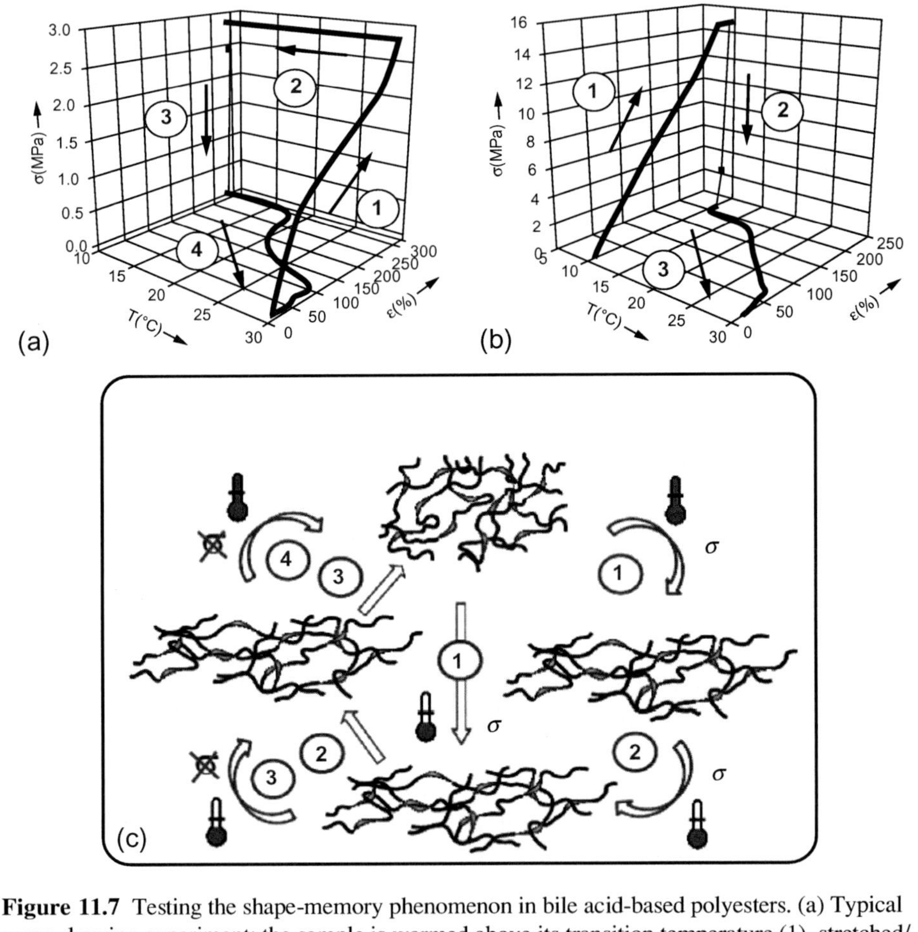

Figure 11.7 Testing the shape-memory phenomenon in bile acid-based polyesters. (a) Typical warm drawing experiment: the sample is warmed above its transition temperature (1), stretched/deformed to the desired temporary shape (2), the temperature is dropped to fix the temporary shape (3), and shape recovery is triggered by warming the sample above its transition temperature (4). (b) Cold drawing experiment: the sample is directly stretched below its transition temperature (1) and the remaining steps are as for the warm drawing. (c) Shape-memory effect in warm and cold drawing modes. The cold drawing cycle is shorter, which simplifies its use and application in devices. The numbers correspond to the thermo-mechanical steps depicted in (a) and (b).
Reprinted from Gautrot and Zhu (2009a), with permission. Copyright 2012 American Chemical Society.

polyesters, where the shape memory has been suggested to arise from the chain entanglements and the formation of ordered domains (Gautrot and Zhu, 2009a; Thérien-Aubin et al., 2010). The samples have been tested below and above the glass transition temperature (T_g + 10 °C and T_g − 10 °C). Typical shape recovery ratios of SMPs are in the range of 80–99% (Wagermaier et al., 2010), while the shape fixities may depend on the testing protocol (Gautrot and Zhu, 2009a). In addition, three-point flexural tests, material shrinkage measurements, or simple bending tests are used to examine the shape-memory behavior (Wagermaier et al., 2010). Some of the tests have been tailored for intended applications, such as testing the actuation rate and shape-recovery of fabricated devices (Buckley et al., 2006; Baer et al., 2007; Yakacki et al., 2007).

11.3.3 Tailoring the thermo-mechanical properties

The moduli of soft tissues are in the range 0.2–350 MPa, while those of hard tissues range from 10 to 1500 MPa (Bettinger et al., 2007; Barrett and Yousaf, 2009). Hence, the stiffness of the material should be tailored for the desired biomedical applications. For example, the shape change may be triggered by body heat when the activation temperature is close to body temperature. The thermo-mechanical properties of SMPs can be tailored by varying the crosslinking density or the chain backbone stiffness by the choice of monomers. For example, the T_g and the toughness of (meth)acrylate networks can be independently adjusted using such parameters, yielding T_gs ranging from −29 to 112 °C and moduli from 2.8 to 129.5 MPa (Safranski and Gall, 2008). At low cross-link densities, the structure of the comonomers, such as bulky side groups or α-methyl groups in the backbone, has a profound effect on the material toughness (Safranski and Gall, 2008; Yakacki et al., 2008). In another example, the copolymerization of flexible ricinoleic acid with a more rigid bile acid-based monomer (Figure 11.3) allows the fine-tuning of the mechanical properties of the resulting SMP. The effects of comonomer content on T_g and Young's modulus of a lithocholate-based copolymer at 37 °C are demonstrated in Figure 11.8 (Gautrot and Zhu, 2008, 2009a). In addition, minor changes in the bile acid monomer structure, such as replacing lithocholic acid with cholic acid bearing two additional hydroxyls or replacing part of the ester groups with amides, have a drastic effect on the chain stiffness, increasing both the T_g and the Young's modulus of the homopolymers. As a result, the combined strategies of tailored monomer synthesis and copolymerization yield bile acid-based copolymers with T_gs close to body temperature (36–42 °C), tunable Young's moduli (6–75 MPa at 37.5 °C), and excellent shape-memory properties (shape recoveries R_r = 95–99%; shape fixities R_f = 91–94%, depending on the testing protocol) (Gautrot and Zhu, 2009a). In addition to tuning the thermo-mechanical properties, introducing hydrolyzable comonomers can enhance the degradation rate of the materials, such as glycolide in PLA- or PCL-based shape-memory networks (Choi and Lendlein, 2007; Kelch et al., 2007). The thermal transitions can also be controlled by additives. For example, the T_g of starch and thus the transition temperature of the corresponding shape-memory materials can be controlled in a temperature range from 10 to 100 °C by the addition of a plasticizer, such as glycerol or sorbitol

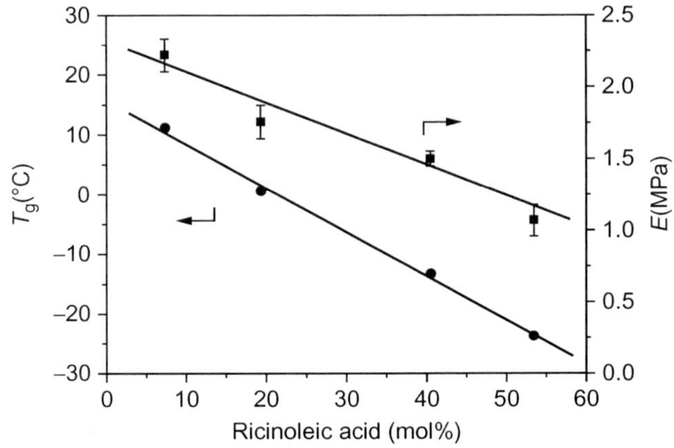

Figure 11.8 Variation of T_g (circles) and Young's modulus (squares) of the copolymers of lithocholate-based monomer and ricinoleic acid (structure in Figure 11.3) as a function of ricinoleic acid content.
Reproduced from Gautrot and Zhu (2008) with permission. Copyright 2012 Royal Society of Chemistry.

(Lourdin et al., 1997; Chaunier and Lourdin, 2009). These materials are highly sensitive to water, which decreases the T_g, leading to a shape recovery in a high-humidity atmosphere (Chaunier and Lourdin, 2009; Véchambre et al., 2010a). The shape-memory effect of the amorphous starch-based material was assigned to the local molecular orientation and a deformation-induced mesophase between amorphous and crystalline state that disappears when the sample relaxes and recovers its initial shape (Véchambre et al., 2010b, 2011).

11.4 Biodegradation and biomedical applications

11.4.1 Requirements for biomaterials

A definition of a biomaterial is a "nonviable material used in a medical device, intended to interact with biological systems" (Ratner et al., 2004). These materials need to be biocompatible, which means the ability of the material to perform with an appropriate host response in the desired applications (Ratner et al., 2004), such as implants, surgical instruments, extracorporeal devices, wound covers, or controlled drug-delivery systems, which are common applications for polymeric biomaterials (Lendlein et al., 2010). Some examples of appropriate host responses include resistance to blood clotting or to bacterial colonization, and uncomplicated healing process (Ratner et al., 2004). *In vitro* tests are commonly used for evaluating the cytotoxicity, cytocompatibility, cell adhesion, genotoxicity, hemocompatibility, and cell proliferation for the materials, their degradation products, as well as possible contaminants (catalysts, monomers, solvents, endotoxins), while *in vivo* tests are used to estimate the local and systemic interactions of host tissues with implant materials and their components (Lendlein et al., 2010). Both types of tests have also their disadvantages. *In vitro* tests on cell cultures cannot represent the complexity of the whole organisms, they may sometimes lead to false negatives due to the specific sensitivity, or they may be restricted by the choice of cell type. In addition, adequate information on the biomaterial degradation involving the host–biomaterial interactions can only be obtained *in vivo*, although the degradation rates and erosion mechanisms under physiological conditions can be evaluated (Silva et al., 2005). Nevertheless, *in vivo* tests on a single animal species cannot represent a general model for the human species (Lendlein et al., 2010).

Biodegradability of biomaterials, for example in sutures or surgical staples, may be required to support wound healing or tissue regeneration as long as required, after which the material would break down into nontoxic degradation products and become excreted or metabolized without removal or surgical revision. The materials should be processable, have suitable degradation times and mechanical properties for the intended use, and not cause a sustained inflammatory response (Ulery et al., 2011). In addition, the sterilization of medical devices prior to their implantation is necessary to minimize the risk of infection. Ideally, the sterilization process should not alter the physical, mechanical, and biological properties of the material (Lendlein et al., 2010). This brings an additional challenge for thermoplastics and particularly for the temperature-actuated shape-memory devices, which cannot be treated at high temperatures. Therefore, steam sterilization (autoclave) cannot be used. Low-temperature sterilization methods include γ- or e-beam irradiation, hydrogen peroxide (H_2O_2) vapor, ethylene oxide treatment, and low-temperature plasma technique. Some of these methods may change the material properties through cross-linking or degradation reactions, or due to the changes in functional groups, which need to be studied for the polymers intended for medical devices (Lendlein et al., 2010).

11.4.2 Degradation studies on SMPs

The biodegradability of SMPs can be achieved by introducing weak hydrolyzable bonds that cleave under physiological conditions. The degradation of polymeric biomaterials depends not only on the degradation rate of labile bonds, listed in Table 11.1, but also on factors such as water diffusion, monomer solubility and diffusion, material homogeneity, processing technique, and device geometry and size (Azevedo and Reis, 2005; Lyu and Untereker, 2009; Ulery et al., 2011). In addition to tuning the chemical composition of the polymer, blending and surface modification can be used to adjust the degradation (Azevedo and Reis, 2005). Biodegradable polymers are typically classified into bulk- and surface-eroding polymers. Bulk degradation is characterized by the hydrolysis of chemical bonds at the center of material, leading to a nonlinear degradation profile, as the diffusion of water in the material becomes much faster than the degradation. In surface erosion, the loss of material occurs on the surface only, as the mass relief at the water-material interface is much greater than the diffusion of water into the bulk of the material. This leads to linear, well-predictable mass loss profiles; the surface-eroding devices get smaller but keep their geometric shape. Bulk-eroding materials, such as PLA, allow the hydrolytic diffusion and permeability useful in tissue engineering applications (Ulery et al., 2011). Surface erosion, such as in the case of polyanhydrides and polyorthoesters, is beneficial in providing constant drug-release kinetics and maintaining the mechanical and structural integrity of the material with degradation. Enzyme-catalyzed degradation may follow a surface erosion mechanism, especially if the material is highly crystalline and hydrophobic, because the enzymes with high hydrodynamic volume cannot penetrate the tightly packed structure of certain polymers. The enzymatic action may be enhanced through the degradation-induced surface roughening and, thus, increase in the surface area (Azevedo and Reis, 2005). The degradation can be monitored through water absorption, mass loss, decrease in molar mass, changes in crystallinity, surface morphology, surface chemistry and sample dimensions, deterioration of mechanical properties, and analysis of degradation products (Azevedo and Reis, 2005).

The more hydrophilic domains of shape-memory copolymers show faster hydrolytic degradation than the more hydrophobic ones. Degradation is often accompanied by a change in macroscopic properties of the materials from elastic to brittle, change in the shape-memory characteristics, and/or an increase in surface roughness (Pretsch et al., 2009). Examples of SMP systems where the degradation behavior depends on the hydrophobicity of the material and can thus be adjusted include PCL-polydepsipeptide multiblock copolymers, where PCL is the more hydrophobic and thus slower degrading domain (Feng et al., 2009); copolymer networks based on oligo(L-lactide-*co*-glycolide)dimethacrylates or on oligo(ε-caprolactone-*co*-glycolide)dimethacrylates copolymerized with butyl acrylate, where the higher glycolide content increases the water uptake of the materials and accelerates the degradation, but butyl acrylate or methacrylate moieties decrease these characteristics (Choi and Lendlein, 2007; Kelch et al., 2007); P(DLLA-*co*-GA)-POSS network, where higher poly(silsesquioxane) (POSS) content induces slower degradation (Knight et al., 2009); and poly diol citrates, where the use of more hydrophobic diols with longer alkyl chains leads to slower degradation (Serrano et al., 2011). Relatively hydrophobic lithocholate-ricinoleide-copolymers (Figure 11.3) degrade slowly in phosphate-buffered saline solution above the T_g (25% relative weight loss in 5 months), and the varying amounts of ricinoleide comonomer do not significantly change the degradation process occurring via surface erosion mechanism (Gautrot and Zhu, 2008). While rapidly degrading materials are potential candidates for drug-delivery systems, slower degradation is desirable in applications requiring long-term performance, such as in orthopedic or cardiovascular devices.

As enzymes can alter the hydrolytic degradation profile, selective enzymatic degradation has been observed when comparing the hydrolytic and enzymatic degradation rates of multiblock shape-memory copolymers composed of PCL and PPDO segments. While hydrolytic degradation behavior is governed by the PPDO segments, *Pseudomonas cepacia* lipase is capable of attacking both crystalline and amorphous PCL, accelerating significantly the degradation occurring through random chain scission and surface erosion mechanism. Several other lipases, such as *Rhizopus delemar*, *Rhizopus arrhizus*, and *Humicola lanuginose* lipases as well as lipase *AK*, have also been reported to accelerate the degradation of PCL (Kulkarni et al., 2007, 2008), and while porcine pancreatic lipase has been reported to be less effective in the degradation of PCL homopolymer (Gan et al., 1997), it has provided fast degradation of SMPs based on the inclusion complexes of α-cyclodextrin and PCL (Luo et al., 2010).

In drug-loaded shape-memory poly(lactide-*co*-glycolide)urethane networks, the hydrophilicity and the acidity of the drug may influence the hydrolytic degradation rate: for instance, aspirin- or enoxacin-loaded materials degrade faster or have higher water uptake due to the local acidity that catalyzes ester bond cleavage (Wischke et al., 2009, 2010; Feng et al., 2011). On the other hand, incorporating excipients that neutralize the hydrolysis products has been shown to retard the degradation (Azevedo and Reis, 2005). The mechanical properties of the drug-loaded network deteriorated faster upon degradation compared with the drug-free network (Wischke et al., 2009). In addition, high drug loading has been demonstrated to alter the thermo-mechanical properties of SMP networks. Incorporating high amounts (20 wt%) of theophylline in branched oligo(ε-caprolactone)-derived networks weakened the mechanical strength and network elasticity of the SMP and, as a result, no shape-memory programming could be conducted (Nagahama et al., 2009). However, the number of reports on this effect is limited and extensive studies with a wider range of materials and drugs would be required.

11.4.3 Biomedical applications of biodegradable SMPs

Polymeric shape-memory materials are interesting for biomedical applications owing to features such as lightness, low cost, easy processability, high recoverable strains, tailored thermo-mechanical properties and shape-recovery temperature range, and the possibility for different and even multiple stimuli as well as for remote actuation (Sun et al., 2012). Therefore, an attractive application area is active medical devices. These include self-tightening and self-retaining sutures, surgical fasteners, intraluminal stents in vascular, urogenital and gastrointestinal applications, anchoring cannulas, orthopedic fixations, expandable implants for reconstructive or aesthetic surgery, and craniofacial meshes and plates (Yakacki and Gall, 2010; Lendlein et al., 2010; Serrano, 2012). The shape-memory feature would allow minimally invasive surgery, requiring smaller incisions for inserting the compressed medical devices in the body and causing less surgical stress. Degradable SMPs loaded with drugs can be employed in these applications or as injectable or implantable self-anchoring implant rods that enable special fixation for localized drug release (Wischke et al., 2009, 2010). Sometimes the observed shape memory of surgical implants has been unintended, such as in the case of PLA-based craniofacial plates that were programmed by heating and bending to a desired shape but which lost that shape at body temperature (Losken et al., 1994).

SMPs can be used in wound closure devices, such as self-tightening or tissue-anchoring sutures and surgical fasteners, including self-tightening staples. Proper wound closure is essential to allow tissue regeneration and avoid scarring, while the removal of sutures or fasteners by biodegradation is desirable. Hence, SMP-based smart degradable sutures have been created that are capable of tying themselves in conjunction with minimally invasive surgical approaches (Lendlein and Langer, 2002).

A self-untying property has also been demonstrated (Huang et al., 2012). A self-anchoring suture consists of a filament that has retainers on its surface to engage and retain tissue without knots, and the shape of the suture, including the retainers, will change upon the stimulus (Goraltchouk et al., 2011). As an example of smart surgical fasteners, the temperature-induced self-tightening of a bioabsorbable PLA/PGA-copolymer-based subcuticular staple has been demonstrated in Figure 11.9. The use of shape-memory material-based fasteners reduces the need for staples of different sizes and provides gentle force to close the wound (Huang et al., 2012). As surgical aids during minimally invasive procedures, cannulas are utilized to provide an access port for surgical instruments and a channel for introducing insufflation gases into the body cavities. After inserting the cannula, it can be prevented from migrating or slipping out through the incision using SMP-based anchoring structures on the distal portion of the cannula that can expand upon heating (Sung, 2009).

In the search of alternative materials for intraluminal stents, SMPs are attractive candidates for the next generation of stents, which could combine the tissue anchoring capability with self-expandability, biodegradability and, if necessary, controlled drug release. An example of a simulated ureteral stent combining these features is shown in Figure 11.10. Here, the stent is composed of a degradable oligo[(ε-caprolactone)-*co*-glycolide]dimethacrylate network, which has been tested for shape memory and drug-release properties when loaded with model drugs ethacridine lactate and enoxacin (Neffe et al., 2009). Ureteral stents are temporary implants that need to be fixed in their position to prevent obstruction of the ureter and to restore the flow of urine to

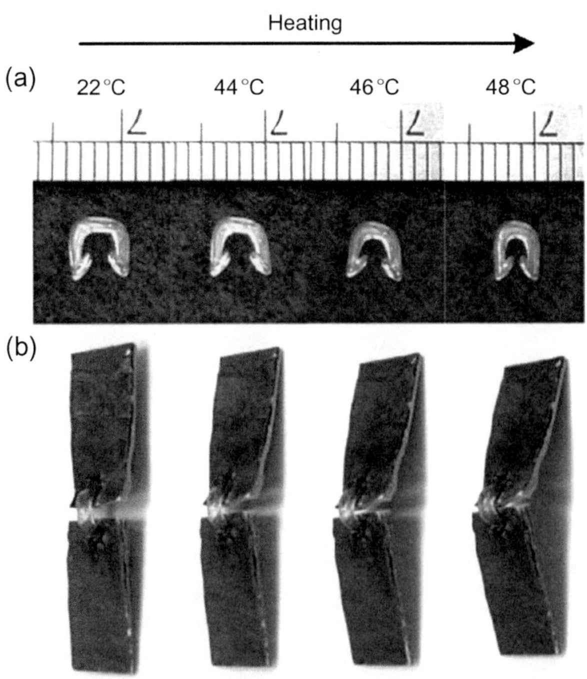

Figure 11.9 Temperature-induced self-tightening of a PLA/PGA-copolymer-based Insorb® staple. (a) Shrinking of the staple upon heating; (b) tightening of staple upon heating to demonstrate wound closure.
Reproduced from Huang et al. (2012), with permission. Copyright 2012 Elsevier.

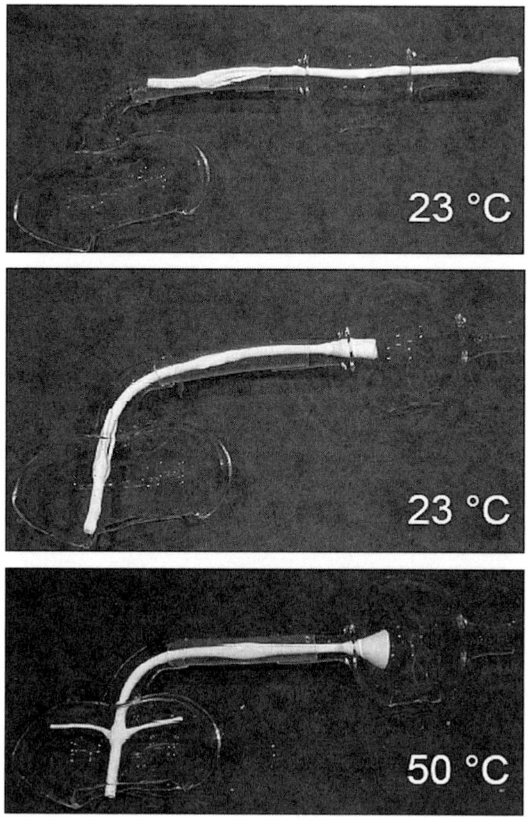

Figure 11.10 Principle of a self-anchoring drug-eluting (ureteral) stent based on a biodegradable oligo [(ε-caprolactone)-*co*-glycolide] dimethacrylate network. The inner diameter of the demonstration object (stent) is 2 mm, the outer diameter is 4 mm, and the diameter of the polyethylene tube simulating a ureter between the glass substitutes representing a bladder and a kidney is 9 mm. The shape change is stimulated by rinsing with water at 50 °C. Reprinted from Supporting Information of Neffe et al. (2009), with permission. Copyright 2012 John Wiley and Sons.

the bladder. Another class of stents exploiting the shape-memory effect is vascular stents, which are small tubular scaffolds used to maintain the luminal size of an artery and widely used in the treatment of arterial stenosis (narrowing of the lumen) (Baer et al., 2007). As metallic stents based on shape-memory alloys (SMAs) are too stiff for complex navigation through tortuous vessels and show a compliance mismatch with the arterial walls, which may lead to an abnormal stress concentration initiating an adaptive response in the vascular tissue, SMP-based stents have been introduced to overcome these challenges. For example, degradable PCL-based polyurethane/ester blends with tunable melting points were prepared and a PU/PCL (70/30) blend with the shape-memory activation temperature of 37 °C was used for molding a vascular stent. The performance of the stent was demonstrated in a femoral vein (*in vitro*) and the material showed excellent biocompatibility, indicated by the *in vitro* adhesion and proliferation of bone marrow mesenchymal stem cells (Ajili et al., 2009). As an example of gastrointestinal stents, a biodegradable SMP stent based on P(CL-*co*-DLLA) with a monomer ratio 10/90 and T_g of 37 °C was developed for the treatment of esophageal stenosis and tested for *in vitro* degradation as well as *in vivo* for the intended application. The rigidity of the stent material increased with degradation leading to a loss of shape memory in 3 weeks at 37 °C. The fast-expanding stent kept its shape well in the esophagus but maintained its position only for 7 days due to the device design, which needs improvement (Yu et al., 2012).

Transparency is a desirable feature in orthodontic applications and the use of PCL-based shape-memory polyurethanes for archwires in realigning the teeth has been demonstrated. A melt-spun polymer wire was stretched and installed in a dental model with metal brackets. Heating above the transition temperature (40 °C) displaced misaligned teeth during a 1 h period; although the shape-recovery force decreased exponentially during the first 2 h, equilibrium was reached after 20 days. The possible biodegradation of the wires was not tested in this study. Constant shape-recovery force on the teeth could be provided over a long period of time (nearly 3 months) in contrast to usual elastomers; hence, SMPs together with their aesthetically appealing appearance have high potential as novel orthodontic materials (Jung and Cho, 2010).

Soft-tissue reconstructions, such as repairing ligament or tendon damages, are commonly based on screw devices. Biodegradable polymers have provided the advantage of initially bearing the mechanical load and upon degradation, gradually transferring the load to the repaired tissue. Although their degradability was not shown, biocompatible SMPs based on methyl methacrylate and PEG dimethacrylate were studied as possible high-strength shape-memory biomaterials for soft-tissue fixation, where the shape-memory function would offer the advantage of easy insertion and subsequent expansion. The fixation force could be tuned by crosslinking density, which would also allow the design of patient-specific devices according to the bone quality of the patient (Yakacki et al., 2008; Yakacki and Gall, 2010).

In principle, tissues could be grown *in vitro* on collapsible SMP scaffolds, delivered into the body by minimally invasive techniques, and implanted to initiate repair or reconstruction of tissues or organs (Small et al., 2007). For example, a PCL-based shape-memory network was cytocompatible on different cell types, supporting cell viability and proliferation (Neuss et al., 2009). In addition, the differentiation of mesenchymal stem cells was supported by the network, and the temperature-induced activation of shape-memory effect did not affect the majority of adherent cells, although caution should be used on high shear forces. The results on mesothelial cells that line the serous cavities and internal organs give promise to materials for abdominal repair or even regeneration diminishing adhesions, while those on mesenchymal stem cells capable of differentiating to osteoblasts or adipocytes suggest applications as a scaffold for bone regeneration or for the production of adipose tissue (Neuss et al., 2009). For example, a stem cell-seeded porous scaffold or matrix based on biodegradable SMPs was proposed as an implant and delivery system for the repair or augmentation of a breast tissue defect in a patient (Quijano et al., 2007).

11.5 Discussion and future perspectives

The field of "smart" materials and SMPs is developing rapidly; the current research focus is on material design and on extending the ranges of applicable stimuli and device technologies. From the viewpoint of biomedical applications, SMPs have several advantages over SMAs, including low density, transparency, low cost, biodegradability, possibility for surface or bulk functionalization or incorporation of active substances, and tailorability of mechanical properties and transition temperatures. There is a constant demand for SMPs that can be actuated by different stimuli than heat—for example, by UV light. The recent advances in the multi-SMPs capable of sequential shape changes, the application of multiple stimuli, and the indirect and remote actuation methods give promise to novel stimulus-responsive materials interesting not only for medical technologies, but also for the textile industry and aircraft and spacecraft applications. The shape-memory effect based on reversible chemical bonding and/or directed interactions such as hydrogen bonding or inclusion complexation also provides unforeseen possibilities in building degradable SMPs and tailoring the material properties.

One of the challenges of polymer-based shape-memory biomaterials is the medical device sterilization process: the currently available methods may alter the chemical and physical characteristics of the SMPs, which may lead to shifting the actuation temperature or hampering the shape-memory effect. Hence, changes in the material properties as well as in the biocompatibility either due to the chemical modifications in the process or the sterilizing agent residues require further testing. Drug-loaded SMPs are a new field of research, and the studies so far have shown that the drugs embedded in the polymer matrix may influence the degradation and drug-release profiles as well as the shape-memory behavior; thus, the processes of drug loading and material shaping need to be established. Even in the absence of drugs, the changes in material performance upon degradation should be taken into consideration. In most applications exploiting the shape memory of biodegradable materials, this property plays an important role at the initial stage of application, for example, in the insertion of a medical device, where the device takes first a temporary shape and then a permanent shape after it is placed in the body. After this, biodegradability becomes the most important feature, where the chemical and physical changes upon degradation are inevitable, but should be known. Additional challenges in biomedical applications of SMPs are brought about by the nanoscale approaches used for remote or indirect actuation, as the issue of nanotoxicology is under growing debate.

Biodegradable SMPs are an important class of stimuli-responsive materials designed for biomedical applications, and research in this field is progressing rapidly. Bio-based strategies give promise to materials with higher biocompatibility, and multifunctionality is a feature in great demand. Despite the regulatory and commercial barriers, the arrival of biodegradable SMP-based medical technologies to market is greatly anticipated, and many interesting innovations are expected in the future.

References

Ajili, S.H., Ebrahimi, N.G., Soleimani, M., 2009. Polyurethane/polycaprolactane blend with shape memory effect as a proposed material for cardiovascular implants. Acta Biomater. 5, 1519–1530.

Arditti, S.J., Avedikian, S.Z., Bernstein, B.S., (Radiation Applications Inc.), 1971. Articles with polymeric memory and method of constructing same. US patent application 3,563,973, February 16.

Azevedo, H.S., Reis, R.L., 2005. Understanding the enzymatic degradation of biodegradable polymers and strategies to control their degradation rate. In: Reis, R.L., San Roman, J. (Eds.), Biodegradable Systems in Tissue Engineering and Regenerative Medicine. CRC Press, Taylor & Francis Group, Boca Raton, FL, pp. 177–201.

Baer, G.M., Small, W., Wilson, T.S., Benett, W.J., Matthews, D.L., Hartman, J., Maitland, D.J., 2007. Fabrication and in vitro deployment of a laser-activated shape memory polymer vascular stent. BioMed. Eng. OnLine 6, 43–51.

Barrett, D.G., Yousaf, M.N., 2009. Design and applications of biodegradable polyester tissue scaffolds based on endogenous monomers found in human metabolism. Molecules 14, 4022–4050.

Barrett, D.G., Yousaf, M.N., 2010. Thermosets synthesized by thermal polyesterification for tissue engineering applications. Soft Matter 6, 5026–5036.

Behl, M., Lendlein, A., 2007a. Shape-memory polymers. Mater. Today 10, 20–28.

Behl, M., Lendlein, A., 2007b. Actively moving polymers. Soft Matter 3, 58–67.

Behl, M., Ridder, U., Feng, Y., Kelch, S., Lendlein, A., 2009. Shape-memory capability of binary multiblock copolymer blends with hard and switching domains provided by different components. Soft Matter 5, 676–684.

Behl, M., Zotzmann, J., Lendlein, A., 2010. Shape-memory polymers and shape-changing polymers. Adv. Polym. Sci. 226, 1–40.

Behl, M., Zotzmann, J., Schroeter, M., Lendlein, A., 2011. Biodegradable shape-memory polymers. In: Lendlein, A., Sisson, A. (Eds.), Handbook of Biodegradable Polymers: Synthesis, Characterization and Applications. Wiley-WCH, Weinheim, Germany, pp. 195–216.

Bettinger, C.J., Borenstein, J.T., Langer, R., 2007. Micro- and nanofabricated scaffolds. In: Lanza, R.P., Langer, R., Vacanti, J. (Eds.), Principles of Tissue Engineering, third ed. Elsevier Academic Press, London, UK, pp. 341–358.

Buckley, P.R., McKinley, G.H., Wilson, T.S., Small, W., Benett, W.J., Bearinger, J.P., McElfresh, M.W., Maitland, D.J., 2006. Inductively heated shape memory polymer for the magnetic actuation of medical devices. IEEE Trans. Biomed. Eng. 53, 2075–2083.

Cai, W., Liu, L., 2007. Shape-memory effect of poly(glycerol-sebacate) elastomer. Mater. Lett. 62, 2171–2173.

Chaunier, L., Lourdin, D., 2009. The shape memory of starch. Starch–Stärke 61, 116–118.

Chen, M.C., Tsai, H.W., Chang, Y., Lai, W.Y., Mi, F.L., Liu, C.T., Wong, H.S., Sung, H.W., 2007. Rapidly self-expandable polymeric stents with a shape-memory property. Biomacromolecules 8, 2774–2780.

Chen, Y., Zhou, S., Li, Q., 2011. Mathematical modeling of degradation for bulk-erosive polymers: applications in tissue engineering scaffolds and drug delivery systems. Acta Biomater. 7, 1140–1149.

Cho, C.G., 2010. Shape memory material. In: Cho, G. (Ed.), Smart Clothing: Technology and Applications. CRC Press, Taylor & Francis Group, Boca Raton, FL, pp. 189–228.

Cho, J.W., Kim, J.W., Jung, Y.C., Goo, N.S., 2005. Electroactive shape-memory polyurethane composites incorporating carbon nanotubes. Macromol. Rapid Commun. 26, 412–416.

Choi, N.Y., Lendlein, A., 2007. Degradable shape-memory polymer networks from oligo [(L-lactide)-*ran*-glycolide]dimethacrylates. Soft Matter 3, 901–909.

Choi, N.Y., Kelch, S., Lendlein, A., 2006. Synthesis, shape-memory functionality and hydrolytical degradation studies on polymer networks from poly(rac-lactide)-b-poly(propylene oxide)-b-poly(rac-lactide) dimethacrylates. Adv. Eng. Mat. 8, 439–445.

Feng, Y., Guo, J., 2009. Biodegradable polydepsipeptides. Int. J. Mol. Sci. 10, 589–615.

Feng, Y., Behl, M., Kelch, S., Lendlein, A., 2009. Biodegradable multiblock copolymers based on oligodepsipeptides with shape-memory properties. Macromol. Biosci. 9, 45–54.

Feng, Y., Lu, J., Behl, M., Lendlein, A., 2010. Progress in depsipeptide-based biomaterials. Macromol. Biosci. 10, 1008–1021.

Feng, Y., Zhang, S., Wang, H., Zhao, H., Lu, J., Guo, J., Behl, M., Lendlein, A., 2011. Biodegradable polyesterurethanes with shape-memory properties for dexamethasone and aspirin controlled release. J. Control. Release 152, e21–e23.

Fini, A., Roda, A., 1987. Chemical properties of bile acids. IV. Acidity constants of glycine-conjugated bile acids. J. Lipid Res. 28, 755–759.

Gan, Z., Liang, Q., Zhang, J., Jing, X., 1997. Enzymatic degradation of poly(ε-caprolactone) film in phosphate buffer containing lipases. Polym. Degr. Stability 56, 209–213.

Gautrot, J.E., Zhu, X.X., 2006a. Biodegradable polymers based on bile acids and potential biomedical applications. J. Biomater. Sci. Polymer Edn. 17, 1123–1139.

Gautrot, J.E., Zhu, X.X., 2006b. Main-chain bile acid based degradable elastomers synthesized by ring-opening metathesis polymerization. Angew. Chem. 118, 7026–7028.

Gautrot, J.E., Zhu, X.X., 2008. High molecular weight bile acid and ricinoleic acid-based copolyesters via entropy-driven ring-opening metathesis polymerisation. Chem. Commun., 1674–1676.

Gautrot, J.E., Zhu, X.X., 2009a. Shape memory polymers based on naturally-occurring bile acids. Macromolecules 42, 7324–7331.

Gautrot, J.E., Zhu, X.X., 2009b. Macrocyclic bile acids: from molecular recognition to degradable biomaterial building blocks. J. Mater. Chem. 19, 5705–5716.

Goraltchouk, A., Lai, J., Herrmann, R.A., (Angiotech Pharmaceuticals Inc.), 2011. Shape-memory self-retaining sutures, methods of manufacture and methods of use. US patent application US 2011/0125188 A1, May 26.

Guo, B., Chen, Y., Lei, Y., Zhang, L., Zhou, W.Y., Rabie, A.B.M., Zhao, J., 2011. Biobased poly(propylene sebacate) as shape memory polymer with tunable switching temperature for potential biomedical applications. Biomacromolecules 12, 1312–1321.

Heuwers, B., Quitmann, D., Katzenberg, F., Tiller, J.C., 2012. Stress-induced melting of crystals in natural rubber: a new way to tailor the transition temperature of shape memory polymers. Macromol. Rapid. Commun. 33 (18), 1517–1522. http://dx.doi.org/10.1002/marc.201200313.

Hoffmann, A.F., 1999. Bile acids: the good, the bad and the ugly. News Physiol. Sci. 14, 24–29.

Huang, W.M., Yang, B., An, L., Li, C., Chan, Y.S., 2005. Water-driven programmable polyurethane shape memory polymer: demonstration and mechanism. Appl. Phys. Lett. 86, 114105-1–114105-3.

Huang, W.M., Song, C.L., Fu, Y.Q., Wang, C.C., Zhao, Y., Purnawali, H., Lu, H.B., Tang, C., Ding, Z., Zhang, J.L., 2012. Shaping tissue with shape memory materials. Adv. Drug Deliv. Rev. 65 (4), 515–535. http://dx.doi.org/10.1016/j.addr.2012.06.004.

Iordanskii, A.L., Rudakova, T.E., Zaikov, G.E., 1994. Interaction of Polymers with Bioactive and Corrosive Media. VSP, Utrecht, Netherlands, p. 196.

Jung, Y.C., Cho, J.W., 2010. Application of shape memory polyurethane in orthodontic. J. Mater. Sci. Mater. Med. 21, 2881–2886.

Jung, Y.C., So, H.H., Cho, J.W., 2006. Water-responsive shape memory polyurethane block copolymer modified with polyhedral oligomeric silsesquioxane. J. Macromol. Sci. Part B: Phys. 45, 453–461.

Kelch, S., Steuer, S., Schmidt, A.M., Lendlein, A., 2007. Shape-memory polymer networks from oligo[(ε-hydroxycaproate)-*co*-glycolate]dimethacrylates and butyl acrylate with adjustable hydrolytic degradation rate. Biomacromolecules 8, 1018–1027.

Knight, P.T., Lee, K.M., Chung, T., Mather, P.T., 2009. PLGA-POSS end-linked networks with tailored degradation and shape memory behavior. Macromolecules 42, 6596–6605.

Koerner, H., Price, G., Pearce, N.A., Alexander, M., Vaia, R.A., 2004. Remotely actuated polymer nanocomposites – stress-recovery of carbon-nanotube-filled thermoplastic elastomers. Nat. Mater. 3, 115–120.

Kulkarni, A., Reiche, J., Kratz, K., Kamusewitz, H., Sokolov, I.M., Lendlein, A., 2007. Enzymatic chain scission kinetics of poly(ε-caprolactone) monolayers. Langmuir 23, 12202–12207.

Kulkarni, A., Reiche, J., Hartmann, J., Kratz, K., Lendlein, A., 2008. Selective enzymatic degradation of poly(ε-caprolactone) containing multiblock copolymers. Eur. J. Pharm. Biopharm. 68, 46–56.

Kumar, M.N.V., Muzzarelli, R.A.A., Muzzarelli, C., Sashiwa, H., Domb, A.J., 2004. Chitosan chemistry and pharmaceutical perspectives. Chem. Rev. 104, 6017–6084.

Lee, K.M., Knight, P.T., Chung, T., Mather, P.T., 2008. Polycaprolactone-POSS chemical/physical double networks. Macromolecules 41, 4730–4738.

Lendlein, A., Kelch, A., 2002. Shape-memory polymers. Angew. Chem. Int. Ed. 41, 2034–2057.

Lendlein, A., Langer, R., 2002. Biodegradable, elastic shape-memory polymers for potential biomedical applications. Science 296, 1673–1676.

Lendlein, A., Jiang, H., Jünger, O., Langer, R., 2005a. Light-induced shape-memory polymers. Nature 434, 879–882.

Lendlein, A., Schmidt, A.M., Schroeter, M., Langer, R., 2005b. Shape-memory polymer networks from oligo(ε-caprolactone)dimethacrylates. J. Polym. Sci. Part A: Polym. Chem. 43, 1369–1381.

Lendlein, A., Behl, M., Hiebl, B., Wischke, C., 2010. Shape-memory polymers as a technology platform for biomedical applications. Expert Rev. Med. Devices 7, 357–379.

Li, J., Lewis, C.L., Chen, D.L., Anthamatten, M., 2011. Dynamic mechanical behavior of photo-cross-linked shape-memory elastomers. Macromolecules 44, 5336–5343.

Li, G., Fei, G., Xia, H., Han, J., Zhao, Y., 2012. Spatial and temporal control of shape memory polymers and simultaneous drug release using high intensity focused ultrasound. J. Mater. Chem. 22, 7692–7696.

Liu, Y., Leng, J., 2010. Applications of shape-memory polymers in aerospace. In: Leng, J., Du, S. (Eds.), Shape-Memory Polymers and Multifunctional Composites. CRC Press, Taylor & Francis Group, Boca Raton, FL, pp. 234–266.

Liu, P., Long, Y., Wang, X., Li, D., Chen, L., Li, X., 2010. Glass transition temperatures of starches with different amylose/amylopectin ratios. J. Cereal Sci. 51, 388–391.

Losken, H.W., Tschakaloff, A., Vonoepen, R., Mooney, M.P., Moritz, O., Michaeli, W., Lalikos, J., Losken, A., 1994. Memory of DL-polylactic acid biodegradable plates. Ann. Plast. Surg. 32, 606–611.

Lourdin, D., Coignard, L., Bizot, H., Colonna, P., 1997. Influence of equilibrium relative humidity and plasticizer concentration on the water content and glass transition of starch materials. Polymer 38, 5401–5406.

Lowe, J.R., Tolman, W.B., Hillmyer, M.A., 2009. Oxidized dihydrocarvone as a renewable multifunctional monomers for the synthesis of shape memory polyesters. Biomacromolecules 10, 2003–2008.

Lu, X.L., Sun, Z.J., Cai, W., Gao, Z.Y., 2008. Study on the shape memory effects of poly (L-lactide-co-ε-caprolactone) biodegradable polymers. J. Mater. Sci. Mater. Med. 19, 395–399.

Luo, H., Liu, Y., Yu, Z., Zhang, S., Li, B., 2008. Novel biodegradable shape memory material based on partial inclusion complex formation between α-cyclodextrin and poly(ε-caprolactone). Biomacromolecules 9, 2573–2577.

Luo, H., Meng, X., Cheng, C., Dong, Z., Zhang, S., Li, B., 2010. Enzymatic degradation of supramolecular materials based on partial inclusion complex formation between α-cyclodextrin and poly(ε-caprolactone). J. Phys. Chem. B 114, 4739–4745.

Lyu, S.P., Untereker, D., 2009. Degradability of polymers for implantable biomedical devices. Int. J. Mol. Sci. 10, 4033–4065.

Maitland, D.J., Metzger, M.F., Schumann, D., Lee, A., Wilson, T.S., 2002. Photothermal properties of shape memory polymer micro-actuators for treating stroke. Lasers Surg. Med. 30, 1–11.

Marin, J.J.G., 2009. Bile acids: chemistry, physiology, and pathophysiology. World J. Gastroenterol. 15, 804–816.

Martina, M., Hutmacher, D.W., 2007. Biodegradable polymers applied in tissue engineering research: a review. Polym. Int. 56, 145–157.

Migneco, F., Huang, Y.C., Birla, R.K., Hollister, S.J., 2009. Poly(glycerol-dodecanoate), a biodegradable polyester for medical devices and tissue engineering scaffolds. Biomaterials 30, 6479–6484.

Mitrus, M., Wojtowicz, A., Moscicki, L., 2009. Biodegradable polymers and their practical utility. In: Janssen, L., Moscicki, L. (Eds.), Thermoplastic Starch: A Green Material for Various Industries. Wiley-WCH, Weinheim, Germany, pp. 1–33.

Mohr, R., Kratz, K., Weigel, T., Lucka-Gabor, M., Moneke, M., Lendlein, A., 2006. Initiation of shape-memory effect by inductive heating of magnetic nanoparticles in thermoplastic polymers. Proc. Natl. Acad. Sci. U. S. A. 103, 3540–3545.

Mukhopadhyay, S., Maitra, U., 2004. Chemistry and biology of bile acids. Curr. Sci. 87, 1666–1683.

Nagahama, K., Ueda, Y., Ouchi, T., Ohya, Y., 2009. Biodegradable shape-memory polymers exhibiting sharp thermal transitions and controlled drug release. Biomacromolecules 10, 1789–1794.

Neffe, A.T., Hanh, B.D., Steuer, S., Lendlein, A., 2009. Polymer networks combining controlled drug release, biodegradation, and shape memory capability. Adv. Mater. 21, 3394–3398.

Neuss, S., Blomenkamp, I., Stainforth, R., Boltersdorf, D., Jansen, M., Butz, N., Perez-Bouza, A., Knüchel, R., 2009. The use of a shape-memory poly(e-caprolactone)dimethacrylate network as a tissue engineering scaffold. Biomaterials 30, 1697–1705.

Pretsch, T., Jakob, I., Müller, W., 2009. Hydrolytic degradation and functional stability of a segmented shape memory poly(ester urethane). Polym. Degrad. Stab. 94, 61–73.

Quijano, R.C., Nguyen, T.T., Williams, K.J., Tu, H., Carter, R.L., 2007. Breast augmentation system. US patent application US 2007/0104693 A1, May, 10.

Rainer, W.C., Barrington, R.I., Redding, E.M., Hitov, J.J., Sloan, A.W., Stewart, W.D. (W.R. Grace & Co), 1964. Polyethylene product and process. US patent application 3,144,398, August 11.

Ratner, B.D., Hoffmann, A.S., Schoen, F.J., Lemons, J.E., 2004. Biomaterials science: a multidisciplinary endeavor. In: Ratner, B.D., Hoffmann, A.S., Schoen, F.J., Lemons, J.E. (Eds.), Biomaterials Science: An Introduction to Materials in Medicine. second ed. Elsevier Academic Press, London, UK, pp. 1–9.

Rodriguez-Galan, A., Franco, L., Puiggali, J., 2011. Degradable poly(ester amide)s for biomedical applications. Polymers 3, 65–99.

Sabir, M.I., Xu, X., Li, L., 2009. A review on biodegradable polymeric materials for bone tissue engineering applications. J. Mater. Sci. 44, 5713–5724.

Safranski, D.L., Gall, K., 2008. Effect of chemical structure and crosslinking density on the thermo-mechanical properties and toughness of (meth)acrylate shape memory polymer networks. Polymer 8, 4446–4455.

Serrano, M.C., Carbajal, L., Ameer, G.A., 2011. Novel biodegradable shape-memory elastomers with drug-releasing capabilities. Adv. Mater. 23, 2211–2215.

Shao, Y., Lavigueur, C., Zhu, X.X., 2012. Multishape memory effect of norbornene-based copolymers with cholic acid pendant groups. Macromolecules 45, 1924–1930.

Silva, G.A., Marques, A.P., Gomes, M.E., Coutinho, O.P., Reis, R.L., 2005. Cytotoxicity screening of biodegradable polymeric systems. In: Reis, R.L., San Roman, J. (Eds.), Biodegradable Systems in Tissue Engineering and Regenerative Medicine. CRC Press, Taylor & Francis Group, Boca Raton, FL, pp. 339–353.

Small, W., Singhal, P., Wilson, T.S., Maitland, D.J., 2007. Biomedical applications of thermally activated shape memory polymers. J. Mater. Chem. 20, 3356–3366.

Strandman, S., Gautrot, J.E., Zhu, X.X., 2011. Recent advances in entropy-driven ring-opening polymerizations. Polym. Chem. 2, 791–799.

Sun, L., Huang, W.M., Ding, Z., Zhao, Y., Wang, C.C., Purnawali, H., Tang, C., 2012. Stimulus-responsive shape memory materials: a review. Mater. Design 33, 577–640.

Sung, J. (Tyco Healthcare Group LP), 2009. Access port using shape memory anchor. US patent application US 2009/0105691 A1, April 23.

Tamminen, J., Kolehmainen, E., 2001. Bile acids as building blocks for supramolecular hosts. Molecules 6, 21–46.

Thérien-Aubin, H., Gautrot, J.E., Shao, Y., Zhu, X.X., 2010. Shape memory properties of main chain bile acids polymers. Polymer 51, 22–25.

Tschan, M.J.-L., Brulé, E., Haquette, P., Thomas, C.M., 2012. Synthesis of biodegradable polymers from renewable resources. Polym. Chem. 3, 836–851.

Tsuji, H., 2005. Poly(lactide) stereocomplexes: formation, structure, properties, degradation, and applications. Macromol. Biosci. 5, 569–597.

Ulery, B.D., Nair, L.S., Laurencin, C.T., 2011. Biomedical applications of biodegradable polymers. J. Polym. Sci. Part B: Polym. Phys. 49, 832–864.

Véchambre, C., Chaunier, L., Lourdin, D., 2010a. Novel shape-memory materials based on potato starch. Macromol. Mater. Eng. 295, 115–122.

Véchambre, C., Buléon, A., Chaunier, L., Jamme, F., Lourdin, D., 2010b. Macromolecular orientation in glassy starch materials that exhibit shape memory behavior. Macromolecules 43, 9854–9858.

Véchambre, C., Buléon, A., Chaunier, L., Gauthier, C., Lourdin, D., 2011. Understanding the mechanisms involved in shape memory starch: macromolecular orientation, stress recovery and molecular mobility. Macromolecules 44, 9384–9389.

Venkatraman, S.S., Tan, L.P., Joso, J.F.D., Boey, Y.C.F., Wang, X., 2006. Biodegradable stents with elastic memory. Biomaterials 27, 1573–1576.

von Burkersroda, F., Schedl, L., Göpferich, A., 2002. Why degradable polymers undergo surface erosion or bulk erosion. Biomaterials 23, 4221–4231.

Wagermaier, W., Kratz, K., Heuchel, M., Lendlein, A., 2010. Characterization methods for shape-memory polymers. Adv. Polym. Sci. 226, 97–145.

Wang, R., Xie, T., 2010. Shape memory- and hydrogen bonding-based strong reversible adhesive system. Langmuir 26, 2999–3002.

Wang, Y., Ameer, G.A., Sheppard, B.J., Langer, R., 2002. A tough biodegradable elastomer. Nat. Biotechnol. 20, 602–606.

Wang, W., Ping, P., Chen, X., Jing, X., 2007. Biodegradable polyurethane based on random copolymer of L-lactide and ε-caprolactone and its shape-memory property. J. Appl. Polym. Sci. 104, 4182.

Wang, Y., Huang, M., Luo, Y., Li, Y., 2010. In vitro degradation of poly(lactide-co-p-dioxanone)-based shape memory poly(urethane-urea). Polym. Degrad. Stab. 95, 549–556.

Wischke, C., Neffe, A.T., Steuer, S., Lendlein, A., 2009. Evaluation of a degradable shape-memory polymer network as matrix for controlled drug release. J. Control. Release 138, 243–250.
Wischke, C., Neffe, A.T., Lendlein, A., 2010. Controlled drug release from biodegradable shape-memory polymers. Adv. Polym. Sci. 226, 177–205.
Wong, Y.S., Xiong, Y., Venkatraman, S.S., Boey, F.Y.C., 2007. Shape memory in un-cross-linked biodegradable polymers. J. Biomater. Sci. Polymer Edn. 19, 175–191.
Wu, L., Jin, C., Sun, X., 2011. Synthesis, properties, and light-induced shape memory effect of multiblock polyesterurethanes containing biodegradable segments and pendant cinnamamide groups. Biomacromolecules 12, 235–241.
Xie, T., 2010. Tunable polymer multi-shape memory effect. Nature 464, 267–270.
Xu, S., Zhang, M., 2007. Synthesis and characterization of a novel polyurethane elastomer based on CO_2 copolymer. J. Appl. Polym. Sci. 104, 3818–3826.
Xue, Z., Mayer, M.F., 2009. Entropy-driven ring-opening olefin metathesis polymerizations of macrocycles. Soft Matter 5, 4600–4611.
Xue, L., Dai, S., Li, Z., 2009. Synthesis and characterization of three-arm poly(ε-caprolactone)-based poly(ester-urethanes) with shape-memory effect at body temperature. Macromolecules 42, 964–972.
Yakacki, C.M., Gall, K., 2010. Shape-memory polymers for biomedical applications. Adv. Polym. Sci. 226, 147–175.
Yakacki, C.M., Shandas, R., Lanning, C., Rech, B., Eckstein, A., Gall, K., 2007. Unconstrained recovery characterization of shape-memory polymer networks for cardiovascular applications. Biomaterials 28, 2255–2263.
Yakacki, C.M., Shandas, R., Safranski, D., Ortega, A.M., Sassaman, K., Gall, K., 2008. Strong, tailored, biocompatible shape-memory polymer networks. Adv. Funct. Mater. 18, 2428–2435.
Yakacki, C.M., Nguyen, T.D., Likos, R., Lamell, R., Guigou, D., Gall, K., 2011. Impact of shape-memory programming on mechanically-driven recovery in polymers. Polymer 52, 4947–4954.
Yang, K.J., Wang, X.L., Wang, Y.Z., 2002. Poly(p-dioxanone) and its copolymers. J. Macromol. Sci. Part C: Polym. Rev. C42, 373–398.
Yang, B., Huang, W.M., Li, C., Lee, C.M., Li, L., 2004. On the effects of moisture in a polyurethane shape memory polymer. Smart Mater. Struct. 13, 191–195.
Yang, B., Huang, W.M., Li, C., Li, L., 2006. Effects of moisture on the thermomechanical properties of a polyurethane shape memory polymer. Polymer 47, 1348–1356.
Yu, X., Wang, L., Huang, M., Gong, T., Li, W., Cao, Y., Ji, D., Wang, P., Wang, J., Zhou, S., 2012. A shape memory stent of poly(ε-caprolactone-co-DL-lactide) copolymer for potential treatment of esophageal stenosis. J. Mater. Sci. Mater. Med. 23, 581–589.
Zhang, J.W., Zhu, X.X., 2009. Biomaterials made of bile acids. Sci. China Ser. B: Chem. 52, 849–861.
Zhao, Y., 2007. Facial amphiphiles in molecular recognition: from unusual aggregates to solvophobically driven foldamers. Curr. Opin. Colloid Interface Sci. 12, 92–97.
Zhu, X.X., Nichifor, 2002. Polymeric materials containing bile acids. Acc. Chem. Res. 35, 539–546.
Zini, E., Scandola, M., Dobrzynski, P., Kasperczyk, J., Bero, M., 2007. Shape memory behavior of novel (L-lactide-glycolide-trimethylene carbonate) terpolymers. Biomacromolecules 8, 3661–3667.

Part Three

Biomedical applications of shape-memory polymers

Shape-memory polymers for vascular and coronary devices

12

R. Rath, M.K. Gupta, S.W. Crowder, H.-J. Sung
Vanderbilt University, Nashville, TN, USA

12.1 Introduction: Key principles

Shape-memory polymers (SMPs) undergo reversible changes from a *temporary* to a *permanent shape* in response to a defined external stimulus (Pretsch, 2010). SMPs are classified by both the type of stimulus that triggers this change (i.e., temperature, ion concentration, pH, etc.) (Aguilar et al., 2007) and the exact point of stimuli parameter at which the shape change occurs (i.e., transition temperature, etc.) (Lendlein and Langer, 2002). Because of their ability to rapidly and automatically respond to changes in the environment, SMPs are considered to be "smart" materials. Their shape-memory (SM) functions can be fine-tuned by altering the material properties (Zhang et al., 2012). Although SMPs have been applied to a variety of applications, this chapter focuses on the potential of thermo-responsive SMPs in developing vascular and coronary devices.

12.2 Background

Thermo-responsive SMPs are a class of SMPs that use temperature to trigger a shape change. They are of particular interest in developing vascular devices because of their self-expanding properties (Schmidt et al., 2010). By programming a SMP with a small, collapsed *temporary shape* that expands to a larger *permanent shape*, the physical dimensions of the device can be minimized to allow for less invasive surgical procedures (Schmidt et al., 2010). This in turn reduces the chance for potential damage to the blood vessel, thereby preventing restenosis (re-narrowing of the blood vessel).

Additionally, because each thermo-responsive SMP has a transition temperature that can be finely tuned, only a modest change in temperature is needed to trigger the shape change. The example of shape change includes self-assembly of free-floating polymers into micelles for controlled drug delivery and reversible gelation of *in situ* forming polymer scaffolds for vascular grafts (Liu et al., 2009). While other types of SMPs that respond to pathological parameters (e.g., pH and redox status) often exploit theoretical shape changes due to unpredictable variations in the physiological environment, thermo-responsive SMPs can undergo a reliable change from a *temporary* to a *permanent* shape by a programmed response to a change in

Shape Memory Polymers for Biomedical Applications. http://dx.doi.org/10.1016/B978-0-85709-698-2.00012-X

temperature, for example, from 25 to 37 °C. This *transition temperature* (T_s) can be defined as a critical solution temperature (lower or upper) at which thermo-responsive polymers undergo a change in their phase behavior (phase change from one phase to two phases or *vice versa*) (Ward and Georgiou, 2011).

In general, the classification of thermo-responsive SMPs falls into one of two categories: (1) lower critical solution temperature (LCST) SMPs, or (2) upper critical solution temperature (UCST) SMPs. A LCST SMP is delivered to the body at a temperature *below* T_s and heated *above* the LCST to make its recovery to a permanent shape. A UCST SMP is delivered at a temperature *above* T_s and cooled *below* the UCT to assume its permanent shape. For endovascular applications, LCST SMPs are more common, because T_s can be tailored such that, as stated before, a switch from room temperature (25 °C) to physiological temperature (37 °C) activates the shape-change behavior, thereby facilitating the pre-implantation process at room temperature (Ping et al., 2005; Aguilar et al., 2007).

12.3 Applications

12.3.1 Stents

The major types of thermo-responsive SMPs currently used to develop vascular and coronary devices are composite metal alloy/polymer materials. Their main application area includes endovascular stents and clot removal devices. Stents have been employed for several decades as a means to open occluded blood vessels caused by lesion formation (Dotter, 1969). As Dotter explained, the major function of a stent is operated by a principle of forced "shape expansion." Traditionally, this shape expansion is accomplished via the inflation of a saline-filled balloon that is placed inside a collapsed metal stent that is delivered to the body by an endovascular catheter (Figure 12.1). However, this method is invasive and inherently risky, with common complications such as arterial damage and restenosis (Rogers et al., 1999). SM metals alloys and SMPs reduce these risks significantly due to their innate ability to automatically expand, removing the need to introduce an additional device for shape expansion.

The best-known metal alloy for SM stent applications is Nitinol (Machado and Savi, 2003). Nitinol, a nickel/titanium alloy, has excellent biocompatibility relative to other metal alloy stents. Being composed of titanium, the most biocompatible metal, the alloy is able to withstand corrosion by body fluids, stay inert in the human body, and be compatible with cell growth (Shabalovskaya, 1996; Putters et al., 1992). Additionally, even though nickel has been shown to have some degree of cytotoxicity to mammalian cells, nickel can decrease thrombogenicity (causing coagulation of blood and forming a thrombus or clot) by forming an oxide layer on the surface of the implant (Ryhänen et al., 1997).

Furthermore, the super-elastic properties of Nitinol allow for full recovery to an original shape in response to a small deforming force that causes up to an 8% change in size and shape (Dotter et al., 1983). Most natural elastic materials require up to 10%

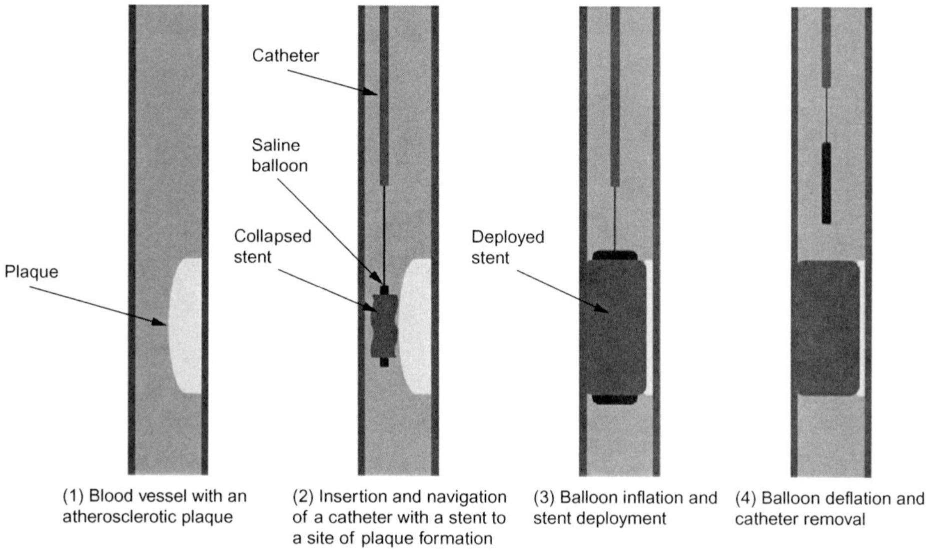

Figure 12.1 Shape transition of balloon angioplasty during deployment procedure.

deformation strain and elongate/compress in a nonlinear way (Fontaine et al., 1993). Unlike other elastic materials, Nitinol enables elongation and compression linearly proportional to the applied force (Duerig et al., 1999). As shown in Figure 12.2, biological materials require the unique range of stress–strain hysteresis. In particular, the changed ranges of stress and strain in bone are covered by the area of Nitinol. This property match was found to improve physiological similarity, thereby promoting bone in-growth and proper healing. Nitinol exhibits this super-elastic property because its crystalline structure changes as a result of stress-induced phase transformation (Duerig et al., 2000). As described by Duerig, when a stress is applied to Nitinol, after a slight elastic deformation, the material yields to the applied stress and changes its crystalline structure and stores the mechanical energy as potential energy in its new bonds. By storing the energy, Nitinol is able to linearly deform without causing any permanent deformation. Once the stress is removed, the stored energy in the bonds is released, and the material returns to its original shape.

The SM function of Nitinol is operated by a similar mechanism to stress-induced phase transformation but via a completely separate process known as thermal phase transformation (Stoeckel et al., 2004; Duerig et al., 1999). Described by Stoeckel and Duerig, when Nitinol is cooled below its T_s, its crystalline structure is changed accordingly. Unlike the stress-induced phase change, this thermal change in crystalline structure does not require any external force. Even though no force is applied, a change in temperature still induces phase transformation in its crystalline structure. Once the material is cooled, mechanical force can then be applied to generate a temporary shape. The material retains this temporary deformed shape until it is reheated; it returns to its original, pre-cooled shape upon reheating.

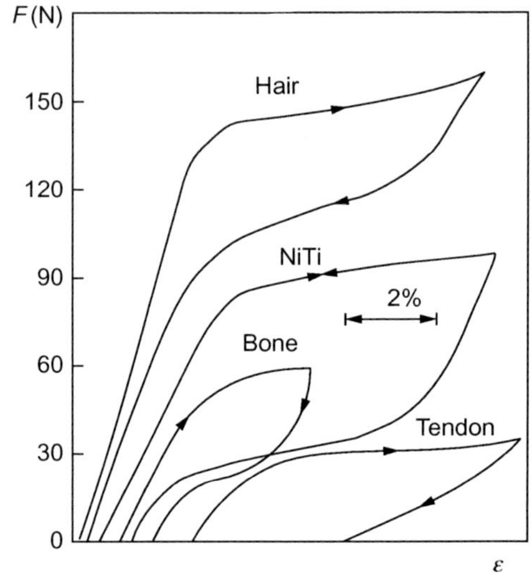

Figure 12.2 Hysteresis diagrams for living tissues and NiTi alloy. Each of hair, tendon, and bone exhibits a unique stress–strain profile. Strain accumulated as a result of applied stress is partially recovered after the stress is released. Bone exhibits 2% recoverable strain as well as hysteresis in the loading–unloading cycle. NiTi exhibits super-elastic behavior with 9–10% recoverable strain (Shabalovskaya, 1996).
Figure modified from Duerig et al. (1999).

Due to its unique self-expansion and programmable shape-transition properties, Nitinol is considered as an excellent stent material and has shown significant improvement in the treatment of narrowed blood vessels (Schillinger et al., 2006). In spite of these advantages, Nitinol still has issues associated with immune rejection and inflammation (Hara et al., 2006). As described by Hara, in order to reduce the various host responses to bare metal stents, drug-eluting composite stents have been developed as a platform for local drug delivery. Several designs over the past decade, including Johnson & Johnson's Cypher and Medtronic's Endeavor (Roiron et al., 2006), have already proven to be more effective than bare metal and metal alloy stents. Through drug embedding with biodegradable polymer coatings, both Johnson & Johnson's Cypher and Medtronic's Endeavor stents release drugs to inhibit the proliferation of vascular smooth muscle cells, thereby limiting subsequent neointimal hyperplasia (or thickening of the blood vessel) and consequent restenosis (Maeng et al., 2012). The biodegradable polymer coating additionally helps the stent material reduce immune rejection and inflammation (Maeng et al., 2012).

Despite better performance in clinical trials compared to bare metal stents, these drug-eluting stents still exhibit long-term side effects, such as impaired healing and late thrombosis following drug release (Joner et al., 2006; Waksman and Pakala, 2010). Because of these drawbacks, there has been recent renewed interest in fully biodegradable polymeric stents. Because of an ability to enable burst or sustained release of drugs to a target site (Ramcharitar and Serruys, 2008; Garg and Serruys, 2009) and complete removal of stent materials from the body, a variety of biodegradable polymers have been investigated for stent design, including polyesters, polycarbonates, and bacteria-derived polymers (Waksman and Pakala, 2010). Unlike metals, polymeric stents can be functionalized with bioactive molecules on the material surface and/or engineered to tightly control drug-release kinetics through modification of polymer composition, molecular weight, and/or surface area (e.g., pore generation) (Liechty et al., 2010; Qiu and Bae, 2006).

12.3.1.1 Thermoplastic polyurethane

The first polymeric thermo-responsive SMP stent was developed in 2003 by Wache et al. and was made up of a thermoplastic polyurethane that underwent shape transition at body temperature (Wache et al., 2003). Wache et al. demonstrated that this polyurethane SMP stent had several advantages over Nitinol and other bare metal stents, including large drug-loading capability and low cost. The group further emphasized the mechanical properties of polyurethane stent, which enable size expansion by more than 200% axially and more than 100% in diameter relative to the original dimensions (Figure 12.3). Further investigation into this material revealed additional advantages of easy fabrication into different shapes and dimensions by injection molding, extrusion, and immersion (Baer et al., 2007b).

12.3.1.2 Neurovascular stent for aneurysm therapy

In 2002, Maitland et al. used a thermoplastic SMP stent to treat stroke, cerebrovascular aneurysms, and abnormal arterial widening (Maitland et al., 2002). A loss of blood supply to the brain accounts for approximately 87% of the 795,000 reported cases of stroke (Members et al., 2012). Currently, one of the two approved therapies for an acute ischemic stroke is intravenous treatment of recombinant tissue plasminogen activator (tPa) (Pierre Gobin et al., 2004). Because tPa is a protein involved in dissolving blood clots and is delivered systemically (not locally), there is a risk of severe internal and intracranial bleeding (Xian et al., 2012). Furthermore, tPa must be delivered within 3–4.5 h upon bleeding to have any noticeable effects on the initial stroke incident (Wardlaw et al., 2012). Therefore, an alternative solution to treat ischemic

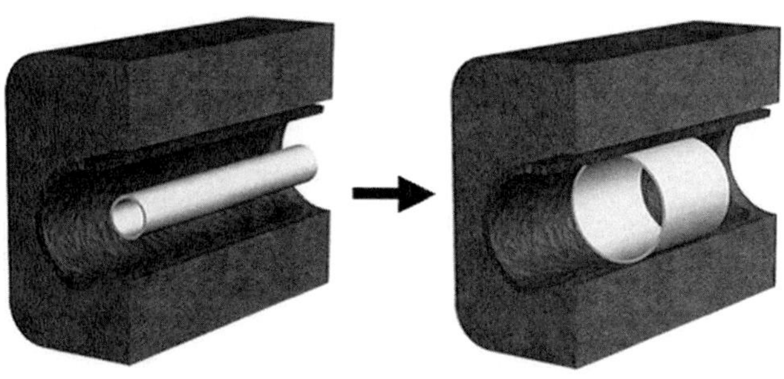

Figure 12.3 Principle of the SM effect: prior to stimulation (left) and after reset (right) (Wache et al., 2003).

stroke would be to use a stent that can deliver a drug locally at any point after an artery is clotted. Unlike other endovascular stents, neurovascular stents must be more flexible due to the increased complexity of vessel networks in the brain. The size of neurovascular stents must also be smaller than those of other endovascular stents, due to the diameter of the neurovasculature. Moreover, stent expansion to an exact size is required for neurovascular deployment. In order to meet this need, the Maitland group used a laser to selectively heat the local area and activate a SMP function instead of relying on body temperature, which may result in premature activation of the neurovascular stent (Maitland et al., 2002). The thermo-responsive polymeric stent was able to expand up to 2.7 times its size with only 1% axial shortening (Figure 12.4). This material was also shown to withstand collapses above an average pressure in the brain due to robust mechanical properties. Some challenges that still remain to be overcome include addressing issues with wide-necking of the stent (4 mm or dome-to-neck ratio <2). Also fusiform aneurysms can be formed with undefined dome-to-neck ratios, making it difficult to ensure that the deployed stent will remain safely within the aneurysm sac and not obstruct blood flow to neighboring vasculature (Higashida et al., 2005).

12.3.2 Clot removal

Besides the use of tPa, another method that is clinically approved to remove clots is embolectomy (the mechanical removal of embolus using a corkscrew-like catheter system) (Pierre Gobin et al., 2004) (Figure 12.5). This mechanical system is composed of a tapered wire with five helical loops of descending diameter. To perform embolectomy, an interventional radiologist threads a wire into a microcatheter, causing the helical wire to straighten out. Using a separate balloon-guided catheter, the radiologist then inserts the device into the clotted artery. Guided by angiography (a medical imaging technique to visualize the inside of blood vessels), the radiologist feeds the retriever into the carotid artery until it reaches the clot. The radiologist inserts the microcatheter with the wire until it reaches the clot and pushes the wire out, resulting in a shape change of the wire to the corkscrew shape. The radiologist then ensnares the embolus, capturing it in the net-like mesh. Once the clot is captured, the radiologist

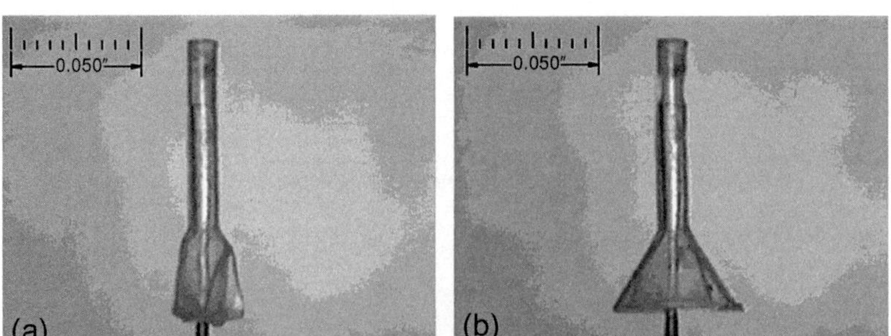

Figure 12.4 Operational demonstration of the umbrella microactuator (a) before and (b) after its shape transition for deployment (Maitland et al., 2002; Metzger et al., 2002).

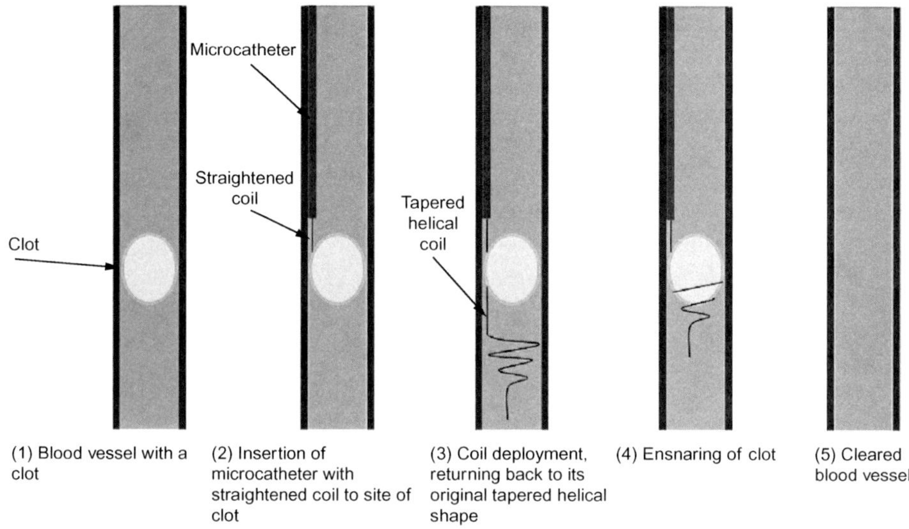

Figure 12.5 Procedure of mechanical removal of embolus.

inflates the balloon near the femoral artery, temporarily stopping blood flow while the clot is pulled through the catheter. As soon as the clot has been completely removed from the artery, the balloon is deflated and normal blood flow is returned to neighboring vessels. Because the device has a fixed shape, the clot can be essentially trapped in a net and carefully removed from the hosting artery. This method requires multiple catheters and has an inherent risk of failing to fully entangle the clot due to early formation of the corkscrew-like shape before the capture of clot. If this situation happens, the leftover clot can be dislodged and gets stuck further downstream. To address these issues, Dr. Jonathan Hartman at the University of California-Davis School of Medicine developed a microactuator composed of a thermosetting polyurethane shell cast around a Nitinol (Hartman et al., 2007). In this design, the microactuator is attached to copper lead wires that are capable of delivering current. At physiological temperature, the thermosetting polyurethane shell assumes a brittle, glassy state, forcing the Nitinol to straighten and enabling the user to locally place the device to a site of clot. Once positioned distal to the occlusion, the user then applies a current to the copper wires, heating both the polyurethane shell and the Nitinol wire. Acting as an UCST SMP, the polyurethane shell undergoes property transition into a low modulus rubbery state, allowing the Nitinol to return to its pre-programmed corkscrew-like shape. The clot that is trapped within the coiled wire can be drawn into the sheath of the delivery catheter and safely removed from the body.

Challenges with the mechanical removal of clots are similar to those described for neurovascular stents. Concerns about not properly ensnaring a clot can result in the clot traveling downstream and blocking a neighboring vessel. The mechanical removal of embolus is also dependent on the user's (surgeon) skill and experience with the device.

12.4 Tailoring the shape-memory properties

Due to the complex nature of vasculature, designing SMPs for vascular applications has specific constraints that must be considered through the stepwise characterization of material properties. In recent years, various polymer designs have been approached to tailor SM functions by modification of cross-linking density, monomer type, and/or co-monomer ratio (Yakacki et al., 2010). These modifications are intended to tune T_s, to widen a T_s range and to achieve multiple points of T_s (Messori et al., 2013).

In 2007, Yakacki et al. tailored the thermo-mechanical cycle of vascular SMP stents by varying the contents and molecular weight of bifunctional dimethacrylate cross-linking monomers poly(ethylene glycol) dimethacrylate (PEGDMA) and di (ethylene glycol) dimethacrylate (DEGDMA) (Yakacki et al., 2007). In particular, the storage, deployment, and subsequent deformation characteristics of SMP stents that are associated with glass transition temperature, cross-linking density, and mechanical design were investigated. In this study, six sets of polymer networks were prepared with 10, 20, and 40 wt% cross-links with two glass transition temperatures (T_g: 52 and 55 °C) and evaluated their recovery rates. Among the six tested stent materials, the material with 40 wt% cross-links and 52 °C T_g showed the fastest rate of recovery (Figure 12.6a). To test the recovery rate at different temperatures, the 10 wt% cross-linked material with 52 °C T_g was deformed at either room or body temperature and allowed for shape changes. The material deformed from a permanent to temporary shape faster at 25 °C (below body temperature) (Figure 12.6b) but recovered from a temporary shape back to permanent shape faster at 42.5 °C (above body temperature) (Figure 12.6c). The results indicate that tuning T_g by altering the polymer design plays a key role in controlling the shape recovery rate within the physiological range of temperature.

In another study, the same group investigated step-by-step alternations in thermomechanics and SM responses of polymer networks for cardiovascular applications (Yakacki et al., 2008). In their study, copolymers of methyl methacrylate (MMA) and PEGDMA were used to create networks with varying T_g and modulus; and the effect of polymer network structure on shape recovery was studied (Figure 12.7). Based on the amount and molecular weight of the PEGDMA cross-linkers, the group was able to alter the polymer's T_g and modulus. The group found that free-strain recovery (recovery without strain) was highly dependent on the T_g of the networks but was negligibly influenced by the cross-link density. On the other hand, fixed-strain recovery (generating stress against its external constraints) was highly dependent on the cross-link density but was negligibly influenced by T_g.

Hu et al. investigated a dependency between SM properties and thermo-mechanical cycling conditions in polyurethane (Hu et al., 2005). The group demonstrated that strain-recovery ratios increased as the deformation speed increased or the maximum strain decreased. When the polyurethane was deformed at a high temperature and rapidly cooled below its T_g into a frozen state (T_g −20), the shape recovery ratio increased, compared to when slowly cooled.

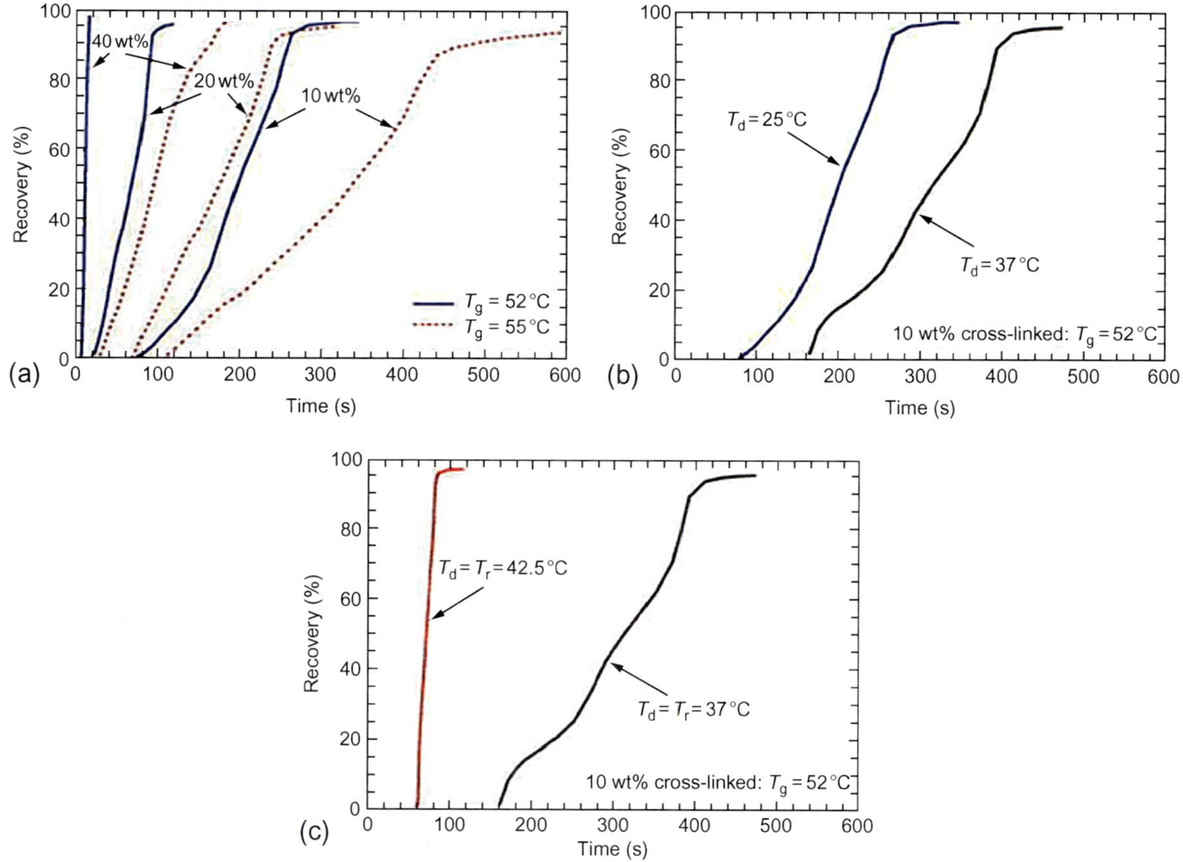

Figure 12.6 Performance assessment of polymer stents. (a) Recovery of stent shape with various cross-linking densities (10, 20, and 40 wt%) and T_g of 52 or 55 °C when deformed at room temperature and recovered at body temperature; (b) room temperature recovery of stent shape with 10 wt% cross-linking and 52 °C T_g, when deformed either at room or body temperature; (c) recovery of stent shape with 10 wt% cross-linking and 52 °C T_g, when deformed and recovered at either 37 and 42 °C, respectively (Yakacki et al., 2008).

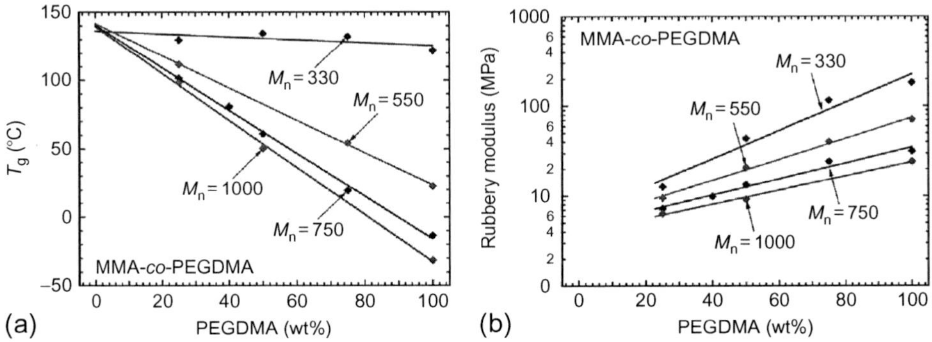

Figure 12.7 Tailoring SM properties. (a) T_g and (b) rubbery modulus. These properties were altered by varying wt% and molecular weight PEGDMA in MMA-*co*-PEGDMA polymers (Yakacki et al., 2008).

In similar studies, T_s of polyurethanes was tuned to body temperature by incorporation of oligomeric biodegradable polyester diols of poly(ε-caprolactone) (PCL) (Ping et al., 2005) and polylactic acid (PLA) (Wang et al., 2006). Wang et al. prepared a series of segmented polyurethanes with PLA soft-segments and HDI–BDO (hexane diisocyanate/butanediol) hard segments. In their study, they observed that T_s could be adjusted to near body temperature by altering the molecular weight of the PLA diol and the ratio of the hard-to-soft segments (Wang et al., 2006). In a similar way, Ping et al. were able to control T_s (37–42 °C) by preparing a series of segmented PCL polyurethanes by altering the molecular weight and content of PCL-diol (Ping et al., 2005).

12.5 Interface considerations

As with other biomaterials, biomedical applications of SMPs require a substantial degree of biocompatibility, including maintenance of cell viability and immune tolerance. In a physiological environment, degradation products from biodegradable SMPs should be either bioresorbable (digested by cells) or easily cleared from the host. Degrading SMPs should maintain their bulk mechanical properties despite being weakened. Specific to vascular biomaterials, blood protein aggregation and dysfunctional cell activation must be minimized to prevent restenosis and keep the vessel lumen clear of obstructions. It is essential that suitable stent materials and surfaces take these physico-chemical properties into design consideration to prevent stent rejection (Karagkiozaki et al., 2012). Disregarding these issues may trigger activation of platelets and blood coagulation pathways, leading to immune rejection, including inflammation, clot formation on the stent surface, and arterial occlusion. Additionally, the ideal vascular biomaterial should encourage healthy phenotypes for vascular cells with which the material interacts. For example, Crowder et al. demonstrated that a block copolymer composed of PEG and PCL could influence the phenotype and oxidative status of the primary human smooth muscle and endothelial cells with which it interacted (Crowder et al., 2012), suggesting that this material could be used as a potential stent coating.

12.6 Strengths and limitations

In recent years, SMPs have been used to overcome shortcomings associated with the use of shape-memory alloys (SMAs) for vascular applications (Sokolowski et al., 2007). The SM effect of vascular devices can be tailored by altering polymer structure and/or polymer morphology with advanced processing and programming technologies (Lendlein et al., 2010). Considering the nature of polymeric materials, SMPs have certain strengths and limitations (Table 12.1) that can be exploited or that will need to be addressed for future applications.

A major strength of SMPs is their capacity to recover a wide range of strains resulting from large mechanical deformation upon a small change in temperature (Gall et al., 2005). This special property allows SMP devices to be assembled to a temporary shape with a size much smaller than the size of permanent shape so that the temporary shape enables device delivery via small catheters, which has been challenging when SMAs are used. The delivery via small catheters offers a less-invasive deployment of SMP devices. After being inserted into a patient, the SMP devices can undergo shape recovery upon stimuli, such as an increase in temperature supplied either by the body or an external device (Baer et al., 2009).

Moreover, SMP devices can be prepared using simple standard techniques such as extrusion, molding, and conventional or computer numerical control (CNC) machining (Liu et al., 2007). The biodegradability, lower mass, low cost, and biocompatibility of these materials provide an extra advantage over SMAs (Table 12.1). Similarly, the thermo-mechanical cycle of SMP vascular devices can be optimized to work in physiological conditions, as modulus, viscoelastic properties, and damping coefficient can be altered accordingly (Messori et al., 2013). These properties can be modified to enable continuous size expansion as the vessel diameter increases, thereby allowing the device to grow with the patient. This property is especially useful for pediatric applications (Mather et al., 2009). These devices may be utilized for delivery of

Table 12.1 Major strengths and limitations of using SMP devices for vascular applications

S.N.	Strengths	Limitations
1.	Tunable thermo-chemical properties	Short life time
2.	Good recovery strain	Fatigue susceptibility
3.	Easy processing	Low recovery force
4.	Cheap and lightweight	Poor electrical conductivity
5.	Biodegradable, biocompatible, and non-toxic	Poor mechanical properties

significant quantities of anti-thrombogenic, anti-inflammatory, or other drugs packaged within the device for sustained release over longer periods of time (Baer et al., 2007a).

Although SMPs provide tremendous advantages over other SM materials for use in constrained environments (Rousseau, 2008), several tasks still remain in SMP development, including (i) to improve recovery force, stiffness, and strength; (ii) to accelerate recovery time; and (iii) to improve the efficiency of triggering SM functions (Rousseau, 2008). It is difficult for SMPs to provide the same radial force and recoil structure that SMAs can provide. The bulkiness inherited from general polymeric properties could limit applications for small vessels (Gall et al., 2005). The biodegradability of polymers also generates additional challenges in long-term performance, as SMPs loses their mechanical integrities over time. The packaging, storage, and shipping of the devices along with proper activation of SM functions are also issues to address (Yakacki et al., 2010). Overall, despite the limitations, significant progress has made in SMP development as the next generation of materials for vascular and coronary applications (Serrano and Ameer, 2012).

12.7 Future trends

The future of smart polymers lies in advancing current materials or developing new SMP materials with new or more efficient activation mechanisms. This concept can be exemplified by the dialysis needle proposed by Ortega et al. (2007). The proposed needle was made of thermoset SM polyurethane that, unlike the aforementioned thermoset stents, could undergo reversible transition at body temperature. This polyurethane needle was used to connect an artery and a vein to allow rapid blood flow for hemodialysis by adapting the shape of an arteriovenous graft or a synthetic graft inserted into a patient's arm. In this way, the needle could minimize hemodynamic stress or internal forces acting within blood. The deploying device had a tube-like shape with a distal end larger than the needle diameter. Upon exposure to body temperature, the SMP needle expanded and generated a funnel whose maximum radius was equal to the radius of the deploying tube. Following dialysis, the SMP needle could be retracted through the delivery tube, thereby reducing abnormal shear stress related to a change in blood flow. However, the paper demonstrated only a proof of concept model using computer simulation of the results. Due to the multifaceted stimuli needed for activation of the SM needle function, such a material is not currently available. In order to fulfill the SM function, the needle should undergo shape transition at body temperature, adapt to flow in the tube while maintaining mechanical integrity, and, once the dialysis treatment is complete, fold safely back into the catheter from which it was delivered.

The smart function of SMPs to recover a programmed shape on controlled external stimulation has motivated polymer scientists to design various types of SMPs with different properties (Yakacki et al., 2010). Even though outstanding progress has been made to apply SMPs for various vascular applications, such as vascular stents

(Baer et al., 2007a), clot removal (Metzger et al., 2002; Maitland et al., 2002), and embolic aneurysm treatment (Koebbe et al., 2006), the field is still far from mature and requires more efforts to develop advanced SMPs that can make accurate shape recovery at an upper or a lower transition temperature. Moreover, the SMP design needs to be specified for a defined application; and the storage and maintenance of SMPs should be carefully considered depending on T_s (above or below the body temperature) (Lendlein and Langer, 2002).

Regardless of SMP type, a potential risk resulting from localized cell damage at the target of deployment should be considered (Metzger et al., 2002). Another important issue in current SMP research is a lack of adequate understanding about the structure–function relationships between polymer type and SM function (Gall et al., 2005). Thermo-mechanical properties related to shape storage and recovery of SMPs with lower transition temperature versus upper transition temperature should be thoroughly characterized and understood. Mechanical modeling of accurate time-dependent and finite-strain SM phenomena could help predict the balanced biodegradability and long-term storage stability of vascular and coronary SMP devices (Mather et al., 2009).

The current development of vascular SMPs with tunable properties is promising. However, continuous progress should be made by employing new activation mechanisms, such as pH (Han et al., 2012), temperature, specific enzymes (Stuart et al., 2010), or ROS (Sung et al., 2005; Yu et al., 2011). The next generation of SMPs should enable accurate, robust shape recovery with a controlled rate at desired T_s in a target site of the body.

12.8 Sources of further information

1. Lendlein, A. (2010) Shape-Memory Polymers, Springer.
2. Otsuka, K., Wayman, C. M. (1999) Shape Memory Materials, Cambridge University Press.
3. Xu, J., Song, J. (2011) Thermal Responsive Shape Memory Polymers for Biomedical Applications, Biomedical Engineering—Frontiers and Challenges, Reza Fazel-Rezai (Ed.), ISBN: 978-953-307-309-5, InTech.
4. Huang, W. M., Yang, B., Fu, Y. Q. (2011) Polyurethane Shape Memory Polymers, Taylor & Francis.
5. Leng, J. (2009) Shape-Memory Polymers and Multifunctional Composites, Taylor & Francis.

References

Aguilar, M.R., Elvira, C., Gallardo, A., Vázquez, B., Román, J.S., 2007. Smart polymers and their applications as biomaterials. In: Ashammakhi, N., Reis, R., Chiellini, E. (Eds.), Topics in Tissue Engineering, CiteSeer.

Baer, G., Small, W., Wilson, T., Benett, W., Matthews, D., Hartman, J., Maitland, D., 2007a. Fabrication and in vitro deployment of a laser-activated shape memory polymer vascular stent. Biomed. Eng. Online 6, 43.

Baer, G., Wilson, T.S., Matthews, D.L., Maitland, D.J., 2007b. Shape-memory behavior of thermally stimulated polyurethane for medical applications. J. Appl. Polym. Sci. 103, 3882–3892.

Baer, G.M., Wilson, T.S., Small, W., Hartman, J., Benett, W.J., Matthews, D.L., Maitland, D.J., 2009. Thermomechanical properties, collapse pressure, and expansion of shape memory polymer neurovascular stent prototypes. J. Biomed. Mater. Res. B Appl. Biomater. 90B, 421–429.

Crowder, S.W., Gupta, M.K., Hofmeister, L.H., Zachman, A.L., Sung, H.J., 2012. Modular polymer design to regulate phenotype and oxidative response of human coronary artery cells for potential stent coating applications. Acta Biomater. 8 (2), 559–569.

Dotter, C.T., 1969. Transluminally-placed coilspring endarterial tube grafts: long-term patency in canine popliteal artery. Investig. Radiol. 4, 329–332.

Dotter, C.T., Buschmann, R.W., Mckinney, M.K., Rösch, J., 1983. Transluminal expandable nitinol coil stent grafting: preliminary report. Radiology 147, 259–260.

Duerig, T., Pelton, A., Stöckel, D., 1999. An overview of nitinol medical applications. Mater. Sci. Eng. A 273–275, 149–160.

Duerig, T.W., Tolomeo, D.E., Wholey, M., 2000. An overview of superelastic stent design. Minim. Invasive Ther. Allied Technol. 9, 235–246.

Fontaine, A.B., Dake, M.D., Tschang, T.-P., Guertin, S., Stabbe, M.T., Dos Passos, S., 1993. Tantalum balloon-expandable stent: in vivo swine studies. J. Vasc. Interv. Radiol. 4, 749–752.

Gall, K., Yakacki, C.M., Liu, Y., Shandas, R., Willett, N., Anseth, K.S., 2005. Thermomechanics of the shape memory effect in polymers for biomedical applications. J. Biomed. Mater. Res. A 73A, 339–348.

Garg, S., Serruys, P., 2009. Biodegradable stents and non-biodegradable stents. Minerva Cardioangiol. 57, 537–565.

Han, X.-J., Dong, Z.-Q., Fan, M.-M., Liu, Y., Li, J.-H., Wang, Y.-F., Yuan, Q.-J., Li, B.-J., Zhang, S., 2012. pH-induced shape-memory polymers. Macromol. Rapid Commun. 33, 1055–1060.

Hara, H., Nakamura, M., Palmaz, J.C., Schwartz, R.S., 2006. Role of stent design and coatings on restenosis and thrombosis. Adv. Drug Deliv. Rev. 58, 377–386.

Hartman, J., Small, W., Wilson, T.S., Brock, J., Buckley, P.R., Benett, W.J., Loge, J.M., Maitland, D.J., 2007. Embolectomy in a rabbit acute arterial occlusion model using a novel electromechanical extraction device. Am. J. Neuroradiol. 28, 872–874.

Higashida, R.T., Halbach, V.V., Dowd, C.F., Juravsky, L., Meagher, S., 2005. Initial clinical experience with a new self-expanding nitinol stent for the treatment of intracranial cerebral aneurysms: the Cordis Enterprise stent. Am. J. Neuroradiol. 26, 1751–1756.

Hu, J.L., Ji, F.L., Wong, Y.W., 2005. Dependency of the shape memory properties of a polyurethane upon thermomechanical cyclic conditions. Polym. Int. 54, 600–605.

Joner, M., Finn, A.V., Farb, A., Mont, E.K., Kolodgie, F.D., Ladich, E., Kutys, R., Skorija, K., Gold, H.K., Virmani, R., 2006. Pathology of drug-eluting stents in humans: delayed healing and late thrombotic risk. J. Am. Coll. Cardiol. 48, 193–202.

Karagkiozaki, V., Karagiannidis, P.G., Kalfagiannis, N., Kavatzikidou, P., Patsalas, P., Georgiou, D., Logothetidis, S., 2012. Novel nanostructured biomaterials: implications for coronary stent thrombosis. Int. J. Nanomedicine 7, 6063–6076.

Koebbe, C.J., Veznedaroglu, E., Jabbour, P., Rosenwasser, R.H., 2006. Endovascular management of intracranial aneurysms: current experience and future advances. Neurosurgery 59 (5 Suppl. 3), S93–S102. http://dx.doi.org/10.1227/01.NEU.0000237512.10529.58.

Lendlein, A., Langer, R., 2002. Biodegradable, elastic shape-memory polymers for potential biomedical applications. Science 296, 1673–1676.

Lendlein, A.B.M., Hiebl, B., Wischke, C., 2010. Shape-memory polymers as a technology platform for biomedical applications. Expert Rev. Med. Devices 7, 357–379.

Liechty, W.B., Kryscio, D.R., Slaughter, B.V., Peppas, N.A., 2010. Polymers for drug delivery systems. Annu. Rev. Chem. Biomol. Eng. 1, 149–173.

Liu, C., Qin, H., Mather, P.T., 2007. Review of progress in shape-memory polymers. J. Mater. Chem. 17, 1543–1558.

Liu, R., Fraylich, M., Saunders, B., 2009. Thermoresponsive copolymers: from fundamental studies to applications. Colloid Polym. Sci. 287, 627–643.

Machado, L.G., Savi, M.A., 2003. Medical applications of shape memory alloys. Braz. J. Med. Biol. Res. 36, 683–691.

Maeng, M., Tilsted, H.-H., Jensen, L.O., Kaltoft, A., Kelbæk, H., Abildgaard, U., Villadsen, A. B., Krusell, L.R., Ravkilde, J., Hansen, K.N., Christiansen, E.H., Aarøe, J., Jensen, J.S., Kristensen, S.D., Bøtker, H.E., Madsen, M., Thayssen, P., Sørensen, H.T., Thuesen, L., Lassen, J.F., 2012. 3-Year clinical outcomes in the randomized SORT OUT III superiority trial comparing zotarolimus- and sirolimus-eluting coronary stents. J. Am. Coll. Cardiol. Intv. 5, 812–818.

Maitland, D.J., Metzger, M.F., Schumann, D., Lee, A., Wilson, T.S., 2002. Photothermal properties of shape memory polymer micro-actuators for treating stroke. Lasers Surg. Med. 30, 1–11.

Mather, P., Luo, X., Rousseau, I., 2009. Shape memory polymer research. Annu. Rev. Mater. Res. 39, 445–471.

Members, W.G., Roger, V.L., Go, A.S., Lloyd-Jones, D.M., Benjamin, E.J., Berry, J.D., Borden, W.B., Bravata, D.M., Dai, S., Ford, E.S., Fox, C.S., Fullerton, H.J., Gillespie, C., Hailpern, S.M., Heit, J.A., Howard, V.J., Kissela, B.M., Kittner, S.J., Lackland, D.T., Lichtman, J.H., Lisabeth, L.D., Makuc, D.M., Marcus, G.M., Marelli, A., Matchar, D.B., Moy, C.S., Mozaffarian, D., Mussolino, M.E., Nichol, G., Paynter, N.P., Soliman, E.Z., Sorlie, P.D., Sotoodehnia, N., Turan, T.N., Virani, S.S., Wong, N.D., Woo, D., Turner, M.B., 2012. Heart disease and stroke statistics—2012 update. Circulation 125, e2–e220.

Messori, M., Degli Esposti, M., Paderni, K., Pandini, S., Passera, S., Riccò, T., Toselli, M., 2013. Chemical and thermomechanical tailoring of the shape memory effect in poly(ε-caprolactone)-based systems. J. Mater. Sci. 48 (1), 424–440. http://link.springer.com/article/10.1007%2Fs10853-012-6757-8.

Metzger, M.F., Wilson, T.S., Schumann, D., Matthews, D.L., Maitland, D.J., 2002. Mechanical properties of mechanical actuator for treating ischemic stroke. Biomed. Microdevices 4, 89–96.

Ortega, J.M., Small, W., Wilson, T.S., Benett, W.J., Loge, J.M., Maitland, D.J., 2007. A shape memory polymer dialysis needle adapter for the reduction of hemodynamic stress within arteriovenous grafts. IEEE Trans. Biomed. Eng. 54, 1722–1724.

Pierre Gobin, Y., Starkman, S., Duckwiler, G.R., Grobelny, T., Kidwell, C.S., Jahan, R., Pile-Spellman, J., Segal, A., Vinuela, F., Saver, J.L., 2004. MERCI 1. Stroke 35, 2848–2854.

Ping, P., Wang, W., Chen, X., Jing, X., 2005. Poly(ε-caprolactone) polyurethane and its shape-memory property. Biomacromolecules 6, 587–592.

Pretsch, T., 2010. Review on the functional determinants and durability of shape memory polymers. Polymers 2, 120–158.

Putters, J.L.M., Kaulesar Sukul, D.M.K.S., De Zeeuw, G.R., Bijma, A., Besselink, P.A., 1992. Comparative cell culture effects of shape memory metal (Nitinol®), nickel and titanium: a biocompatibility estimation. Eur. Surg. Res. 24, 378–382.

Qiu, L., Bae, Y., 2006. Polymer architecture and drug delivery. Pharm. Res. 23, 1–30.

Ramcharitar, S., Serruys, P.W., 2008. Fully biodegradable coronary stents: progress to date. Am. J. Cardiovasc. Drugs 8, 305–314.

Rogers, C., Tseng, D.Y., Squire, J.C., Edelman, E.R., 1999. Balloon-artery interactions during stent placement—a finite element analysis approach to pressure, compliance, and stent design as contributors to vascular injury. Circ. Res. 84, 378–383.

Roiron, C., Sanchez, P., Bouzamondo, A., Lechat, P., Montalescot, G., 2006. Drug eluting stents: an updated meta-analysis of randomised controlled trials. Heart 92, 641–649.

Rousseau, I.A., 2008. Challenges of shape memory polymers: a review of the progress toward overcoming SMP's limitations. Polym. Eng. Sci. 48, 2075–2089.

Ryhänen, J., Niemi, E., Serlo, W., Niemelä, E., Sandvik, P., Pernu, H., Salo, T., 1997. Biocompatibility of nickel-titanium shape memory metal and its corrosion behavior in human cell cultures. J. Biomed. Mater. Res. 35, 451–457.

Schillinger, M., Sabeti, S., Loewe, C., Dick, P., Amighi, J., Mlekusch, W., Schlager, O., Cejna, M., Lammer, J., Minar, E., 2006. Balloon angioplasty versus implantation of nitinol stents in the superficial femoral artery. N. Engl. J. Med. 354, 1879–1888.

Schmidt, D., Dijkman, P.E., Driessen-Mol, A., Stenger, R., Mariani, C., Puolakka, A., Rissanen, M., Deichmann, T., Odermatt, B., Weber, B., Emmert, M.Y., Zund, G., Baaijens, F.P.T., Hoerstrup, S.P., 2010. Minimally-invasive implantation of living tissue engineered heart valves: a comprehensive approach from autologous vascular cells to stem cells. J. Am. Coll. Cardiol. 56, 510–520.

Serrano, M.C., Ameer, G.A., 2012. Recent insights into the biomedical applications of shape-memory polymers. Macromol. Biosci. 12 (9), 1156–1171.

Shabalovskaya, S.A., 1996. On the nature of the biocompatibility and on medical applications of NiTi shape memory and superelastic alloys. Biomed. Mater. Eng. 6, 267–289.

Sokolowski, W., Metcalfe, A., Hayashi, S., Yahia, L., Raymond, J., 2007. Medical applications of shape memory polymers. Biomed. Mater. 2, S23–S27.

Stoeckel, D., Pelton, A., Duerig, T., 2004. Self-expanding nitinol stents: material and design considerations. Eur. Radiol. 14, 292–301.

Stuart, M.A.C., Huck, W.T.S., Genzer, J., Muller, M., Ober, C., Stamm, M., Sukhorukov, G.B., Szleifer, I., Tsukruk, V.V., Urban, M., Winnik, F., Zauscher, S., Luzinov, I., Minko, S., 2010. Emerging applications of stimuli-responsive polymer materials. Nat. Mater. 9, 101–113.

Sung, H.-J., Eskin, S., Sakurai, Y., Yee, A., Kataoka, N., Mcintire, L., 2005. Oxidative stress produced with cell migration increases synthetic phenotype of vascular smooth muscle cells. Ann. Biomed. Eng. 33, 1546–1554.

Wache, H.M., Tartakowska, D.J., Hentrich, A., Wagner, M.H., 2003. Development of a polymer stent with shape memory effect as a drug delivery system. J. Mater. Sci. Mater. Med. 14, 109–112.

Waksman, R., Pakala, R., 2010. Biodegradable and bioabsorbable stents. Curr. Pharm. Des. 16, 4041–4051.

Wang, W., Ping, P., Chen, X., Jing, X., 2006. Polylactide-based polyurethane and its shape-memory behavior. Eur. Polym. J. 42, 1240–1249.

Ward, M.A., Georgiou, T.K., 2011. Thermoresponsive polymers for biomedical applications. Polymers 3, 1215–1242.

Wardlaw, J.M., Murray, V., Berge, E., Del Zoppo, G., Sandercock, P., Lindley, R.L., Cohen, G., 2012. Recombinant tissue plasminogen activator for acute ischaemic stroke: an updated systematic review and meta-analysis. Lancet 379, 2364–2372.

Xian, Y., Liang, L., Smith, E.E., et al., 2012. RIsks of intracranial hemorrhage among patients with acute ischemic stroke receiving warfarin and treated with intravenous tissue plasminogen activator. JAMA 307, 2600–2608.
Yakacki, C.M., Shandas, R., Lanning, C., Rech, B., Eckstein, A., Gall, K., 2007. Unconstrained recovery characterization of shape-memory polymer networks for cardiovascular applications. Biomaterials 28, 2255–2263.
Yakacki, C.M., Shandas, R., Safranski, D., Ortega, A.M., Sassaman, K., Gall, K., 2008. Strong, tailored, biocompatible shape-memory polymer networks. Adv. Funct. Mater. 18, 2428–2435.
Yakacki, C., Gall, K., Lendlein, A., 2010. Shape-memory polymers for biomedical applications. In: Shape-Memory Polymers. Springer, Berlin/Heidelberg.
Yu, S.S., Koblin, R.L., Zachman, A.L., Perrien, D.S., Hofmeister, L.H., Giorgio, T.D., Sung, H.-J., 2011. Physiologically relevant oxidative degradation of oligo(proline) cross-linked polymeric scaffolds. Biomacromolecules 12, 4357–4366.
Zhang, Q., Song, S., Feng, J., Wu, P., 2012. A new strategy to prepare polymer composites with versatile shape memory properties. J. Mater. Chem. 22, 24776–24782.

Shape-memory polymers for dental applications

13

R.O. do Nascimento, N. Chirani
École Polytechnique, Montréal, QC, Canada

13.1 Introduction

Dental treatments are the most common intervention performed by human beings. The range of treatment types varies from aesthetic interventions and plaque removal to teeth reconstruction and implants. Dental materials vary according to their application and most recently, to their biocompatibility (Wataha, 2012).

Dental materials can be generated by different sources and include metal alloys, ceramic and cement materials, and polymer-associated substances, among others. The region of application, purpose of use, biocompatibility, degradation ratios, resistance, and aesthetic applications are factors in determining which materials will be selected for dental applications. In this respect, this chapter will present a general overview of the materials used in dental applications; it will focus on shape-memory polymers (SMPs), describing their important physical and chemical properties, interface interactions, strengths, and limitations. We will also describe the new generation of SMP composites and nanocomposites.

13.2 Dental materials

Polymers, ceramic materials, cement materials, and metal alloys are examples of dental materials in use nowadays. The selection of such materials depends on the region, the intended application, and the cost for the patient.

13.2.1 Metal alloys—amalgam

Amalgam is a metal alloy that has been used most often until today for total restoration and fillings: compared with other materials, it has considerable durability and successful application even in difficult operative circumstances (Hørsted-Bindslev and Arenholt-Bindslev, 2009). On the other hand, the amalgam presents undesirable effects generated by the diffusion of mercury, copper, zinc, or silver. The corrosion of these metals, mercury in particular, presents toxic effects for the organism. The release of these compounds could be increased by intensive brushing, mastication, and saliva (Hørsted-Bindslev and Arenholt-Bindslev, 2009). In this respect, Okabe

Shape Memory Polymers for Biomedical Applications. http://dx.doi.org/10.1016/B978-0-85709-698-2.00013-1

et al. (2003) related a study describing amalgam degradation by mercury dissolution in liquids such as artificial saliva, static conditions, and different pH from neutral to acid. Indeed, it was observed that the dissolution of the mercury decreases exponentially with time. However, in samples with high-copper amalgam, the release of mercury was higher at pH = 1.0 than at deionized water. These results suggest that the chronic concentration of mercury at the body, from an amalgam source, can be influenced by the pH of the patient's mouth. In this respect, Pizzichini et al. (2002) studied the correlation between the mercury release from the dental amalgam and the total antioxidant activity of saliva. Indeed, the release of significant amounts of mercury in the saliva could represent a source of oxidative damage for the tissues of the mouth. According to Pizzichini et al. (2002), the small increase of salivary Hg level is enough to produce significant decreases in salivary antioxidant capacity, which could mean less resistance to further oxidative injury.

The risk for dentists who manipulate the amalgam is also considerable. Cooley et al. (1985) reported the risks of contamination by the manipulation and sterilization of amalgam-contaminated materials. Contamination through the generation of Hg vapor occurs when the materials are heated during the sterilization process.

The Minamata Convention (Mackey et al., 2014) on Mercury is a new global health and environment treaty that has as its objective to monitor, quantify, and minimize the impacts of contamination of health and the environment by products that contain mercury, including the amalgam. In this respect, the convention focuses on the wide application of amalgam as a dental filling material and its potential risks to human health and damage to the environment through the emission of Hg and improper waste-water management. Indeed, it has identified several sources of contamination by Hg. However, there is no recommendation or rules to be followed to decrease the Hg release and accumulation for humans or the environment at this point.

To avoid the problems related with the release or aspiration of mercury during the preparation of amalgam, new amalgams have been developed, replacing mercury with gallium, indium, and tin (Hørsted-Bindslev and Arenholt-Bindslev, 2009). Today, several formulations of Hg-free amalgam are available, such as mixtures of 50–60% Ag, 25–28% Sn, 11–15% Cu, 2–9% Pd, and, eventually 0.3% Zn and 0.05% Pt; 62–65% Ga, 19–25% In, 13–16% Sn, and 0.05% Bi. However, these new alloys have a greater tendency for cracks and crevices. New materials such as polymers, resins, and mercury-free amalgam to replace the traditional amalgam are now in the market.

13.2.2 Cements and ceramics materials

With some exceptions, cements and ceramics are essentially inorganic, nonmetallic, and hydrophilic materials. Cements are powder–liquid systems that are obtained by chelate or salt formation. To achieve the desired form, they should be fired, cast, or pressed under heat (Stanley and Schmalz, 2009).

The composition of some cements present polyacrylic acid or eugenol as a liquid phase, and zinc oxide or silicon dioxide as a powder phase. Additionally, calcium hydroxide is also considered to be a cement. Furthermore, calcium phosphates are a new generation of solid-phase cements and are considered osteoinductive and osteoconductive; however, they have limited application because of their poor mechanical properties and washing-out effects. The principal cements are silicate cements, zinc phosphate cements, silicophosphate cements, polycarboxylate cements, glass ionomer cement (GIC), and zinc oxide and eugenol cement (Stanley and Schmalz, 2009).

Silicate cements are common filling materials; however, they are associated with pulp damage when applied without a cavity base. Nevertheless, this type of damage has been also associated with bacteria, which proliferate in cement surfaces.

Silicophosphate cements are a combination of silicate and zinc phosphate cement. They have been used as a filling material and for indirect restoration material as an alternative to amalgam.

Polycarboxylate cements have good pulp compatibility; however, they may cause pain after their application. In this respect, the zinc phosphate cements do not present this type of reaction and are less toxic to cells than the silicophosphate cements.

GICs can be used as a filling material for cavity bases and root canal fillings, among others. GICs are also doped with some metals, such as silver, which could minimize the proliferation of bacteria on the surface of the cement. Indeed, a huge number of composites have been developed using the combination of cements, metals ions, and resin-based materials. These composites could present better adhesion properties and mechanical resistance and aim to decrease the release of their components that may cause damage for the patient. Indeed, for the development of new composites of GICs, new substances such as cellulose have been added. In this regard, Silva et al. (2013) studied the influence of cellulose fibers on the physical and chemical properties of GICs. Furthermore, the influence of different concentrations of cellulose fibers improved the water absorption capacity of the composite with similar solubility in water, as a traditional matrix of GICs. The samples doped with eucalyptus cellulosic fibers also presented higher compressive strength, resistance to abrasion, and bond strength when compared with the GIC matrix.

New generations of GICs made with polymers have been developed. In this regard, Howard et al. (2014) developed new star-shaped polyacid dental GICs. The synthesis of these composites of GICs was used as a chain-transfer radical polymerization technique. The prepared samples presented low viscosity and better mechanical strength compared with similar cements with linear chain, even after aging tests.

The cements can be used to seal a space or cement two or more components together in crowns and bridges and as filling materials. Indeed, the two most important properties of cements in the retention of fixed restorations are their solubility and mechanical properties. The high solubility of the cement in water or liquid solutions with the same characteristics of saliva can induce the release and degradation of the cement. In these cases, there may be a loss of the cement needed and the generation of plaque-retention sites. The release of the components from the cement could create a growth of bacteria. Moreover, the released materials could cause allergies or inflammations (Forss et al., 1991) such as pulp reactions (Costa et al., 2003) (Figure 13.1).

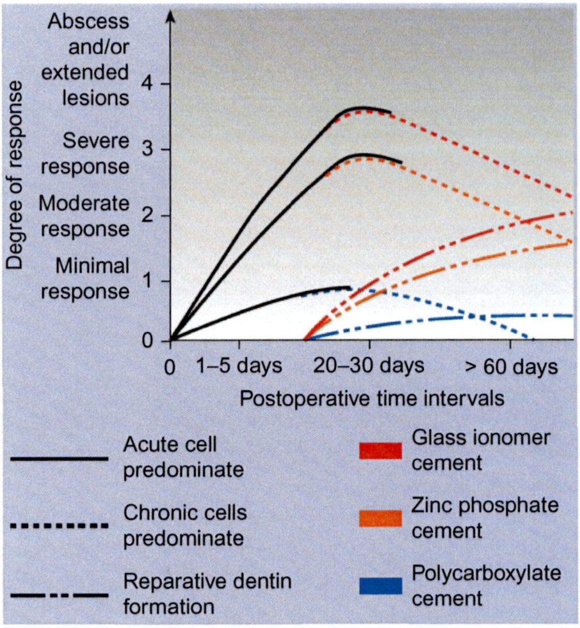

Figure 13.1 Types of pulp reactions from cement materials per time of exposition; data has been collected from the literature without statistical significance. The GICs presented stronger reaction than zinc phosphate and polycarboxylate cements (Stanley, 1996).

13.2.3 Resin-based materials

Resin-based materials are a mixture of polymers, monomers, initiators, and filler particles. These particles could consist of silica or barium-glasses, among others. Resin-based materials have as a principle the application of light to initiate the curing process, which means the polymerization begins by the bonding of the monomers in linear chains or with presence of cross-linked chains. Resin-based materials are used in filling materials, bonding of brackets, orthodontic bands, filling canals, and temporary bridges, among others (Schmalz, 2009). Despite their high biocompatibility, resin-based materials could present adverse reactions by the presence of residual monomers or nonbiocompatible products of degradation. Resins can be divided into groups of components such as filler particles, matrix resins and catalyst materials, and coupling agents. The filler particles normally consist of ground boron silicate, quartz, lithium-aluminum silicate glasses, or silicon dioxide. Indeed, the size of these particles varies from some microns until nanometers. The physical–chemical properties of resin-based materials are dependent on the size and distribution of the filler particles.

The matrix resin is a mixture of monomers. In fact, monomers of triethyleneglykol dimethacrylate, urethane dimethacrylate, and bisphenol a-diglycidyl dimethacrylate, among others, are the main compounds used in the matrix resin.

The coupling agents mainly consist of "silanes" (compounds with Si–OH as the principal functional group). These agents are responsible for the bonding of the components of matrix resin and filler particles. The resin materials could also be divided according to their application. Indeed, in the dental area, resin materials are classified as adhesives, luting resin-based composites, fissure sealants, auxiliary substances, and light-curing units. The polymerization of resin materials is more frequently initiated by light through the opening of the double bonds of the methacrylate residues of the monomers. The conversion rate is determined by the number of double bonds opened during the process. This number can vary from 35% to 75% of the total double bonds present. Because of this fact, some patients present adverse reactions from resin-based materials. In fact, their application in special patients, such as children, requires attention. According to Donly and García-Godoy (2002), the resin-based materials are the main components of pediatric restorative dentistry today. The most common infections in children are caries, which are the main application of resin-based materials in those patients. The authors described the application of those materials as hypoallergenic and advise complete isolation of the tooth; otherwise, the region can be contaminated by saliva. In the same regard, the limitation of the application of these materials consists also of the patient's history; the presence of multiple caries may be associated with the demineralization of the tooth.

The degradation of resin-based materials could appear after the initial polymerization. In this case, the production of degradation products from resin-based materials could last as long as the service life of the material (Bakopoulou et al., 2009).

13.2.4 Nanomaterials for dental applications

Nanomaterials or nanocomposites are those that present at least one type of nanoparticle in their composition. Indeed, some dental materials have been developed with nanocellulose (NC), silver nanoparticles (AgNPs), and gold nanoparticles (AuNPs), among others. Those nanoparticles could bring about improvements in the mechanical properties (Choi et al., 2013) of dental materials, antibacterial activity (Beyth et al., 2014), sustained release (Hook et al., 2014), and osteo-integration (Chien et al., 2013). Although dental materials present a huge diversity, improvement is imperative because of the increase in cases of multiresistant bacteria strains (MRSs). Indeed, bacteria are able to generate biofilms (Besinis et al., 2014), a mechanism of survival that is responsible for furthering the infections' reach. In fact, caries are the biofilm-dependent oral disease most responsible for tooth destruction caused by the acid attack of bacteria (Fejerskov and Kidd, 2008). Although caries are caused by microorganisms such as *Streptococcus mutans*, *Streptococcus sobrinus*, and *Lactobacillus spp.*, they are also a result of an imbalance between mineral ions and dental plaque (demineralization and remineralization processes). Therefore, a way to prevent the formation of caries is to control bacteria and biofilm. According to Melo et al. (2008), nanomaterials such as AgNPs and zinc nanoparticles (ZiNPs) could be applied to the prevention of caries. In fact, those nanoparticles could prevent the biofilm damage caused by the intracellular mechanisms of bacteria. Indeed, AgNPs are applied in implant coating (Cheng et al., 2013), wound dressing (Fan et al., 2014), cosmetic products (Keller et al., 2014), and antimicrobial fabrics (Busila et al., 2014), among others. However, their mechanism of action against bacteria is not well known. The antibacterial effects of AgNPs may be related to the synergistic effect between the free-Ag ions and AgNPs, which have small size and high surface area to interact with the cell

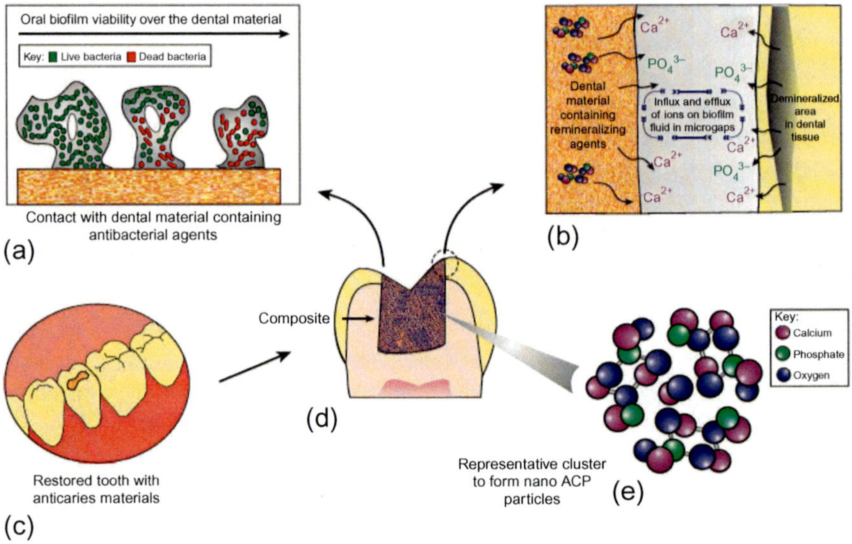

Figure 13.2 Schematic representation of anticaries products, showing the antibacterial properties to mitigate the formation of biofilm (a) as well as the diffusion of calcium and phosphate ions into teeth environment (b). Moreover, (c) represents the clinical application of those materials, (d) a schematic representation of the longitudinal section of restored tooth, and (e) schematic representation of the calcium phosphate cluster (Melo et al., 2008).

wall or cell membrane of bacteria (Chaloupka et al., 2010). These nanoparticles could also prevent the replication of bacterial DNA (Espinosa-Cristobál et al., 2012) by interaction with sulfhydryl groups. Furthermore, the AgNPs >50 nm decreased the bacteria invasion in dentinal tubules (microscopic channels of dentin, a major component of the teeth) (Cheng et al., 2012a). The calcium phosphate nanoparticles are more soluble than other compounds of calcium used for remineralization process. The amorphous calcium phosphate nanofillers (NACPs) have been used to release calcium and phosphate ions into the oral environment (Figure 13.2). The advantage of these NACPs in dental resins is that they promote remineralization with the loss of the mechanical characteristics of microfill composite resins (Cheng et al., 2012b). Indeed, the application of NACPS and nanoparticles with antibacterial properties in adhesive systems may reach a fortunate combination of anticaries and antibacterial capabilities in the same material (Figure 13.2).

13.3 Shape-memory polymers (SMPs) in dental materials

SMPs can change their previous shape to another in a controlled way with an external stimulus such as light (Lendlein et al., 2005), temperature (Tsukada et al., 2014), the application of a magnetic field (Yakacki et al., 2009), or mechanical strength (Ratna and Kocsis, 2008). SMPs are classified as smart materials (SMs), which include some metal alloys, composites, and nanocomposites. In fact, SMPs have been used in biomedical and dental fields. Indeed, SMPs are used as restorative dental materials (McCabe et al., 2011) for anticaries as well as composites with antibacterial activity (Zhuo et al., 2011).

Indeed, SMPs should present two useful properties: a network structure that determines the permanent structure (memory) and a switching part that provides significant changes in the mobility of the polymer network (transitory shape) (Mather and Lou, 2013).

Briefly, some strategies are useful to obtain SMPs (Mather and Lou, 2013): one-step polymerization of monomers/prepolymers and cross-linking agents, chemical cross-linking of high M_w thermoplastic polymer, directing blending of different polymers, and one-step synthesis of phase-segregated block copolymers.

The biosmart materials (BSMs) and SMPs have been used in dentistry as alternatives for traditional materials (Ahuja and Badami, 2014). Indeed, one of the principal characteristics of these materials is related to the control of thermally induced volumetric changes. In fact, these materials should present expansion and contraction properties similar of tooth substances to decrease the gap formation at the interface, thus the microleakage (Bullard et al., 1988). Indeed these changes should be also investigated in wet conditions to improve dental applications.

SMPs have been used in smart obturation to prevent the formations of new caries (Highgate and Frankland, 1986). Furthermore, the well filling of root canals aims to prevent reinfections, biofilm formation, and periradicular diseases. This objective could be achieved by the application of three–dimensional filling of dead spaces, main canals, and accessory canals. The C point system (Lloyd and Highgate, 2007) is an available technology in which the C points are the deformable endodontic points. These points have the ability to expand laterally without axial expansions, by absorption of residual water presented in the instrumented canal (main canal of obturation). This C point system is formed by nylon polymers cross-linked by acrylonitrile and vinylpolyrrol. Indeed, the lateral expansion of C points is nonuniform and depends on the hydrophilic polymer. However, this nonisotropic property enhances the sealing ability of the material, which decreases the reinfections in the tooth.

The polyurethane block copolymer (PU) is used to prepare a shape-memory wire in orthodontic applications (Jung and Cho, 2010). SMPU presents hard and soft segments that, when combined, improve the flexibility and mechanical resistance of orthodontic wires to correct misaligned teeth through thermal heating from body temperature (Figure 13.3).

Hyperbranched PU was prepared with ε-caprolactone (PCL) using the A_2+B_3 approach (Sivakumar and Nasar, 2009). Furthermore, the presence of PCL improves the biocompatibility of the material, as well as, its high-shape recovery. In fact, the composite made of PU and PCL presents a recovery temperature (RT) close to that of the human body. Moreover, such composite could be indicated for dental applications, dental implants in particular, inasmuch as the material presents low degradation rates, and high biocompatibility. Furthermore, the PU and PCL SMPs tested presented antibacterial and antifungal activities against *Pseudomonas aeruginosa*, *Escherichia coli*, *Klebsiella pneumonia*, and *Bacillus subtilis*. These results suggest that the

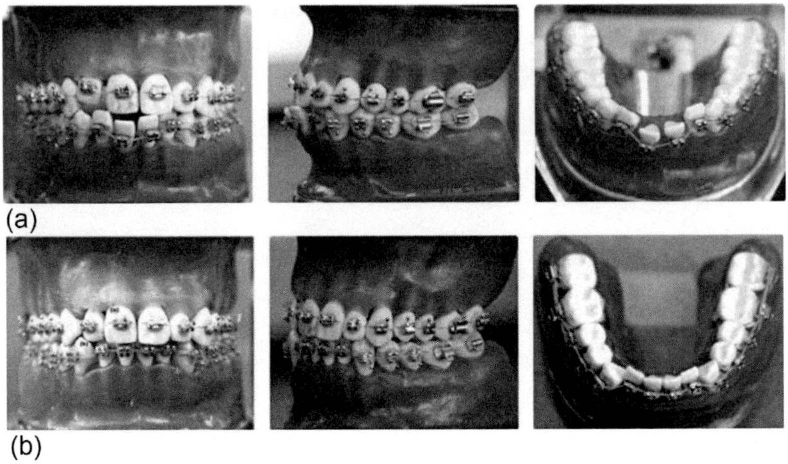

Figure 13.3 Photographs of appliance before (a) and after (b) orthodontic treatment using PUSPM wire (Jung and Cho, 2010).

application of PU and PCL shape-memory composites could avoid or decrease the biofilm formation, decreasing the rate of secondary infections associated with the implants.

The SMPs could improve the sustained release of drugs to prevent opportunist infections and caries dissemination. Although the mouth is exposed to considerable change in temperature and pH caused by food, the SMPs should maintain their shape and mechanical properties to be applied as dental materials. The SMPs made with cyclodextrin (Han et al., 2012) and alginates have been used for sustained release in medical and dental materials.

Composites and nanocomposites made by SMPs are a strong tool in the dental area to decrease the application or replace traditional dental materials. Indeed, gold nanoparticles (AuNPs) have been used as heat absorbers to induce the permanent shape of SMPs (Hribar et al., 2009). Moreover, other nanoparticles, superparamagnetic iron nanoparticles (SPIONs), cellulose nanofibers (CNFs), and silver nanoparticles (AgNPs) have been used as agents to improve the biocompatibility, controlled and sustained release, mechanical properties, and antibacterial activity of SMPs in dental materials. However, these materials need to be approved by health regulatory agencies, such as the U.S. FDA, Health Canada, and European Union, among others.

13.4 Dental implant process

A missing tooth can be replaced surgically by inserting a prosthetic device resembling the absent root and supporting the prosthetic crown. Such a device is called a dental implant. After insertion, the wound-healing process creates a firm, stable, and long-lasting connection between the bone and the implant, a process called osseo-integration (Villar et al., 2011), that comprises the acceptance of the implant by the living tissues and the formation of the viable bone over the implant surface. However, proper healing of the bone–dental implant interface depends on several biological and patient-related factors (Albrektsson and Johansson, 2001), including the implant design and surface (Milleret et al., 2001), the load distribution between bone and implant (Gapski et al., 2003), and the surgical procedure used for the implant placement (Fragiskos and Alexandridis, 2007).

Bone healing at the bone–dental implant interface is a complex biological process involving several types of cells and molecules (Polimeni et al., 2006). However, the chain of events can be summarized in four different and sequential stages, each one with a specific biological outcome. The process starts with damage caused during implant placement. The insertion of the implant is performed with a surgical drill and some mechanical force to introduce the implant body into the jaw bone. As a consequence of the insertion, intact blood vessels are damaged and bleeding commences. Although implantation procedures and implant designs have been improved to reduce trauma during placement, bleeding is inevitable because intact tissues are displaced and disrupted by the presence of the implant itself. After bleeding, blood clotting begins (stage 1), reducing the spilled blood into a fibrillar structure that detains the blood loss (Eyres and Gamlin, 2010). This fibrillar structure is then cleaned by macrophages and neutophils (stage 2) and reduced to an initial fibrillar scaffold. Using these fibers as support, immature bone cells start to migrate toward the damaged area (stage 3) (Davis, 2003). At the same time, the damaged blood vessels are repaired, and a new vascular network sprouts along the scaffold fibers to provide nutritional support to the new tissues. Finally, mature bone cells initiate the formation of a new bone matrix (stage 4), which is subsequently remodeled several times before getting the final biomechanical structure of the surrounding intact jaw bone (Sikavitsas et al., 2001).

A successful formation of stable and functional bone at the bone–dental implant interface cannot be obtained in the absence of a proper initial stability of the implant. Although mechanical factors dominate this initial stability, it is accepted that controlled bleeding and suitable formation of soft tissues at the interface keep the implant in place.

Control of blood clot formation is achieved typically by using chemical reactions that accelerate the clotting phase (Butenas and Mann, 2002). However, findings on the electrical behavior of blood elements have shown that blood clot formation can be also induced by the application of an external electric signal (Erol et al., 2010). The experimental evidence shows that the electrical stimulus increases the rate of bone formation over a dental implant (Shayestech et al., 2007).

While during past years, research and development of dental implant biomaterials have been focused on osseo-integration, soft tissue integration is one of the frontiers in dental implant research today, as dental implants require a soft-tissue barrier to prevent bacterial penetration (Rompen et al., 2006) and to inhibit epithelial down-growth (Chehroudi et al., 1992). After installation of a dental implant, fibroplasts from the oral connective tissue (gingival fibroblasts) are the preferred cells to form a healthy and collagen-rich connective tissue to repopulate the wound and attach to the abutment of the implant.

Titanium–zirconium (TiZr) alloys have shown increased corrosion resistance (Khan et al., 1999); improved tensile and fatigue strength (Thomas et al., 2011); similar biocompatibility (Grandin et al., 2012); higher integrin-β3 expression in comparison with titanium (Ti), the gold standard in implantology (Steinemann, 1998); and have been suggested as potential clinical candidates to improve soft-tissue integration.

The tremendous success of dental implants has been tempered in some prosthetic applications by complications such as screw loosening, screw fracture, gold cylinder fracture, framework fracture, and infrequently, implant fracture (Zarb and Schmitt, 1990). In order to avoid such a problematic design, the main objective of a successful dental implant should be to ensure that it can support biting forces and deliver them safely to interfacial tissues over the long term (Brunski, 1992).

Computational methods, such as the finite element method (FEM), have been widely used in dental and orthopedic biomechanics and have become an important tool in the design and analysis of different types of implants. There is no doubt that FEM is the most general and widely accepted technique in this field and has been applied to analyze different restorative techniques (Maceri et al., 2007) and implant applications, investigating the influence of implant and prosthesis design, magnitude and direction of loads, bone mechanical properties, and different bone–implant interface conditions.

Previous analyses were deterministic and resulted in a quantitative evaluation of the stresses on the implant and its surrounding bone, neglecting the potential impact of many individual factors in variability such as geometry, material properties, and component alignment or loading conditions on the overall approach of the model (Bah et al., 2011). The combined effects to variability in individual parameters can dramatically affect component performance.

Recently, studies have taken a probabilistic approach to assess the structural integrity of orthopedic implants: cervical spine components, tibial components, knee replacement, uncemented hip implants, cemented hip implants, and dental implants (Guda et al., 2008).

Pretie and Williams (2007) examined the influence of bone properties and loading variability on peri-implant crestal and cancellous bone strains.

Bone quality is well accepted as one of the key factors affecting the long-term success of dental implants. Several studies have suggested that poor bone quality exhibits the greatest failure rates because of a thin cortical bone and low-density cancellous bone with a poor capability to react properly to stresses generated by occlusal loads and is especially correlated with cases of single implants and high crown-root ratios (Jaffin and Berman, 1991).

In contrast to natural teeth, there is no periodontal ligament between a dental implant and the surrounding bone, and the poor capacity for detection of biting forces may increase the tendency for occlusal overloading, which can result in peri-implant bone loss and implant failure. Occlusal overloading is usually caused by premature contact between the implant-retained crown and opposing natural teeth or even implant prostheses. Some animal studies investigated the influence of occlusal overloading on the bone around dental implants. Results of these studies revealed that occlusal overloading could be a very important factor in loss of osseo-integration of dental implants.

Another interesting issue is the prosthetic concept of platform switching, which has been introduced to the market recently and has been studied histologically in both animals and humans (Becker et al., 2007).

13.5 Future trends

SMPs are important materials in biomedical applications, in particular dental applications. In fact, SMPs could be applied in caries treatments, orthodontics, reparations, implants, and infection control, among others. Furthermore, the new composites made by the cross-linking of branched polymeric chains improve the mechanical properties as well as the interface between the SMPs and the teeth material.

Indeed, the new SMP composites and nanocomposites come into play in the multifunctional application of smart materials to promote the sustained release of drugs to combat local established infections, prevent biofilm formation, and create better adhesion of the materials onto the surface of teeth.

References

Ahuja, B., Badami, V., 2014. Biosmart materials: breaking new ground of dentistry. Sci. World J. 2014, Article ID 986912, 7 pp.

Albrektsson, T., Johansson, C., 2001. Osteoinduction, osteocondustion and osseointegration. Eur. Spine J. 10, S96–S101.

Bah, M.T., Nair, P.B., Taylor, M., Browne, M., 2011. Efficient computational method for assessing the effects of implant positioning in cementless total hip replacements. J. Biomech. 44, 1417–1422.

Bakopoulou, A., Papadopoulos, T., Garefis, P., 2009. Molecular toxicology of substances released from resin-based dental restorative materials. Int. J. Mol. Sci. 10, 3861–3899.

Becker, J.J., Ferrari, D., Herten, M., Kirsh, A., Schaer, A., Schwarz, F., 2007. Influence of platform switching on crestal bone changes at non-submerged titanium implants: a histomorphometrical study in dogs. J. Clin. Periodontol. 34, 1089–1096.

Besinis, A., De Peralta, T., Handy, R.D., 2014. Inhibition of biofilm formation and antibacterial properties of a silver nano-coating on human dentine. Nanotoxicoloy 8, 1–10.

Beyth, N., et al., 2014. Antibacterial dental resin composites. React. Funct. Polym. 75, 81–88.

Brunski, J.B., 1992. Biomechanical factors affecting the bone-dental implant interface. Clin. Mater. 10, 153–201.

Bullard, R.H., Leinfelder, K.F., Russell, C.M., 1988. Effect of coefficient of thermal expansion on microleakage. J. Am. Dent. Assoc. 116, 871–874.

Busila, M.I., et al., 2014. Photocatalytic and antimicrobial Ag/ZnO nanocomposites for functionalization of textile fabrics. J. Alloys Compd. 610, 244–249.

Butenas, S., Mann, K., 2002. Blood coagulation. Biochemistry 67, 3–12.

Chaloupka, K., Malam, Y., Seifalian, A.M., 2010. Nanosilver as a new generation of nanoproduct in biomedical applications. Trends Biotechnol. 28, 580–588.

Chehroudi, B., Gould, T.R., Brunette, D.M., 1992. The role of connective tissue in inhibiting epithelial domngrowth on titanium-coated percutaneous implants. J. Biomed. Mater. Res. 26, 493–515.

Cheng, L., et al., 2012a. Anti-biofilm dentin primer with quaternary ammonium and silver nanoparticles. J. Dent. Res. 91, 598–604.
Cheng, L., et al., 2012b. Antibacterial and physical properties of calcium–phosphate and calcium–fluoride nanocomposites with chlorhexidine. Dent. Mater. 28, 573–583.
Cheng, H., et al., 2013. Long-lasting in vivo and in vitro antibacterial ability of nanostructured titania coating incorporated with silver nanoparticles. J. Biomed. Mater. Res. A 102, 3488–3499.
Chien, C.Y., et al., 2013. Dopamine-assisted immobilization of hydroxyapatite nanoparticles and RGD peptides to improve the osteoconductivity of titanium. J. Biomed. Mater. Res. A 101A, 740–747.
Choi, A.H., Ben-Nissan, B., Matilinna, J.P., Conway, R.C., 2013. Calcium phosphate nanocoatings and nanocomposite coatings in dentistry. J. Dent. Res. 92 (10), 853–859. http://dx.doi.org/10.1177/0022034513497754.
Cooley, R.L., Stilley, J., Lubow, R.M., 1985. Mercury vapour produced during the sterelization of amalgam-contaminated instruments. J. Prosthet. Dent. 53, 304–308.
Costa, C.A., Giro, E.M., et al., 2003. Short-term evaluation of the pulp-dentin complex response to a resin-modified glass ionomer cement and a bonding agent applied in deep cavities. Dent. Mater. 19, 739–746.
Davis, J., 2003. Understanding peri-implant endosseous healing. J. Dent. Educ. 67, 932–949.
Donly, K.J., García-Godoy, F., 2002. The use of resin-based composite in children. Pediatr. Dent. 24 (5), 480–488.
Erol, O., Uysal, O., Agaoglu, G., 2010. Percutaneous electrothrombosis: a minimally invasive technique for the treatment of deep hemangiomas. Aesthet. Plast. Surg. 34, 214–217.
Espinosa-Cristobál, L.F., et al., 2012. Antimicrobial sensibility of Streptococcus mutans serotypes to silver nanoparticles. Mater. Sci. Eng. C Mater. Biol. Appl. 32, 896–901.
Eyres, L., Gamlin, F., 2010. Haemostasis, blood platelets and coagulation. Anaesth. Intensive Care Med. 11, 244–246.
Fan, Z., et al., 2014. A novel wound dressing based on Ag/graphene polymer hydrogel: effectively kill bacteria and accelerate wound healing. Adv. Funct. Mater. 24, 3933–3943.
Fejerskov, O., Kidd, E., 2008. Dental Caries: The Disease and Its Clinical Management. Wiley-Blackwell, Australia.
Forss, H., et al., 1991. Fluoride and mutans streptococci in plaque grown on glass ionomer and composite. Caries Res. 25, 454–458.
Fragiskos, F., Alexandridis, C., 2007. Osseointegrated implants. In: Oral Surgery. Springer, Berlin, Heidelberg, pp. 337–348.
Gapski, R., et al., 2003. Critical review of immediate implant loading. Clin. Oral Implants Res. 14, 515–527.
Grandin, H.M., Berner, S., Dard, M., 2012. A review of titanium zirconium (TiZr) alloys for use in endosseous dental implants. Materials 5, 1348–1360.
Guda, T., Ross, T.A., Lang, L.A., Millwater, H.R., 2008. Probabilistic analysis of preload in the abutment screw of a dental implant complex. J. Prosthet. Dent. 100, 183–193.
Han, X.J., et al., 2012. pH-induced shape-memory polymers. Macromol. Rapid Commun. 33, 1055–1060.
Highgate, D.J., Frankland, J.D., 1986. Deformable polymeric compositions. United States patent no. 4,565,722.
Hook, E.R., et al., 2014. Development of a novel antimicrobial-releasing glass ionomer cement functionalized with chlorhexidine hexametaphosphate nanoparticles. J. Nanobiotechnol. 12, 1–9.
Hørsted-Bindslev, P., Arenholt-Bindslev, D., 2009. Dental amalgam. In: Schmalz, G., Arenholt-Bindslev, D. (Eds.), Biocompatibility of Dental Materials. Springer-Verlag, Berlin, Heidelberg.

Howard, L., Weng, Y., Xie, D., 2014. Preparation and evaluation of a novel star-shaped polyacid-constructed dental glass-ionomer system. Dent. Mater. 30, 644–653.
Hribar, K.C., Metter, R.B., Ifkovits, J.L., Troxler, T., Burdick, J.A., 2009. Light-induced temperature transitions in biodegradable polymer and nanorod composites. Small 5, 1830–1834.
Isidor, F., 1996. Loss of osseointegration caused by occlusal load of oral implants. A clinical and radiographic study in monkeys. Clin. Oral Implants Res. 7, 143–152.
Jaffin, R.A., Berman, C.L., 1991. The excessive loss of Branemark fixtures in type IV bone: a 5-year analysis. J. Periodontol. 62, 2–4.
Jung, Y.C., Cho, J.W., 2010. Application of shape memory polyurethane in orthodontic. J. Mater. Sci. Mater. Med. 21, 2881–2886.
Keller, A.A., et al., 2014. Release of engineered nanomaterials from personal care products throughout their life cycle. J. Nanoparticle Res. 16, 2488–2498.
Khan, M.A., Williams, R.L., Williams, D.F., 1999. Conjoint corrosion and wear in titanium alloys. Biomaterials 20, 765–772.
Lendlein, A., et al., 2005. Light-induced shape-memory polymers. Nature 434, 879–882.
Lloyd, D.J., Highgate J.A., 2007. Expandable/contractable composition for surgical or dental use. United States patent no. 7,210,935.
Maceri, F., Martignoni, M., Vairo, G., 2007. Mechanical behavior of endodontic restorations with multiple prefabricated posts: a finite elements approach. J. Biomech. 40, 2386–2398.
Mackey, T.K., Contreras, J.T., Liang, B.A., 2014. The Minamata Convention on Mercury: attempting to address the global controversy of dental amalgam use and mercury waste disposal. Sci. Total Environ. 472, 125–129.
Mather, P., Lou, X., 2013. Design strategies for shape memory polymers. Curr. Opin. Chem. Eng. 2, 103–111.
McCabe, J.F., et al., 2011. Smart materials in dentistry. Aust. Dent. J. 56, 3–10.
Melo, M.A.S., et al., 2008. Nanotechnology-based restorativies materials for dental caries management. Trends Biotechnol. 31, 459–467.
Milleret, V., et al., 2001. Alkali treatment of microrough titanium surfaces affects macrophage/monocyte adhesion, platelet activation and architecture of blood clot formation. Eur. Cell. Mater. J. 21, 430–444.
Okabe, T., et al., 2003. Mercury release from dental amalgams into continuously repleished liquids. Dent. Mater. 19, 38–45.
Pizzichini, M., et al., 2002. Release of mercury from dental amalgam and its influence on salivary antioxidant activity. Sci. Total Environ. 284, 19–25.
Polimeni, G., Xiropaidis, A., Wikesjo, U., 2006. Biology and principles of periodontal wound healing-regeneration. Periodontology 41, 30–47.
Pretie, C.S., Williams, J.L., 2007. Probabilistic analysis of peri-implant strain predictions as influenced by uncertainties in bone properties and occlusal forces. Clin. Oral Implants Res. 18, 611–619.
Ratna, D., Kocsis, J.K., 2008. Recent advances in shape memory polymers and composites: a review. J. Mater. Sci. 43, 254–269.
Rompen, E., et al., 2006. The effect of material characteristics, of surface topography and of implant components and connections on soft tissue integration: a literature review. Clin. Oral Implants Res. 17, 55–67.
Schmalz, G., 2009. Resin based materials. In: Schmalz, G., Arenholt-Bindslev, D. (Eds.), Biocompatibility of Dental Materials. Springer-Verlag, Berlin, Heidelberg.
Shayestech, Y., et al., 2007. The effect of a constant electrical field on osseointegration after immediate implantation in dog mandibles: a preliminary study. J. Prosthodont. 16, 337–342.
Sikavitsas, V., Temenoff, J., Mikos, A., 2001. Biomaterials and bone mechanotransduction. Biomaterials 22, 2581–2593.

Silva, R.M., et al., 2013. Effects of cellulose fibers on the physical and chemical properties of glass ionomer dental restorative materials. Mater. Res. Bull. 48, 118–126.

Sivakumar, C., Nasar, A.S., 2009. Poly(ε-caprolactone)-based hyperbranched polyurethanes prepared via A2+B3 approach and its shape-memory behavior. Eur. Polym. J. 45, 2329–2337.

Stanley, H.R., 1996. Biocompatibility of dental materials. In: Anusavice, K.J. (Ed.), Phillips' Science of Dental Materials. W.B. Saunders, Philadelphia, PA, pp. 75–109.

Stanley, H., Schmalz, G., 2009. Cements and ceramics. In: Arenholt-Bindslev, D., Schmalz, G. (Eds.), Biocompatibility of Dental Materials. Springer-Verlag, Berlin, Heidelberg.

Steinemann, S.G., 1998. Titanium—the material of choice? Periodontology 17, 7–21.

Thomas, D.S., Jones, A.A., Dard, M., Grize, L., Obrecht, M., Cochran, D.L., 2011. Tissue integration of a new titanium-zirconium dental implant: a comparative histologic and radiographic study in the canine. J. Periodontol. 82, 1453–1461.

Tsukada, G., Tokuda, M., Torii, M., 2014. Temperature triggered shape memory effect of transpolyisoprene-based polymer. J. Endod. 40 (10), 1658–1662. http://dx.doi.org/10.1016/j.joen.2014.05.003.

Villar, C., et al., 2011. Wound healing around dental implants. Endod. Top. 25, 44–62.

Wataha, J.C., 2012. Predicting clinical biological responses of dental materials. Dent. Mater. 28, 23–40.

Yakacki, C.M., et al., 2009. Shape-memory polymer networks with Fe_3O_4 nanoparticles for remote activation. J. Appl. Polym. Sci. 112, 3166–3176.

Zarb, G.A., Schmitt, A., 1990. The longitudinal clinical effectiveness of osseointegrated implants: the Toronto study. Part III: problems and complications encountered. J. Prosthet. Dent. 64, 185–194.

Zhuo, H.T., Hu, J.L., Chen, S.J., 2011. Coaxial electrospun polyurethane core-shell nanofibers for shape memory and antibacterial nanomaterials. eXPRESS Polym. Lett. 5, 182–187.

Shape-memory and self-reinforcing polymers as sutures

14

H. Meng[1], G. Li[2]
[1]Southern University, Baton Rouge, LA, USA; [2]Louisiana State University, Baton Rouge, LA, USA

14.1 Introduction: Overview of chapter

Shape-memory polymers (SMPs) can rapidly change their shapes (configuration or dimension) under appropriate stimuli, such as heat (Hu, 2007), moisture/water (Yang et al., 2006), pH value (Feil et al., 1992), electricity (Asaka and Oguro, 2000), light (Jiang et al., 2006), magnetic field (Makhosaxana et al., 2000), and solvents (Siegal and Firestone, 1988). This chapter will briefly introduce the various mechanisms and broad applications of SMPs. Then it will focus on the self-reinforcing shape-memory suture applications of SMPs. The macromolecular design and the application strategies of the SMP are introduced in the chapter. In addition to its present achievements, the future prospects of shape-memory sutures are discussed in the final section of the chapter.

14.2 Various mechanisms of stimuli-active shape-memory polymers (SMPs)

Stimuli-active polymers (Meng and Hu, 2010) significantly change their properties, including shape, mechanical properties, phase separation, surface, permeability, optical properties, and electrical properties, upon a small variation in environmental conditions, such as temperature, electric field, pH value, light, magnetic field, electrical field, sonic field, solvent ions, enzymes, and glucose. Three special issues have been devoted to stimuli-active polymers. The special issue "stimuli-active materials" in Progress in Polymer Science (2010, Vol. 35, issue 1–2) reported significant advances in the recent developments and future trends of stimuli-active polymers (Liu and Urban, 2010; Urban, 2010; Smith et al., 2010; Roy et al., 2010; Chen et al., 2010a,b; Motornov et al., 2010; Agarwal and Hess, 2010; Nandivada et al., 2010; Gabriel et al., 2010). The special issue "stimuli-sensitive polymers" in Advanced Materials (2010, Vol. 22, issue 31) provided a collection of the first class papers on thermal-responsive SMPs (Nguyen et al., 2010; Behl et al., 2010a,b; Zotzmann et al., 2010; Kloxin et al., 2010; Romeo et al., 2010; Ohm et al., 2010; Russew and Hecht, 2010; Tokarev and Minko, 2010; Ji et al., 2010; Sellinger

Shape Memory Polymers for Biomedical Applications. http://dx.doi.org/10.1016/B978-0-85709-698-2.00014-3

et al., 2010). The themed issue "actively moving polymers" in Journal of Materials Chemistry (2010, Vol. 20, issue 17) presented excellent papers on "actively moving polymers" (Lendlein, 2010; Behl et al., 2010a,b; Small et al., 2010; Hollander et al., 2010; Rousseau and Xie, 2010; Xu et al., 2010; Kumar et al., 2010; Behl and Lendlein, 2010; Gunes et al., 2010; Jung et al., 2010; Xiao et al., 2010; Burke and Mather, 2010; Hu and Chen, 2010; Ionov, 2010; Chen et al., 2010a,b; Hmadeh et al., 2010; Simpson et al., 2010; Burmistrova and Klitzing, 2010).

Stimuli-active SMPs, a very important type of SMP, change their shapes or produce mechanical power in response to stimuli (Jiang et al., 2006; Yang et al., 2006). They can "memorize" their original (or permanent) shape and rapidly change from a temporary shape to their original (or permanent) shape under the influence of stimuli. The shape-memory effect has been reported on many polymers since it was found on polynorbornlene in the 1990s. SMPs of different forms are available now, such as solution, emulsion, film, fiber, foam, and bulk (Hu et al., 2007; Tobushi et al., 2006; Marco and Eckhouse, 2006). A few review papers have been published on SMPs (Meng and Hu, 2009; Mather et al., 2009; Gunes and Jana, 2008; Dietsch and Tong, 2007; Tobushi et al., 2007; Hu, 2007; Behl and Lendlein, 2007; Ratna and Karger-Kocsis, 2008; Kim, 2010; Huang et al., 2010; Rousseau and Xie, 2010; Lendlein, 2010; Behl et al., 2010a,b; Yakacki and Gall, 2010; Madbouly and Lendlein, 2010). In general, in comparison with shape-memory alloys, SMPs have the following advantages: (1) low cost, (2) light weight, (3) good processability, (4) high recoverable deformability, (5) tailorable switching temperature, and (6) tailor-able mechanical properties. Due to their polymeric nature, SMPs also have intrinsic disadvantages such as (1) low recovery stress, (2) low mechanical strength, (3) low thermal resistance, and (4) short lifetime.

A polymer stable network and an appropriate reversible switching transition of the polymer are the two prerequisites for the shape-memory effect. The stable network structures could be formed by molecule entanglement, a crystalline phase, chemical cross-linking, or an interpenetrated network (Hu and Mondal, 2005; Hu et al., 2005a,b; Liu et al., 2007; Beloshenko et al., 2005; Voit et al., 2010; Zhang et al., 2008; Yu et al., 2010). The reversible switching transition could be crystallization/melting transition, vitrification/glass transition, anisotropic/isotropic transition, reversible molecule cross-linking, or supramolecular association/disassociation. During the shape-recovery cycle, SMPs are first deformed. If the switch is locked, the deformed polymer cannot recover because of the low mobility of the macromolecules. Also, because the mobility of the macromolecules is restricted by the locks, the internal stress can be partially stored in the cross-linking network. Finally, upon stimulation, the reversible locks are opened by the stimuli. As a result, the SMP recovers, accompanied by the release of internal stress. In addition to a direct trigger to open the reversible locks, other strategies that can significantly change the mobility of the SMP may trigger the shape recovery. These strategies include moisture, water/solvent, light, ultrasonic field, magnetic field, pH, ionic concentration, and electric methods that activate the shape-memory effect (Huang et al., 2010; Li and Nettles, 2010; Nji and Li, 2010; Li and Uppu, 2010).

Several typical SMPs have been commercially produced in large scale in addition to the various SMPs still in lab-scale fabrication. Commercialized SMPS include thermoplastic and thermoset polyurethane (DiAPLEX, SMP Technologies Inc., originally Mitsubishi Heavy Industries), polystyrene-based SMP (Veriflex®, Verilyte™, Veritex™, Cornerstone Research Group, Inc.), aliphatic polyurethane (Tecoflex®, Lubrizol Advanced Materials), epoxy-based SMP (TEMBO®, Composite Technology Development, Inc.), and UV curable thermoset polyurethane (NOA-63, Norland Products Inc.).

The applications of SMPs fall into four categories based on application strategies: shape change, stress generation, modulus change, and vapor permeability change. The applications of SMPs have been extended to many areas, such as intelligent medical instruments and auxiliaries (Lendlein and Langer, 2002; Wache et al., 2004; Langer and Tirrell, 2004; Yakacki and Gall, 2010; Small et al., 2010; Mano, 2008; Lendlein and Behl, 2008; Hampikian et al., 2006; Wischke et al., 2009; Nagahama et al., 2009; Xie and Xiao, 2008), smart textiles and apparels (Li, 2007; Hu and Chen, 2010), heat-shrinkable packaging (Charlesby, 1960, p. 198), micro-electro-mechanical systems (Gall et al., 2002), self-deployable sun sails in spacecrafts (Sokolowski et al., 1999), morphing structures for aerospace vehicles (Vaia and Baur, 2008; Campbell et al., 2006; Eddington and Beebe, 2004; Toensmeier, 2005), miniature manipulators (Smela et al., 1995), damping materials (Yang et al., 2004), self-peeling reversible adhesive (Xie and Xiao, 2008), vehicle components (Lendlein, 2006), toys (Hayashi et al., 2004), micro-systems (Eddington and Beebe, 2004), smart water-vapor permeability materials (Mondal et al., 2006), self-healing (Li and Uppu, 2010; John and Li, 2010; Xiao et al., 2010), hair treatment (Lendlein et al., 2005b; Lendlein and Ridder, 2007), temperature sensors (DiOrio et al., 2011), data-storage media (Wornyo et al., 2009), and chemical feeding in chemical reactions (Laroche et al., 2002).

Medical applications have significantly driven the progress of SMPs (Langer and Tirrell, 2004; Laroche et al., 2002; Yakacki and Gall, 2010; Small et al., 2010; Mano, 2008; Lendlein and Behl, 2008). The tailorable stiffness and biodegradability of SMPs make them especially suitable for medical applications. The Lendlein, Gall, Maitland, and Small research groups have made outstanding contributions and published many papers regarding the biomedical applications of SMPs. The typical medical applications examples of SMPs include self-tightening sutures, laser or magnetically activated devices for cardiovascular stents (Maitland et al., 2002; Buckley et al., 2006; Schmidt, 2006; Small et al., 2007), aneurysm coils for the treatment of intracranial aneurysms (Hampikian et al., 2006), biodegradable intelligent surgery sutures (Langer and Lendlein, 2003), orthodontic appliances (Mather et al., Dec., 2005), self-deployable neuronal electrodes (Sharp et al., 2006), dialysis needle adapters (Ortega et al., 2007), intelligent electrodes, and drug-control-release devices (Wischke et al., 2009; Nagahama et al., 2009). The activation methods to trigger the recovery of biomedical SMPs can be via body temperature, laser remote heating using optical fibers, and remote inductive heating.

14.3 Shape-memory materials for medical and self-reinforcing suture applications

14.3.1 *Macromolecular design*

SMPs for biomedical applications can either be nondegradable or degradable based on their specific application purposes. SMPs as implanted materials with biodegradability can degrade, and a secondary surgery for removal of the material can be avoided after the tissue has healed.

Medshape Solutions, Inc., has done pioneer work on commercializing SMP medical devices such as orthopedic anchors, soft tissue fasteners, and ankle arthrodesis nails. Although not many commercialized medical products have been developed and approved, companies are making great efforts to improve the properties and tackle the engineering challenges of SMPs so that more SMP biomedical products can be brought to market.

Most SMPs for clinical applications need to have a switching transition above physiological temperature, high recovery speed and ratios, suitable elasticity, and tunable degradation rate. Of the engineering challenges, improving the stress recovery, tailoring degradation speed, and remote activation are the most prominent. At a temperature above the switching temperature, the stiffness and recovery stress of SMPs may be too low for many applications. The reported recovery stress of SMPs is normally below 10 MPa, which is far below that of shape-memory alloy. Although remote actuation of SMP has been achieved, there are still safety and regulatory issues. Other problems include degradation speed and that degraded products should not be toxic to the human body.

The biodegradability of SMPs can be achieved by introducing polymer segments with weak, hydrolyzable bonds that can cleave under physiological conditions (Behl and Lendlein, 2007; Storey and Hickey, 1994; Gorna and Gogolewski, 2002). Typical biodegradable SMPs for medical applications are poly(D,L-lactide-*co*-glycolide), cross-linking poly(ε-caprolactone) dimethyacrylate and *N*-butylacrylate (Kelch et al., 2007; Rickert et al., 2003a,b), star-shaped oligoesters of rac-dilactide and diglycolide (Alteheld et al., 2005), multiblock copolyesters from poly(ε-caprolactone), polyethylene glycol and chain extender 4,4′-(adipoyldioxy)dicinnamic acid dichloride (Nagata and Kitazima, 2006), poly(ε-caprolactone)diols or poly(*p*-dioxanone)diols coupled with diisocyanate groups (Lendlein and Langer, 2002; Rickert et al., 2003a,b, 2005; Ping et al., 2005), L-lactide-trimethylene-carbonate-L-lactide block copolymer, multiblock-copolymers containing poly(L-lactide) and polyglycolide-co-(ε-caprotactone) segments (Min et al., 2005), ε-caprolactone-trimethylene-carbonate-ε-caprolactone random copolymer, photocured poly(ε-caprolactone)diol, poly (ethylene glycol), ε-caprolactone-trimethylene-carbonate-L-lactide random copolymer (Wong et al., 2011a,b), cross-linking network of polyhedral oligomeric silsesquioxane functioned with lactides (Xu and Song, 2010), 5-cinnamoyloxyisophthalic acid copolymer (Nagata and Inaki, 2011), cross-linking network of polyhedral oligomeric silsesquioxane functioned with lactides (Xu and Song, 2010), polyurethanes based on 2,6-diisocyanate methyl caproate, poly(ε-caprolactone), polycaprolactone-polyhedral silsesquioxane double networks (Lee et al., 2008), poly(D,L-lactic acid)diol-based polyurethane ureas (Ruan et al., 2012), poly(*b*-amino ester)-*co*-(meth)acrylate monomers (Lakhera et al., 2012), and polyethylene glycol extended with an amino acid chain extender (phenylalanine) (Skarja and Woodhouse, 2000, 2004).

The degradation rate and mechanical properties can be adjusted by copolymerizing different degradable SMPs. Yang et al. (2010) copolymerized lactide with 1,3-trimetylene carbonate to adjust the degradation rate and mechanical properties of the SMPs. 1,3-Trimetylene carbonate degrades by surface erosion without releasing acidic species. Hydrolytic degradation and enzymatic degradation of the copolymers *in vivo* have been investigated (Hua et al., 2009; Yang et al., 2010). Glycolic acid has also been incorporated into lactide to increase degradation rate because of better hydrophilicity (Musumeci et al., 2006). Copolymerization of poly(ethylene glycol) with lactide can also improve flexibility of the degradable SMPs.

In addition to proper degradation speed and mechanical properties, degradation products should not be harmful to the human body. Degradation of polylactic acid polymers can lead to local acidity. This can result in acidity-caused auto-accelerating degradation, which will initiate an inflammatory reaction. Wang et al. (2010) introduced hexamethylene diisocyanate and butanediamine into polylactic SMPs. The hexamethylene diisocyanate and butanediamine not only provided the hard segment to the SMP for better shape-memory performance, but also increased the alkalic group content. The alkali group can thus tune the degradation speed.

Polyhedral oligomeric silsesquioxane nanoparticle core/SMP could have promising medical applications because of its special inorganic/original composite structure. Xu and Song (2010) made an SMP from a polyhedral oligomeric silsesquioxane nanoparticle core grafted with eight polyester arms polylactides (PLAs). The star-shape macromers then reacted with aliphatic diisocyanate to form a spatial cross-linking structure. The abundant reactive groups of the macromer enabled selective end-group functionalization. It was found that the temporary shapes of the SMP could be stable more than 1 year at room temperature. The shape recovery can be completed in a few seconds at a temperature below 51 °C. The versatile structures of the polymer enabled their tunable biodegradability and biofunctionalizability. The degradation profiles and immunogenicity of oligomeric silsesquioxane-SMPs were studied (Filion et al., 2011). Upon implantation, the SMP composite elicited a mild foreign-body-type immune response. Upon degradation *in vivo*, another acute inflammatory response was found to be elicited. The inflammation resolved over time without medical interventions. One year after the implantation of the SMP composite, no pathologic abnormalities were found. The pre-clinical animal studies and full toxicology studies are being studied by this group (Xu and Song, 2010; Filion et al., 2011).

Lee et al. (2008) reported another biodegradable SMP based on polyhedral silsesquioxane. The molecular architecture consisted of a "double network" that features the superposition of a percolative physical network and a covalent network. The covalent network chains featured two polycaprolactone chains tethered to a single oligomeric silsesquioxane moiety by virtue of its use as an initiator for ring-opening polymerization of polycaprolactone. Alvarado-Tenorio et al. (2011) investigated the micro- and nanoscale levels of the biodegradable oligomeric silsesquioxane-polycaprolactone hybrid nanocomposites. It was found that end-capping had a significant impact on oligomeric silsesquioxane crystallization. This finding suggests the possibility of fine-tuning the well-ordered nanostructures from their variable chemical composition and changing the end group reactivity. Feng et al. (2011) synthesized biodegradable SMP multiblock copolymer, which contains polydepsipeptides and poly (ε-caprolactone) or poly(*p*-dioxanone) segments, by coupling their diols using diisocyanate. Polydepsipeptides were used to improve the biocompatibility *in vivo* of the poly(ε-caprolactone)-based polyurethane during the degradation process.

In biomedical applications, the prediction of the shape recovery of an implant after insertion is important. Neffe et al. (2010) studied the shape recovery and mechanical properties of the shape-memory polyurethane networks based on star-shaped precursors of rac-dilactide and diglycolide, *p*-dioxanone, or ε-caprolactone. The thermo-mechanical properties were tailored by changing crosslinking density and co-monomers. Wong et al. (2011a,b) experimentally characterized the shape recovery of the biodegradable shape-memory poly(D,L-lactide-*co*-glycolide), and modeled the shape-recovery behavior of the polymer using a one-dimensional constitutive model. With finely tuned model parameters, the experimental results and molding results showed strong agreement.

14.3.2 SMP fibers

Although there has been much research on SMPs in the past two decades (Hu et al., 2005a,b; Ohki et al., 2004; Yoshihaya et al., 2003; Liu et al., 2002; Lendlein and Kelch, 2002; Lin and Chen, 1998a,b; Kim and Lee, 1998; Tobushi et al., 1998; Kim et al., 1996; Hyashi, 1993), the study of fabricating shape-memory fibers was not started until recently. SMPs with proper processability can be fabricated into shape-memory fibers. Through a wet spinning method, shape-memory fibers were fabricated (Zhu et al., 2006; Ji et al., 2006). Wet spinning of shape-memory fiber is relatively simple in comparison with melt spinning, in that there are no extreme requirements on the processing properties of the SMPs. However, wet spinning of shape-memory polyurethane fibers has problems, as it is a source of environmental pollution and has low manufacturing efficiency and low mechanical properties of the fiber. Therefore, melt spinning of shape-memory polyurethane fibers was developed. Shape-memory polyurethanes for melt spinning should have high thermal stability and relatively high molecular weight to obtain good mechanical properties. Hu et al. (2007, 2008) and Meng et al. (2007) developed different shape-memory polyurethane filaments using polyol as the soft segment and small-size diols and methylene diphenyl diisocyanate as the hard segment by melt spinning. Figure 14.1a shows the SEM image of the shape-memory polyurethane fiber prepared by melt spinning. The diameter of the monofilament is about 50 μm. Figure 14.1b shows the thermo-mechanical properties of the shape-memory polyurethane fiber. The fiber shows good shape-memory effect.

In comparison with its shape-memory film counterparts, shape-memory fibers have higher mechanical strength, higher recovery stress, and better shape-recovery

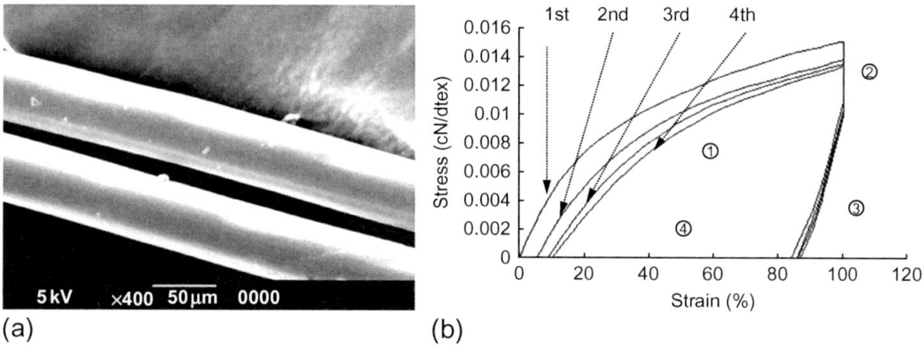

Figure 14.1 (a) The SEM image of the prepared shape-memory polyurethane fiber; (b) the thermo-mechanical properties of the shape-memory fiber.
Copyright by Wiley & Sons. Reprinted with permission, Meng and Hu (2008).

properties as a result of molecular orientation in the fibers brought about by spinning processes. The recovery ratios of shape-memory polyurethane fibers can reach a value of above 100% (Zhu et al., 2006), which means that if the shape-memory fiber is stretched, it can recover to a length shorter than its original length after recovery at a temperature above its switching temperature. In comparison with its elastic counterparts, such as Spandex (a product of Invista, previously a part of DuPont) and XLA (a product of Aquafil, previously of DOW), the shape-memory fiber is more thermal-sensitive with thermal-sensitive recoverability upon stimulation.

14.3.3 SMP filament sutures

SMP monofilament can tie itself into a perfect knot in the human body. This is especially helpful for minimal incision surgeries. One of the biggest challenges in keyhole surgery is how to tie a perfect knot. Traditional delicate stitching is difficult to operate in a confined space after endoscopic keyhole surgery. It is also difficult to achieve a knot with the proper amount of tension on the tissue. Several problems can occur if the stress applied by the suture on the tissue is not adequate. If the stress applied is too high, the surrounding tissue affected by the knot may die. If the stress is too low, scar tissue may form, which can form hernias. Therefore, the incision will not heal well.

Figure 14.2 shows the shape recovery of a thermoplastic elastomer shape-memory suture that is wrapped around a sponge (Huang et al., 2012). The shape-memory suture is able to self-tighten into a knot. The suture was first stretched to achieve a temporary elongated length. Once the suture is heated to a temperature above its switching transition temperature, the suture begins to shrink to achieve a perfect knot.

Biodegradable SMP sutures were prepared by Professors A. Lendlein and R. Langer in 2002 (Lendlein and Langer, 2002; Langer and Lendlein, 2003). The suture was made of a monofilament of SMP. The shape-memory suture was synthesized with oligo(ε-caprolactone)diol and crystallizable oligo(ρ-dioxanone)diol. The thermoplastic SMP is biodegradable; therefore, there is no need to remove the suture after

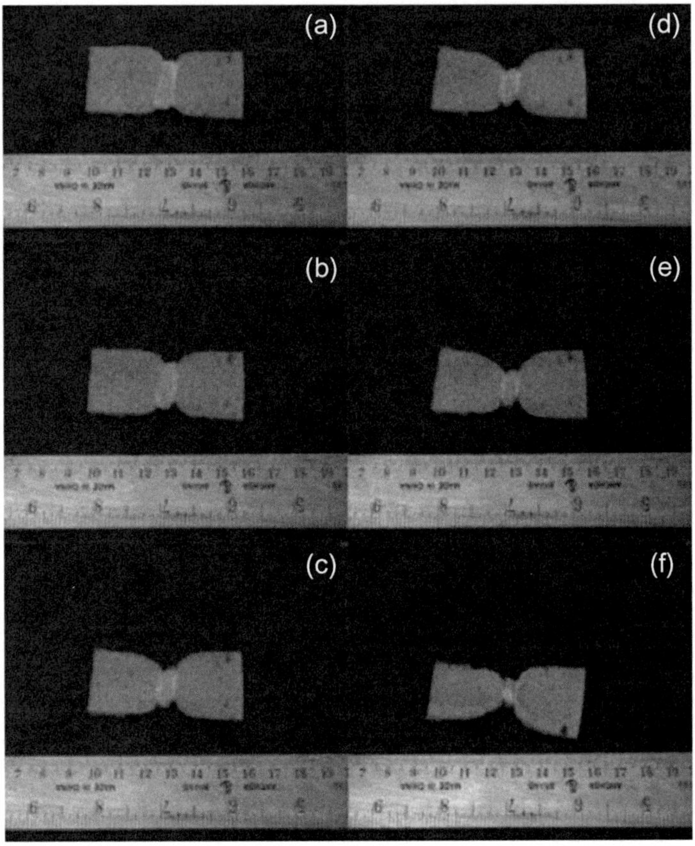

Figure 14.2 Self-tightening of a SMP wire wrapped around a sponge upon heating ((a)–(f)). Copyright by Elsevier. Reprinted with permission, Huang et al. (2012).

the incision is healed. Series experiments have been conducted to demonstrate the feasibility of the novel shape-memory sutures. The applied tension by the shape-memory suture can be tailored by adjusting the stretching conditions such as the strain ratios and molecular structures of the block SMP.

With this suture, the closure of an incision with endoscopic instruments can be easily achieved. The suture is first elongated to a strain of 300% to achieve a temporary shape. The shape-memory suture is applied to close the incision loosely in its temporary shape. After it has been applied in the human body, the heat of the body heats the suture up. Therefore, the shape-memory suture undergoes shape recovery to its original length, which leads to the tightening of the knot. The stress of the suture applied to the tissue can be controlled by the pre-stretching (programming) process. Optimum and even stress can be applied to the incision. Figure 14.3 demonstrates the feasibility of the shape-memory suture to close incision with proper stress. The suture, which is sterilized (ethylene oxide at 45 °C), is stretched to obtain an

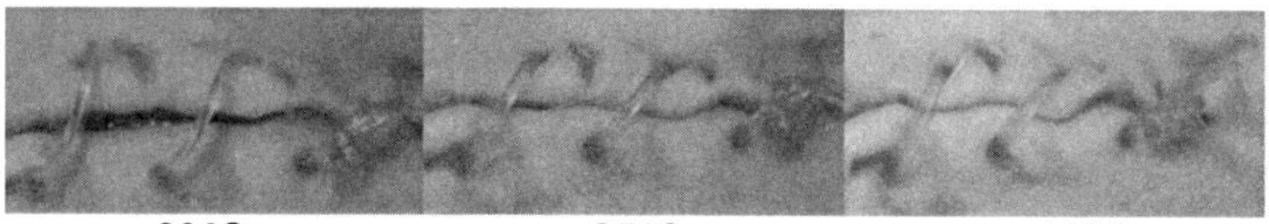

Figure 14.3 Biodegradable SMP suture for wound closure. With increasing temperature, the suture makes a perfect knot on the incision.
Copyright by Elsevier. Reprinted with permission, Behl and Lendlein (2007).

elongated length. The temporary length was fixed by reducing the shape-memory suture to room temperature. The idea is demonstrated by applying the shape-memory suture in a rat belly tissue (Lendlein and Kelch, 2005; Lendlein et al., 2005a). The belly tissue and the abdominal muscle were cut to make an incision. The shape-memory suture was first stretched to an elongation ratio of 200% and the temporary length was fixed. The shape-memory suture is applied to the incision loosely at 20 °C. With increasing temperature, the shape recovery of the shape-memory suture is triggered to make perfect knots. About 0.1 N force is applied to the surrounding tissue. The shape-memory suture is ideal for stitching incisions made during endoscopic surgery.

Reissfelder et al. (2006) applied the shape-memory suture in visceral surgery and evaluated the performance of the biodegradable shape-memory suture. The suturing is a main risk factor in visceral surgery because improper stitching may induce microcirculatory disturbances and/or inadequate adaptation. The mechanical properties, biocompatibility, anastomotic bursting pressure, and shape-memory performance of the shape-memory suture were studied and compared with conventional sutures. The SMP suture was made of block crystallizing oligo(*p*-dioxanone)diol with oligo(ε-caprolactone)diol as the precursor. The oligo(*p*-dioxanone)diol was the hard segment and the oligo(ε-caprolactone)diol acted as the soft segments. The shape-memory properties of the shape-memory suture were evaluated in different solutions (0.9% NaCl, blood, air) at 38 and 45 °C. A comparison was made with conventional suture materials. Biocompatibility testing was conducted using 3T3 fibroblasts, umbilical endothelial cells, and human fibroblasts. It was found that heating the SMP suture could lead to the shrinkage of the suture to 25% in all of the above solutions. The SMP suture tested had no cytotoxic effects according to ISO 10993-5. The SMP suture could provide 33% higher anastomotic bursting pressure than the conventional suture within the first 4 days. This SMP suture material could enable temporarily juxtapositioned self-knotting in the interval.

14.3.4 Shape-memory metallic alloy suture

Different from SMPs, the shape recovery of shape-memory alloys is due to the crystal lattice change of a specific martensite variant to its parent single crystal phase. Nickel–titanium, copper–aluminum–nickel alloys, and copper–zinc–aluminum–nickel are typical shape-memory alloys. During a thermo-mechanical cycle, shape-memory alloys undergo two phase changes, austenite phase (A) with a body-centered cubic structure at high temperature, and martensite phase (M) with tetragonal, orthorhombic, or monoclinic crystal lattice at low temperature. The austenite changes to martensite upon cooling and the martensite changes to austenite upon heating. The phase transformation is not by diffusion of atoms, but by shear lattice distortion. That is why the phase change can finish within a short time. Upon cooling, the austenite transforms to the martensite phase. Several martensitic variants, up to 24 for NiTi, may form. The transformation of the austenite phase to the martensite variants does not induce macroscopic shape change of the materials. If the shape-memory alloy is deformed at a temperature below martensite transformation finish temperature, deformation stress will cause the transformation of other variants of martensite phase into a specific variant of martensite phase accompanied by macroscopic shape changes. If the alloy is heated to a temperature above the start temperature of the austenite phase, the specific martensite variant transforms to the lattice of the original austenite phase, which leads to the one-way shape recovery of the shape-memory alloy.

Shape-memory nitinol can be stretched and becomes soft and flexible. It can be used as shape-memory sutures for stitching. After being heated, the shape-memory nitinol can shrink to its original length, and a proper knot can be achieved. Lamprakis et al. (2009) repaired meniscal using a nitinol suture and evaluated the biomechanical results of the meniscal repair. The performance of the nitinol suture was compared with non-shape-memory suture polyester and nylon. Lamprakis et al. (2009) totally repaired 60 bovine menisci with a vertical longitudinal tear using one horizontal mattress suture. It was found that the shape-memory nitinol suture repair had the highest tensile strength and load to failure. The strength of the shape-memory nitinol suture was significantly stronger than polyester. The research demonstrated the superior load-to-failure and strength of shape-memory nitinol sutures. The shape-memory nitinol suture provided greater efficient primary stability of meniscal repair than that of non-shape-memory suture polyester.

To solve the problem of difficulty suturing during microsurgical procedures, Olson et al. (2012) developed a new injector and a new shape-memory clip that can take the place of conventional sutures. The performance of the injector and clips was assessed and compared with that of conventional suturing. It was found that in the microsurgical scenarios, the new injectable system had 5–20 times greater efficiency. The wound strength was more than three times that of conventional suturing. Another advantage of the shape-memory alloy system is that the shape-memory alloy clips can be forced to open, and then the system recovers to close. Conventional sutures break upon failure.

Lirici et al. (2008) used shape-memory nickel–titanium suture clips in cardiovascular surgery (U-CLIP^{TM}, Medtronic, Minneapolis, MN, U.S.). This suture clip was first used in 2007 to suture the anterior wrap in laparoscopic gastric banding. The research showed that the nitinol clips were safe and that they could facilitate the approximation of tissue in laparoscopic surgery.

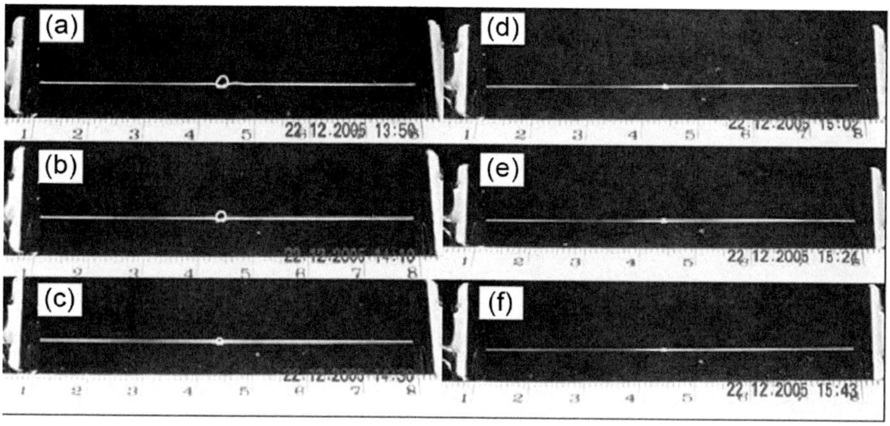

Figure 14.4 Self-tightening of a water-active shape-memory polyurethane suture upon being immersed in water ((a)–(f)).
Copyright by Elsevier. Reproduced with permission, Sun et al. (2012).

14.3.5 Water-active shape-memory sutures

Without using heat, Huang et al. (2012)/Sun et al. (2012) prepared water-sensitive self-tightening shape-memory polyurethane sutures. As can be seen in Figure 14.4a–f, upon immersion into water at room temperature, the suture tightens itself up (Sun et al., 2012). The self-tightening of the suture may be triggered by the fluid in the human body. The maximum recovery stress of the shape-memory suture is in the safe range for human body tissues; therefore, there is no problem of over-tightening. This water-active shape-memory suture made of polyurethane is not biodegradable, and the thermal and hydrolysis degraded products are toxic. If the water-active shape-memory suture were biodegradable, the suture would self-degrade after a certain period of time. More research may be conducted to make the water-stimuli-responsive shape-memory sutures biodegradable and biologically safe.

14.4 Future trends

SMPs provide tremendous current and potential opportunities in medical applications. SMP sutures can self-tighten into a perfect knot with the right amount of tension applied on the tissue. The sutures could be biodegradable, dissolving in the human body after a certain period of time; therefore, a second surgery to remove the suture would be not necessary. By manipulating the programming process and varying the molecular structures of the shape-memory sutures, the mechanical properties and the tension of the suture applied on the tissue can be tailored.

Future research on shape-memory sutures may be as follows. First, specific applications pose specific requirements on the sutures, such as switching temperature, mechanical strength, recovery strength, recovery speed, and degradability speed. Extensive and intensive studies need to be conducted on the relationship between the properties of the shape-memory suture and the requirements of specific applications. Various sutures with various properties that apply to different microsurgery scenarios should be researched and developed.

The shape-memory sutures must have a switching transition temperature above physiological temperature, proper recovery speed, proper recovery ratios, suitable stiffness, and other biological properties. Proper biodegradable speed is very important, so that the suture can dissolve at the right time. These properties cannot impede each other. Though it is claimed that the properties of SMP are tailor-made, it is sometimes difficult to obtain comprehensively good properties for certain applications.

The recovery stress and mechanical strength of SMP sutures is still very low for some applications. Furthermore, at a temperature above the switching temperature of the SMP suture, the materials become too soft. At this temperature, the stress of the suture may relax very soon. The recovery stress and mechanical strength of SMP sutures is far below that of shape-memory alloy sutures. Shape-memory alloy sutures can produce more strength to incisions where high strength is required. The mechanical strength of shape-memory alloys does not relax as it does in the SMP suture. However, the main disadvantage of the shape-memory alloy suture is that it is nondegradable and too stiff for some applications.

SMPs with multiple-step effect have been developed and studied intensively. With this type of SMP, sutures with controllable recovery speed, recovery level, and recovery force at different steps may be developed. The tension on the SMP sutures at different segments may be controlled. These SMP sutures may be more preferable in complicated applications.

14.5 Sources of further information and advice

Institute of Polymer Research in HZG – http://www.hzg.de//institutes_platforms/biomaterial_science/index.php.en

Polymer-based Biomaterials—http://bcrt.charite.de/index.php?id=62

References

Agarwal, A., Hess, H., 2010. Biomolecular motors at the intersection of nanotechnology and polymer science. Prog. Polym. Sci. 35, 252–277.

Alteheld, A., Feng, Y., Kelch, S., Lendlein, A., 2005. Biodegradable, amorphous copolyester-urethane networks having shape memory properties. Angew. Chem. Int. Ed. 44, 1188–1192.

Alvarado-Tenorio, B., Romo-Uribe, A., Mather, P.T., 2011. Microstructure and phase behavior of POSS/PCL shape memory nanocomposites. Macromolecules 44, 5682–5692.

Asaka, K., Oguro, K., 2000. Bending of polyelectrolyte membrane platinum composites by electric stimuli. J. Electroanal. Chem. 480, 186–198.

Behl, M., Lendlein, A., 2007. Shape-memory polymers. Mater. Today 10, 20–28.

Behl, M., Lendlein, A., 2010. Triple-shape polymers. J. Mater. Chem. 20, 3335–3345.
Behl, M., Razzaq, M., Lendlein, A., 2010a. Multifunctional shape-memory polymers. Adv. Mater. 22, 3388–3410.
Behl, M., Zotzmann, J., Lendlein, A., 2010b. Shape-memory polymers and shape-changing polymers. Adv. Polym. Sci. 226, 1–40.
Beloshenko, V.A., Varyukhin, V.N., Voznyak, Y.V., 2005. The shape memory effect in polymers. Russ. Chem. Rev. 74, 265–283.
Buckley, P.R., McKinley, G.H., Wilson IV, T.S., Small, W., Benett, W.J., Bearinger, J.P., McElfresh, M.W., Maitland, D.J., 2006. Inductively heated shape memory polymer for the magnetic actuation of medical devices. IEEE Trans. Biomed. Eng. 53, 2075–2083.
Burke, K.A., Mather, P.T., 2010. Soft shape memory in main-chain liquid crystalline elastomers. J. Mater. Chem. 20, 3449–3457.
Burmistrova, A., Klitzing, R.V., 2010. Control of number density and swelling/shrinking behavior of P(NIPAM/AAc) particles at solid surfaces. J. Mater. Chem. 20, 3502–3507.
Campbell, D., Maji, A., F.Asce, 2006. Failure mechanisms and deployment accuracy of elastic-memory composites. J. Aerosp. Eng. 19, 184–193.
Charlesby, A., 1960. Atomic Radiation and Polymers. Pergamon Press, New York, p. 198.
Chen, T., Chang, D.P., Liu, T., Desikan, R., Datar, R., Thundat, T., Berger, R., Zauscher, S., 2010a. Glucose-responsive polymer brushes for microcantilever sensing. J. Mater. Chem. 20, 3391–3395.
Chen, T., Ferris, R., Zhang, J., Ducker, R., Zauscher, S., 2010b. Stimulus-responsive polymer brushes on surfaces: transduction mechanisms and applications. Prog. Polym. Sci. 35, 94–112.
Dietsch, B., Tong, T., 2007. A review: features and benefits of shape memory polymers (SMPs). J. Adv. Mater. 39, 3–12.
Diorio, A.M., Luo, X., Lee, K.M., Mather, P.T., 2011. A functionally graded shape memory polymer. Soft Matter 7, 68–74.
Eddington, D.T., Beebe, D.J., 2004. Flow control with hydrogels. Adv. Drug Deliv. Rev. 56, 199–210.
Feil, H., Bae, Y.H., Feijen, T., Kim, S.W., 1992. Mutual Influence of pH and temperature on the swelling of ionizable and thermosensitive hydrogels. Macromolecules 25, 5228–5230.
Feng, Y., Lu, J., Behl, M., Lendlein, A., 2011. Degradable depsipeptide-based multiblock copolymers with polyester or polyetherester segments. Int. J. Artif. Organs 34, 103–109.
Filion, T.M., Xu, J., Prasad, M.L., Song, J., 2011. In vivo tissue responses to thermal-responsive shape memory polymer nanocomposites. Biomaterials 32, 985–991.
Gabriel, S., Jérôme, R., Jérôme, C., 2010. Cathodic electrografting of acrylics: from fundamentals to functional coatings. Prog. Polym. Sci. 35, 113–140.
Gall, K., Dunn, M.L., Liu, Y., Finch, D., Lake, M., Munshi, N.A., 2002. Shape memory polymer nanocomposites. Acta Mater. 50, 5115–5126.
Gorna, K., Gogolewski, S., 2002. Biodegradable polyurethanes for implants. II. In vitro degradation and calcification of materials from poly(ε-caprolactone)-poly(ethylene oxide) diols and various chain extenders. J. Biomed. Mater. Res. 60, 592–606.
Gunes, I.S., Jana, S.C., 2008. Shape memory polymers and their nanocomposites: a review of science and technology of new multifunctional materials. J. Nanosci. Nanotechnol. 8, 1616–1637.
Gunes, I.S., Perez-Bolivar, C., Cao, F., Jimenez, G.A., Pavel Anzenbacher, J., Jana, S.C., 2010. Analysis of non-covalent interactions between the nanoparticulate fillers and the matrix polymer as applied to shape memory performance. J. Mater. Chem. 20, 3467–3474.

Hampikian, J.M., Heaton, B.C., Tong, F.C., Zhang, Z., Wong, C.P., 2006. Mechanical and radiographic properties of a shape memory polymer composite for intracranial aneurysm coils. Mater. Sci. Eng. C 26, 1373–1379.

Hayashi, S., Tasaka, Y., Hayashi, N., Akita, Y., 2004. Development of smart polymer materials and its various applications. Mitsubishi Heavy Ind. Ltd. Tech. Rev. 41, 1–3.

Hmadeh, M., Fang, L., Trabolsi, A., Elhabiri, M., Albrecht-Gary, A.-M., Stoddart, J.F., 2010. On the thermodynamic and kinetic investigations of a [c2]daisy chain polymer. J. Mater. Chem. 20, 3422–3430.

Hollander, S.D., Gommes, C.J., Mens, R., Adriaensens, P., Goderis, B., Prez, F.D., 2010. Modeling the morphology and mechanical behavior of shape memory polyurethanes based on solid-state NMR and synchrotron SAXS/WAXD. J. Mater. Chem. 20, 3475–3486.

Hu, J.L., 2007. Shape Memory Polymers and Textiles. Woodhead Publishing, Cambridge.

Hu, J.L., Chen, S., 2010. A review of actively moving polymers in textile applications. J. Mater. Chem. 20, 3346–3355.

Hu, J.L., Mondal, S., 2005. Structural characterization and mass transfer properties of segmented polyurethane: influence of block length of hydrophilic segments. Polym. Int. 54, 764–771.

Hu, J.L., Ji, F.L., Wong, Y.W., 2005a. Dependency of the shape memory properties of a polyurethane upon thermomechanical cyclic conditions. Polym. Int. 54, 600–605.

Hu, J.L., Yang, Z.H., Ji, F.L., Liu, Y.Q., 2005b. Crosslinked polyurethanes with shape memory properties. Polym. Int. 54, 854–859.

Hu, J.L., Meng, Q.H., Zhu, Y., Lu, J., Zhuo, H.T., 2007. Shape memory fibers prepared by wet, reaction, dry, melt, and electro spinning. US Patent 11907012.

Hu, J.L., Meng, Q.H., Zhu, Y., Lu, J., Zhuo, H.T., 2008. Methods for preparing shape memory polyurethanes for textile products. US Patent Office, Pat. No. 61163483.

Hua, J., Gebarowska, K., Dobrzynski, P., Kasperczyk, J., Wei, J., Li, S., 2009. Influence of chain microstructure on the hydrolytic degradation of copolymers from 1,3-trimethylene carbonate and L-lactide. J. Polym. Sci. A Polym. Chem. 47, 3869–3879.

Huang, W.M., Yang, B., Zhao, Y., Ding, Z., 2010. Thermo-moisture responsive polyurethane shape-memory polymer and composites: a review. J. Mater. Chem. 20, 3367–3381.

Huang, W.M., Song, C.L., Fu, Y.Q., Wang, C.C., Zhao, Y., Purnawali, H., Lu, H.B., Tang, C., Ding, Z., Zhang, J.L., 2012. Shaping tissue with shape memory materials. Adv. Drug Deliv. Rev. 65 (4), 515–535. http://dx.doi.org/10.1016/j.addr.2012.06.004.

Hyashi, S., 1993. Properties and applications of polyurethane. Int. Prog. Urethanes 6, 90–115.

Ionov, L., 2010. Actively-moving materials based on stimuli-responsive polymers. J. Mater. Chem. 20, 3382–3390.

Ji, F.L., Zhu, Y., Hu, J.L., Liu, Y., Yeung, L.Y., Ye, G.D., 2006. Smart polymer fibers with shape memory effect. Smart Mater. Struct. 15, 1547–1554.

Ji, Y., Huang, Y.Y., Rungsawang, R., Terentjev, E.M., 2010. Dispersion and alignment of carbon nanotubes in liquid crystalline polymers and elastomers. Adv. Mater. 22, 3436–3440.

Jiang, H.Y., Kelch, S., Lendlein, A., 2006. Polymers move in response to light. Adv. Mater. 18, 1471–1475.

John, M., Li, G., 2010. Self-healing of sandwich structures with a grid stiffened shape memory polymer syntactic foam core. Smart Mater. Struct. 19, Article ID 075013.

Jung, D.H., Jeong, H.M., Kim, B.K., 2010. Organic-inorganic chemical hybrids having shape memory effect. J. Mater. Chem. 20, 3458–3466.

Kelch, S., Steuer, S., Schmidt, A.M., Lendlein, A., 2007. Shape-memory polymer networks from oligo[(ε-hydroxycaproate)-co-glycolate]dimethacrylates and butyl acrylate with adjustable hydrolytic degradation rate. Biomacromolecules 8, 1018–1027.

Kim, B.K., 2010. Editorial corner—a personal view new frontiers of shape memory polymers. eXPRESS Polym. Lett. 4, p. 589.

Kim, B.K., Lee, S.Y., 1998. Polyurethane ionomers having shape memory effects. Polymer 39, 2803–2808.

Kim, B.K., Lee, S.Y., Xu, M., 1996. Polyurethane having shape memory effect. Polymer 37, 5781–5793.

Kloxin, A.M., Kloxin, C.J., Bowman, C.N., Anseth, K.S., 2010. Mechanical properties of cellularly responsive hydrogels and their experimental determination. Adv. Mater. 22, 3484–3494.

Kumar, U.N., Kratz, K., Wagermaier, W., Behl, M., Lendlein, A., 2010. Non-contact actuation of triple-shape effect in multiphase polymer network nanocomposites in alternating magnetic field. J. Mater. Chem. 20, 3404–3415.

Lakhera, N., Laursen, C.M., Safranski, D.L., Frick, C.P., 2012. Biodegradable thermoset shape-memory polymer developed from poly(b-amino ester) networks. J. Polym. Sci. B Polym. Phys. 50, 777–789.

Lamprakis, A., Fortis, A., Kostopoulos, V., Vlasis, K., 2009. Biomedical testing of a shape memory alloy suture in a mensiscal suture model. Arthroscopy 25, 632–638.

Langer, R.S., Lendlein, A., 2003. Biodegradable shape memory polymeric sutures. World Patent WO 2003088818 A2.

Langer, R., Tirrell, D.A., 2004. Designing materials for biology and medicine. Nature 428, 487–492.

Laroche, F.E.F.G., Fiset, M., Mantovani, D., 2002. Shape memory materials for biomedical applications. Adv. Eng. Mater. 4, 91–104.

Lee, K.M., Knight, P.T., Chung, T., Mather, P.T., 2008. Polycaprolactone-POSS chemical/physical double networks. Macromolecules 41, 4730–4738.

Lendlein, A., 2006. Blends of shape memory polymers with thermoplastic polymers. PCT, PCT/EP2006/011420.

Lendlein, A., 2010. Editorial: progress in actively moving polymers. J. Mater. Chem. 20, 3332–3334.

Lendlein, A., Behl, M., 2008. Shape-memory polymers for biomedical applications. Adv. Sci. Technol. 54, 96–102.

Lendlein, A., Kelch, S., 2002. Shape-memory polymers. Angew. Chem. Int. Ed. 41, 2034–2057.

Lendlein, A., Kelch, S., 2005. Shape-memory polymers as stimuli-sensitive implant materials. Clin. Hemorheol. Microcirc. 32, 105–116.

Lendlein, A., Langer, R., 2002. Biodegradable, elastic shape-memory polymers for potential biomedical applications. Science 96, 1673–1676.

Lendlein, A., Ridder, U., 19 Apr. 2007. Method for hair treatment with shape memory polymers. US Patent 2007/0088135 A1.

Lendlein, A., Kratz, K., Kelch, S., Apr. 2005a. Smart implant materials. Med. Device Technol. 16 (3), 12–14.

Lendlein, A., Lang, G., Knitz, K., Krause, T., Kalbfleisch, A., Allwohn, J., Burgliaus, J., Sendelhach, G., Beyer, A., Mallinger, D., Uhl, S., Birkel, S., Duchscherer, A., Hasson, T.A.A., Jiang, H.Y., Morsheim, S., Ghazlan, Y., 3 Nov. 2005b. Method for achieving shape memory effects on hair by combining shape memory polymer with canonic acitive ingredients. US Patent 2005/0244353 A1.

Li, Y.K., 2007. Evaluation of shape memory fabrics. In: Fabrics, E.O.S.M. (Ed.), Institute of Textiles and Clothing. Hong Kong Polytechnic University, Hong Kong.

Li, G., Nettles, D., 2010. Thermomechanical characterization of a shape memory polymer based self-repairing syntactic foam. Polymer 51, 755–762.

Li, G., Uppu, N., 2010. Shape memory polymer based self-healing syntactic foam: 3-D confined thermomechanical characterization. Compos. Sci. Technol. 70, 1419–1427.

Lin, J.R., Chen, L.W., 1998a. Study on shape-memory behavior of polyether-based polyurethanes. II. Influence of soft-segment molecular weight. J. Appl. Polym. Sci. 69, 1575–1586.

Lin, J.R., Chen, L.W., 1998b. Study on shape-memory behavious of polyether-based polyurethanes. I. Influence of the hard-segment content. J. Appl. Polym. Sci. 69, 1563–1574.

Lirici, M.M., Salerno, F., Califano, A., 2008. The use of superelastic suture clips in laparoscopic gastric banding. Minim. Invasive Ther. 17, 176–180.

Liu, F., Urban, M.W., 2010. Recent advances and challenges in designing stimuli-responsive polymers. Prog. Polym. Sci. 35, 3–23.

Liu, J., Ma, D.Z., Li, Z., 2002. FTIR studies on the compatibility of hard-soft segments for polyurethane-imide copolymers with different soft segments. Eur. Polym. J. 38, 661–665.

Liu, C., Qin, H., Mather, P.T., 2007. Review of progress in shape-memory polymers. J. Mater. Chem. 17, 1543–1558.

Madbouly, S.A., Lendlein, A., 2010. Shape-memory polymer composites. Adv. Polym. Sci. 226, 41–95.

Maitland, D.J., Metzger, M.F., Schumann, D., Lee, A., Wilson, T.S., 2002. Photothermal properties of shape memory polymer micro-actuators for treating stroke. Lasers Surg. Med. 30, 1–11.

Makhosaxana, X.P., Filipcsei, G., Zrınyi, M., 2000. Preparation and responsive properties of magnetically soft poly(*N*-isopropylacrylamide) gels. Macromolecules 33, 1716–1719.

Mano, J.F., 2008. Stimuli-responsive polymeric systems for biomedical applications. Adv. Eng. Mater. 10, 515–527.

Marco, D., Eckhouse, S., 2006. Biodegradable self-inflating intragastric implants for curbing appetite. US Patent Office, Pat. No. 0156248.

Mather, P.T., Liu, C., Burstone, C.J., Dec. 2005. Shape memory polymer orthodontic appliances, and methods of making and using the same. European Patent EP1844097, World Patent 2006071520, 2006.

Mather, P.T., Luo, X., Rousseau, I.A., 2009. Shape memory polymer research. Annu. Rev. Mater. Res. 39, 445–471.

Meng, Q., Hu, J., 2008. Study on poly(ε-caprolactone)-based shape memory copolymer fiber prepared by bulk polymerization and melt spinning. Polym. Adv. Technol. 19, 131–136.

Meng, Q., Hu, J., 2009. A review of shape memory polymer composites and blends. Compos. Part A 40, 1661–1672.

Meng, H., Hu, J.L., 2010. A brief review of stimulus-active polymers responsive to thermal, light, magnetic, electric, and water/solvent stimuli. J. Intell. Mater. Syst. Struct. 21, 859–885.

Meng, Q.H., Hu, J.L., Zhu, Y., Lu, J., Liu, Y., 2007. Polycaprolactone-based shape memory segmented polyurethane fiber. J. Appl. Polym. Sci. 106, 2515–2523.

Min, C., Cui, W., Bei, J., Wang, S., 2005. Biodegradable shape-memory polymer—polylactide-co-poly(glycolide-co-caprolactone) multiblock copolymer. Polym. Adv. Technol. 16, 608–615.

Mondal, S., Hu, J.L., Zhu, Y., 2006. Free volume and water vapor permeability of dense segmented polyurethane membrane. J. Membr. Sci. 280, 427–432.

Motornov, M., Roiter, Y., Tokarev, I., Minko, S., 2010. Stimuli-responsive nanoparticles, nanogels and capsules for integrated multifunctional intelligent systems. Prog. Polym. Sci. 35, 174–211.

Musumeci, T., Aventura, C., Giannore, I., 2006. PLA/PLGA nanoparticles for sustained release of docetaxel. Int. J. Pharm. 325, 172–179.
Nagahama, K., Ueda, Y., Ouchi, T., Ohya, Y., 2009. Biodegradable shape-memory polymers exhibiting sharp thermal transitions and controlled drug release. Biomacromolecules 10, 1789–1794.
Nagata, M., Inaki, K., 2011. Biodegradable and photocurable multiblock copolymers with shape-memory properties from poly(ε-caprolactone) diol, poly(ethylene glycol), and 5-cinnamoyloxyisophthalic acid. J. Appl. Polym. Sci. 120, 3556–3564.
Nagata, M., Kitazima, I., 2006. Photocurable biodegradable poly(ε-caprolactone)/poly(ethylene glycol) multiblock copolymers showing shape-memory properties. Colloid Polym. Sci. 284, 380–386.
Nandivada, H., Rossb, A.M., Lahann, J., 2010. Stimuli-responsive monolayers for biotechnology. Prog. Polym. Sci. 35, 141–154.
Neffe, A.T., Tronci, G., Alteheld, A., Lendlein, A., 2010. Controlled change of mechanical properties during hydrolytic degradation of polyester urethane networks. Macromol. Chem. Phys. 211, 182–194.
Nguyen, T.D., Yakacki, C.M., Brahmbhatt, P.D., Chambers, M.L., 2010. Modeling the relaxation mechanisms of amorphous shape memory polymers. Adv. Mater. 22, 3411–3423.
Nji, J., Li, G., 2010. A biomimic shape memory polymer based self-healing particulate composite. Polymer 51, 755–762.
Ohki, T., Ni, Q.-Q., Ohsako, N., Iwamoto, M., 2004. Shape-memory polymers. Compos. Part A 35, 1065–1073.
Ohm, C., Brehmer, M., Zentel, R., 2010. Liquid crystalline elastomers as actuators and sensors. Adv. Mater. 22, 3366–3387.
Olson, J.L., Shandas, R., Erlanger, M., 2012. Development of a minimally invasive, injectable, shape memory suture and delivery system. Ann. Biomed. Eng. 40, 1520–1529.
Ortega, J., Small, W., Wilson, T., Benett, W., Loge, J., Maitland, D., 2007. A shape memory polymer dialysis needle adapter for the reduction of hemodynamic stress within arteriovenous grafts. IEEE Trans. Biomed. Eng. 54, 1722–1724.
Ping, P., Wang, W., Chen, X., Jing, X., 2005. Poly(epsilon-caprolactone) polyurethane and its shape-memory property. Biomacromolecules 6, 587–592.
Ratna, D., Karger-Kocsis, J., 2008. Recent advances in shape memory polymers and composites: a review. J. Mater. Sci. 43, 254–269.
Reissfelder, C., Ritz, J.-P., Kelch, S., Lendlein, A., Buhr, H., 2006. Evaluation of the physical properties of a new fully degradable suture material with a shape memory effect for visceral surgery. In: 47th Annual Meeting May 20-24, Los Angeles, CA.
Rickert, D., Lendlein, A., Schmidt, A.M., Kelch, S., Roehlke, W., Fuhrmann, R., Franke, R.P., 2003a. In vitro cytotoxicity testing of AB-polymer networks based on oligo (ε-caprolactone) segments after different sterilization techniques. J. Biomed. Mater. Res. B Appl. Biomater. 67B, 722–731.
Rickert, D., Moses, M.A., Lendlein, A., Kelch, S., Franke, R.P., 2003b. The importance of angiogenesis in the interaction between polymeric biomaterials and surrounding tissue. Clin. Hemorheol. Microcirc. 28, 175–181.
Rickert, D., Lendlein, A., Kelch, S., Moses, M.A., Franke, R.P., 2005. Expression of MMPs and TIMPs in primary epithelial cell cultures of the upper aerodigestive tract seeded on the surface of a novel polymeric biomaterial. Clin. Hemorheol. Microcirc. 32, 117–128.
Romeo, G., Fernandez-Nieves, A., Wyss, H.M., Acierno, D., Weitz, D.A., 2010. Temperature-controlled transitions between glass, liquid, and gel states in dense p-NIPA suspensions. Adv. Mater. 22, 3441–3445.

Rousseau, I.A., Xie, T., 2010. Shape memory epoxy: composition, structure, properties and shape memory performances. J. Mater. Chem. 20, 3431–3441.

Roy, D., Cambre, J.N., Sumerlin, B.S., 2010. Future perspectives and recent advances in stimuli-responsive materials. Prog. Polym. Sci. 35, 278–301.

Ruan, C., Wang, Y., Zhang, M., Luo, Y., Fu, C., Huang, M., Sun, J., Hu, C., 2012. Design, synthesis and characterization of novel biodegradable shape memory polymers based on poly (D,L-lactic acid) diol, hexamethylene diisocyanate and piperazine. Polym. Int. 61, 524–530.

Russew, M.M., Hecht, S., 2010. Photoswitches: from molecules to materials. Adv. Mater. 22, 3348–3360.

Schmidt, A.M., 2006. Electromagnetic activation of shape memory polymer networks containing magnetic nanoparticles. Macromol. Rapid Commun. 27, 1168–1172.

Sellinger, A.T., Wang, D.H., Tan, L.-S., Vaia, R.A., 2010. Electrothermal polymer nanocomposite actuators. Adv. Mater. 22, 3430–3435.

Sharp, A.A., Panchawagh, H.V., Ortega, A., Artale, R., Richardson-Burns, S., Finch, D.S., Gall, K., Mahajan, R.L., Restrepo, D., 2006. Toward a self-deploying shape memory polymer neuronal electrode. J. Neural Eng. 3, L23–L30.

Siegal, R.A., Firestone, B.A., 1988. pH-dependent equilibrium swelling properties of hydrophobic polyelectrolyte copolymer gels. Macromolecules 21, 3254–3259.

Simpson, B., Nunnery, G., Tannenbaum, R., Kalaitzidou, K., 2010. Capture/release ability of thermo-responsive polymer particles. J. Mater. Chem. 20, 3496–3501.

Skarja, G.A., Woodhouse, K.A., 2000. Structure-property relationships of degradable polyurethane elastomers containing an amino acid-based chain extender. J. Appl. Polym. Sci. 75, 1522–1534.

Skarja, G.A., Woodhouse, K.A., 2004. In vitro degradation and erosion of degradable, segmented polyurethanes containing an amino acid-based chain extender. J. Biomater. Sci. Polym. Ed. 12, 851–873.

Small, W., Wilson, T.S., Buckley, P.R., Benett, W.J., Loge, J.M., Hartman, J., 2007. Prototype fabrication and preliminary in vitro testing of a shape memory endovascular thrombectomy device. IEEE Trans. Biomed. Eng. 54, 1657–1666.

Small, I.W., Singhal, P., Wilson, T.S., Maitland, D.J., 2010. Biomedical applications of thermally activated shape memory polymers. J. Mater. Chem. 20, 3356–3366.

Smela, E., Inganäs, O., Lundström, I., 1995. Controlled folding of micrometer-size structures. Science 268, 1735–1738.

Smith, A.E., Xu, X., McCormick, C.L., 2010. Stimuli-responsive amphiphilic (co)polymers via RAFT polymerization. Prog. Polym. Sci. 35, 45–93.

Sokolowski, W.M., Chmielewski, A.B., Hayashi, S., Yamada, T., 1999. Cold hibernated elastic memory (CHEM) self-deployable structures. In: SPIE International Symposium on Smart Structures and Materials, Newport Beach, CA.

Storey, R.F., Hickey, T.P., 1994. Degradable polyurethane networks based on D,L-lactide, glycolide, e-caprolactone, and trimethylene carbonate homopolyester and copolyester triols. Polymer 35, 830–838.

Sun, L., Huang, W.M., Ding, Z., Zhao, Y., Wang, C.C., Purnawali, H., Tang, C., 2012. Stimulus-responsive shape memory materials: a review. Mater. Des. 33, 577–640.

Tobushi, H., Hashimoto, T., Ito, N., Hayashi, S., Yamada, E., 1998. Shape fixity and shape recovery in a film of shape memory polymer of polyurethane series. J. Intell. Mater. Syst. Struct. 9, 127–136.

Tobushi, H., Hayashi, S., Hoshio, K., Miwa, N., 2006. Influence of strain-holding conditions on shape recovery and secondary-shape forming in polyurethane-shape memory polymer. Smart Mater. Struct. 15, 1033–1038.

Tobushi, H., Hoshio, K., Hayashi, S., Miwa, N., 2007. Shape memory composite of SMA and SMP and its property. Key Eng. Mater. 340-341, 1187–1192.
Toensmeier, P.A., 2005. Shape memory polymers reshape product design. Plast. Eng. 61, 10–11.
Tokarev, I., Minko, S., 2010. Stimuli-responsive porous hydrogels at interfaces for molecular filtration, separation, controlled release, and gating in capsules and membranes. Adv. Mater. 22, 3446–3462.
Urban, M.W., 2010. Guest editorial. Prog. Polym. Sci. 35, 1–2.
Vaia, R., Baur, J., 2008. Adaptive composites. Science 319, 420–421.
Voit, W., Ware, T., Dasari, R.R., Smith, P., Danz, L., Simon, D., Barlow, S., Marder, S.R., Gall, K., 2010. High-strain shape-memory polymers. Adv. Funct. Mater. 20, 162–171.
Wache, H.M., Tartakowska, D.J., Hentrich, A., Wagner, M.H., 2004. Development of a polymer stent with shape memory effect as a drug delivery system. J. Mater. Sci. Mater. Med. 14, 109–112.
Wang, Y., Huang, M., Luo, Y., Li, Y., 2010. In vitro degradation of poly(lactide-co-p-dioxanone)-based shape memory poly(urethaneeurea). Polym. Degrad. Stab. 95, 549–556.
Wischke, C., Neffe, A.T., Steuer, S., Lendlein, A., 2009. Evaluation of a degradable shape-memory polymer network as matrix for controlled drug release. J. Control. Release 138, 243–250.
Wong, Y.S., Stachurski, Z.H., Venkatraman, S.S., 2011a. Modeling shape memory effect in uncrosslinked amorphous biodegradable polymer. Polymer 52, 874–880.
Wong, Y.S., Widjaja, L.K., Li, H., Abadie, M.J.M., Venkatraman, S.S., 2011b. Microstructure—cyclic deformation property relationships of biodegradable di-crystalline triblock copolymers. Polymer 52, 3451–3459.
Wornyo, E., May, G., Gall, K., 2009. Modeling and optimization of the deposition of shape memory polymers for information storage applications. IEEE Trans. Semicond. Manuf. 22, 409–416.
Xiao, X., Xie, T., Cheng, Y.T., 2010. Self-healable graphene polymer composites. J. Mater. Chem. 20, 3508–3514.
Xie, T., Xiao, X., 2008. Self-peeling reversible dry adhesive system. Chem. Mater. 20, 2866–2868.
Xu, J., Song, J., 2010. High performance shape memory polymer networks based on rigid nano-particle cores. Proc. Natl. Acad. Sci. 107, 7652–7657.
Xu, B., Fu, Y.Q., Ahmad, M., Luo, J.K., Huang, W.M., Kraft, A., Reuben, R., Pei, Y.T., Chen, Z.G., Hosson, J.T.M.D., 2010. Thermo-mechanical properties of polystyrene-based shape memory nanocomposites. J. Mater. Chem. 20, 3442–3448.
Yakacki, C.M., Gall, K., 2010. Shape-memory polymers for biomedical applications. Adv. Polym. Sci. 226, 147–175.
Yang, J.H., Chun, B.C., Chung, Y.C., Cho, J.W., Cho, B.G., 2004. Vibration control ability of multilayered composite material made of epoxy beam and polyurethane copolymer with shape memory effect. J. Appl. Polym. Sci. 94, 302–307.
Yang, B., Huang, W.M., Li, C., Li, L., 2006. Effects of moisture on the thermomechanical properties of a polyurethane shape memory polymer. Polymer 47, 1348–1356.
Yang, J., Liu, F., Yang, L., Li, S., 2010. Hydrolytic and enzymatic degradation of poly(trimethylene carbonate-co-D,L-lactide) random copolymers with shape memory behavior. Eur. Polym. J. 46, 783–791.
Yoshihaya, N., Ishihara, H., Yamada, T., 2003. Relationship between segment structutures and elastic properties of segmented poly(urethane-urea) elastic fibers. Polym. Eng. Sci. 43, 1740–1746.

Yu, Z., Liu, Y., Fan, M., Meng, X., Li, B., Zhang, S., 2010. Effects of solvent, casting temperature, and guest/host stoichiometries on the properties of shape memory material based on partial a-CD-PEG inclusion complex. J. Polym. Sci. B Polym. Phys. 48, 951–957.

Zhang, S., Yu, Z., Govender, T., Luo, H., Li, B., 2008. A novel supramolecular shape memory material based on partial a-CD-PEG inclusion complex. Polymer 49, 3205–3210.

Zhu, Y., Hu, J.L., Yeung, L.Y., Liu, Y., Ji, F.L., Yeung, K.W., 2006. Development of shape memory polyurethane fiber with complete shape recoverability. Smart Mater. Struct. 15, 1385–1394.

Zotzmann, J., Behl, M., Hofmann, D., Lendlein, A., 2010. Reversible triple-shape effect of polymer networks containing polypentadecalactone- and poly(epsilon-caprolactone)-segments. Adv. Mater. 22, 3424–3429.

Index

Note: Page numbers followed by *f* indicate figures and *t* indicate tables.

R

S